EIGHTH EDITION

American Health Care Association's

HOW TO BE A NURSE ASSISTANT

A Quality Approach to Long Term Care

Julie Gdowski, RN, BSN, LHNA

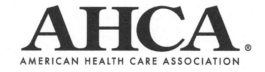

AHCA.®

AMERICAN HEALTH CARE ASSOCIATION

Author/Editor
Julie Gdowski, RN

Designer
Merrifield Graphics & Publishing Service

Cover Designer
Chip Henderson

Cover Photographer
Transcending Dreams Photography

Cover Model
Trang Huynh

Photography & Illustrations
Shutterstock
Imagineeringart.com Inc.

Proofreader
Melissa Rogers

Chief Operating Officer/Senior Vice President, Member Relations
Jennifer Shimer

Marketing and Marketing Research Vice President
Jon-Patrick Ewing

Marketing Director
Chip Henderson

Project Managers
Jon-Patrick Ewing and Chip Henderson

Sales/Customer Service
Lisa Hohenemser

Printer
ASAPfast!

Copyright © 2022
American Health Care Association
1201 L St. NW
Washington DC 20005-4015
web: ahca.org
email: publications@ahca.org

All rights reserved. No part of this publication may be reproduced, stored in a retrieval system, distributed, or transmitted in any form or by any means, including photocopying, recording, or other electronic or mechanical methods, without the prior written permission from the publisher.

EIGHTH EDITION

ISBN 978-1-7923-9588-8

PRINTED IN THE UNITED STATES

Notice to Readers

Great effort has been taken to confirm the accuracy of the information presented and to describe generally accepted practices. However, the author, editors, and publisher are not responsible for errors or omissions or for any consequences from application of the information in this book and make no warranty, expressed or implied, with respect to the currency, completeness, or accuracy of the contents of the publication. Application of this information in a particular situation remains the professional responsibility of the practitioner; the clinical treatments described and recommended may not be considered absolute and universal recommendations.

Ordering Information

How to Be a Nurse Assistant can be ordered directly from the American Health Care Association. Special discounts are available for quantity purchases.

web: ahcapublications.org
phone: 800-321-0343
email: publications@ahca.org

Preface

Welcome and thank you for purchasing **How to Be a Nurse Assistant**. You have chosen a great text to help you learn everything that you will need to know to pass your state nursing competency exam and become a nurse assistant. The text focuses on how to provide quality care to the residents in your care. What makes this book unique is that it goes well beyond the technical skills needed to do the job. You will learn what it really means to care for another human being.

The role of the nurse assistant begins with supporting residents in their activities of daily living (ADLs). The nurse assistant must be the voice for the residents when they cannot communicate, eyes and ears for other interdisciplinary team members when they are not with the residents, and arms and legs for the residents when they cannot move. The nurse assistant must be with residents when they need someone to hold their hands. How the nurse assistant does this is key to whether the residents and their families feel that they are receiving the quality of care needed to enhance their quality of life.

How is this accomplished?

One of the best ways to show that you care is to be aware and understand the people in your care. This text will help you create a culture of caring by introducing the concept of always being aware. Awareness leads to a sense of mindfulness during caregiving activities. You become mindful by being open to change and new ideas as you care for your resident. It is important for nurse assistants to be honest and observant, maintain a positive attitude, and always try to understand what your residents are experiencing. This will help you anticipate what your residents need and build trusting relationships that bring out the best in you and them.

The concept of being aware and understanding are incorporated in the common preparation steps and common completion steps for nearly all the procedures you will need to master as a nurse assistant. A complete list of procedures is listed on page xvii. There are more than 90 step-by-step procedures outlined and illustrated in detail for you in the pages that follow.

The chapter objectives as well as the knowledge and skills you will learn are listed on the first page of each chapter. Key terms are bold and defined in the Glossary in Appendix A. At the end of each chapter, you can check your knowledge with the 10 multiple choice questions designed to help you review the material and prepare for the exam. Answers to these questions are available on your instructor's website.

The 8th edition is published by the American Health Care Association (AHCA). AHCA'S commitment to quality is demonstrated daily through its work on behalf of over a million residents who reside in the more than 14,000 long term and post-acute care facilities that AHCA represents. The very latest information about regulations affecting residents and nurse assistants is included along with everything students need to know to be safe in their practice.

Thank you again for purchasing **How to Be a Nurse Assistant**. I hope that it meets your needs for this important training and that you will continue to use it as a reference tool in the future. It is my hope that you enjoy your learning experience and your career focused on caring for the elderly.

Respectfully,

Julie Gdowski, RN

About the Author

Julie Gdowski is a registered nurse and earned her Bachelor of Science in Nursing from Indiana University. With more than 30 years of experience as a compassionate nurse, certified nurse aide instructor, and licensed nursing home administrator, Julie has held key clinical leadership positions with several provider organizations including Facility Administrator, Medicare Coordinator, and Director of Nursing.

Julie thrives in helping others, especially in caring for our elderly, and values the importance of education as an empowerment tool for everyone to learn and grow. She leads by example and her philosophy of betterment guides her management style and interactions with those she encounters.

Currently, Julie serves on the executive leadership team and is the Director of Clinical Operations for Academic Platforms, an innovative healthcare technology company, which is the parent company of CNAonline. Using **How to Be a Nurse Assistant** curriculum through an exclusive partnership with the American Health Care Association (AHCA), CNAonline develops nurse assistant training courses that are delivered through a hybrid online learning model that combines web-based instruction and hands-on experience in facilities.

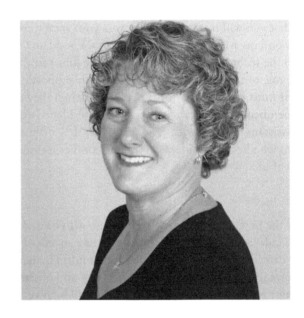

Julie consistently researches, develops, and embraces best practices that can be incorporated into curriculum development. She also leads efforts with state regulators to certify state nurse aide educational programs. Her experience and expertise led AHCA to select Julie as the author and subject matter expert to update the 8th edition of **How to Be a Nurse Assistant**.

Acknowledgments

For 35 years, the American Health Care Association (AHCA) has published **How to Be a Nurse Assistant**, the cornerstone of its educational resources, to provide training for nurse assistants dedicating their career in long term care. AHCA represents more than 14,000 long term and post-acute care facilities across the United States and its **How to Be a Nurse Assistant** curriculum has been developed as a comprehensive set of instruction, guidelines, and procedures based on best practices and industry standards.

The eighth edition of **How to Be a Nurse Assistant** is a collaborative effort involving many dedicated individuals and organizations that share our unwavering commitment and recognition of the significant role of nurse assistants in long term care.

Thank you to the those who contributed their time, expertise, and passion to the continued quality and success of the **How to Be a Nurse Assistant** curriculum.

Reviewers and Advisors

We are grateful to the registered nurses and professional instructors who reviewed this text and provided valuable suggestions and content to improve this edition.

Julie Adair, RN
Vice President, Digital Education and Credentialing, Iowa Health Care Association
Des Moines, Iowa

Jane Garcia, RN, BSN
Nurse Instructor
Louisville, Kentucky

Jasmine Mosdell, RN
Nurse Instructor
Berthoud, Colorado

Annette Werner, RN, BSN
Nurse Instructor
Fairmont, West Virginia

Content Contributor

Michele Mongillo, RN, BSN, MSN, RAC-CT
Senior Clinical Director, First Quality
Bradford, Pennsylvania

Video

AHCA is grateful for Masonic Homes Kentucky and Trasee Whitaker, Sr. VP/Human Resources & Chief Human Resources Officer, for providing the wonderful location to film our **How to Be a Nurse Assistant Skills Video**.

Video Production
Brian Morrison

New to this Edition!

Health care and the role of the nurse assistant in long term care is ever evolving. It is our intent to provide the most current material in our textbook based on the latest information at time of publication

With this eighth edition of **How to Be a Nurse Assistant**, we moved Resident Rights forward to Chapter 4, added procedures, updated key terms, and expanded and enhanced the following content:

- Telephone etiquette
- Sexuality
- Domestic violence
- Alcohol-based hand rub procedure
- Apply and remove PPE
- Asepsis
- Common preparation and completion steps
- Applying a gait belt
- Safety Date Sheets (SDS)
- RACE and PASS acronyms
- Stroke
- Blood pressure classifications
- Procedure for non-contact infrared temperature
- Procedure for electronic blood pressure
- Prone, side-lying (lateral), and sims positions
- Nutrition
- Elimination
- Five food groups
- Gluten free, full liquid and clear liquid diets

- Vegan and vegetarian
- Procedure for measuring output
- Incontinent Associated Dermatitis
- Different types of incontinent products
- Types of urinary incontinence
- Macular degeneration
- Abnormal changes in body functioning
- Intellectual disability
- Down syndrome, cerebral palsy, and autism spectrum disorder
- Mental health and substance abuse disorders
- Insomnia
- Restless leg syndrome
- Sleep apnea
- Physicians Orders for Life-Sustaining Treatment and Do Not Resuscitate
- Long Term Care Survey
- Nurse aide regulations, competency testing, nurse aide registry

Contents

Chapter 11: Aging and Chronic Disease Management

Procedures

1

Your Health Care Career

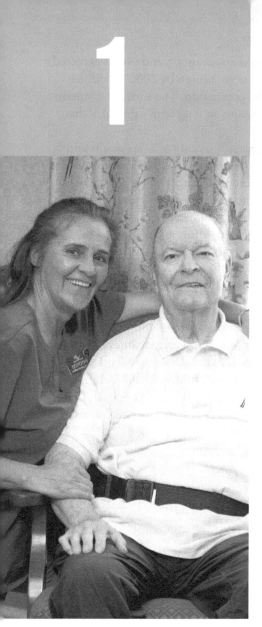

Congratulations on your decision to enter a career in health care! You are entering a growing field with a variety of options for nurse assistants. Long term care is one of the primary areas of health care services. Over the years as patient and client needs have changed, long term care providers have developed a better understanding of how to best serve people as they age. Long term care now involves many diverse specialties, so the role of the nurse assistant continues to evolve and expand.

Today, long term care encompasses many different types of facilities, services, and care. It may include medical care, ongoing skilled nursing care, and care for persons with developmental disabilities or cognitive impairments. Changes in the field have occurred for many reasons. In the United States, the elderly population is growing, and advances in health care allow many to live longer. Our aging population experiences many chronic diseases, so there is an increased need for specialized care. Medical advances and continued research have made it much easier to meet the needs of aging individuals and improve their overall care.

This chapter will introduce you to your career as a health care professional, with a focus on long term care. You will learn about specific types of services and the various settings in which these services are provided. You will learn about the members of the health care team, their roles, and the role you play as part of this team. We will discuss the importance of caring for yourself as you manage a daily work routine and provide guidelines for beginning your new career successfully. Let's get started!

OBJECTIVES:

- Define long term care and list the settings in which this type of care is provided.

- Explain why people enter long term care facilities.

- Describe the services that are offered in long term care facilities and the people and departments that provide them.

- Explain how long term care is paid for and which agencies regulate this care.

- Provide an overview of the primary duties of the nurse assistant.

- Explain the roles of nursing staff and members of the interdisciplinary care team.

- Identify at least three ways to build a good relationship with the charge nurse.

- Identify at least three ways to build a good relationship with coworkers.

- List five main factors that influence how care is delivered.

- Explain how nursing shifts work and how tasks are assigned to nurse assistants.

- Describe time management strategies that are essential for nurse assistants.

- Explain why staying healthy is important for nurse assistants, and list at least three actions you can take to maintain and improve your health.

What Is Long Term Care?

Long term care (LTC) can be defined as health care or personal care services that are provided for an extended period of time. It is a part of our health care system designed to serve people of any age, but it primarily serves the elderly. Long term care meets individuals' medical needs as well as their need for help with **activities of daily living (ADL)**. These activities include bathing, dressing, personal grooming, and eating meals. An overview of the types of services provided by long term care facilities is shown in Table 1-1.

Table 1-1 Types of Services Provided in Long Term Care Facilities

Type of Service	Explanation
Medical and dental care	Care provided by medical professionals that include physicians, physician assistants, nurse practitioners, clinical nurse specialists, and dentists
Nursing and rehabilitative care	Care provided by registered nurses, licensed practical nurses, and physical, occupational, speech, and respiratory therapists
Personal care	Care provided by nurse assistants to assist residents with basic needs such as bathing, dressing, and grooming
Residential care	Services provided to address spiritual, social, and quality-of-life needs; these include services of social workers, activity/recreational therapists, and spiritual advisor
Other services	Dietary, pharmaceutical, laboratory, and diagnostic imaging services

Long term care facilities have staff with many different duties, but most personal care is provided by nurse assistants. As a nurse assistant, you have the opportunity to provide a high quality of care that enhances the quality of life for residents in these facilities.

Long term care is one part of the larger *health care system*, which includes different types of facilities: hospitals, home health agencies, clinics, mental health centers, hospices, alcohol and drug rehabilitation facilities, and individual and group medical practices. Long term care facilities are an important part of this system because of the growing population whose medical, social, personal, and psychological needs require ongoing support. According to the National Center for Chronic Disease Prevention and Health Promotion, by 2030, the number of people in the United States age 65 and over is expected to reach 71 million and 98 million by 2060 — making up almost 25% of the population. There are more opportunities for nurse assistants in long term care today than ever before.

Gerontology is the scientific study of aging adults and the process of aging. This expanding field has proven how important long term care is to a whole system of care. Long term care facilities play an important part in trying to contain growing health care costs. Due to rising costs, new ways of delivering care are being explored, and methods of care are evolving.

Long Term Care Facilities

There are many types of long term care facilities (LTC). These facilities can be stand-alone buildings, or they can be a unit in a hospital. Long term care facilities include nursing facilities, adult day care centers, residential care facilities, assisted living communities, rehabilitation centers, and home-based personal care services. All LTC facilities have the same mission — to provide services to people with special health needs (Figure 1-1).

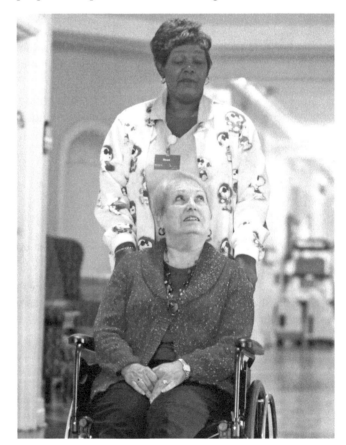

Figure 1-1 As a nurse assistant, you help ensure that residents get the best possible care.

Assisted living facilities (ALF) provide 24-hour supervision in a home-like setting. Support services are based on each resident's personal care needs. Services may include assistance with eating, bathing, dressing, toileting, taking medicine, transportation, laundry, and housekeeping.

Continuing care retirement communities (CCRC) provide a wide range of services based on each resident's needs as they age. A CCRC allows the resident to access multiple levels of care on one campus. These facilities usually offer three main categories of care: *independent living, assisted living,* and *skilled nursing care.* Some CCRC's will offer memory support care as well.

Intermediate care facilities (ICF) provide nursing and supportive care to residents who have a variety of mental or physical disabilities. ICF's are typically for those residents who have a developmental disability. Care focuses on assisting the person to become as independent as possible. Staff members work with each person's skills and build success from his or her starting point. A range of health care services are also available.

Nursing facilities (NF) provide round-the-clock care covering a variety of services depending on the individual residents' needs. Many facilities have post-acute care units that provide specialized care for residents needing a higher level of nursing care or rehabilitation services with the goal of returning residents to the highest level of functioning. These services can be provided for a short period after an injury or hospital stay, or for a longer period to treat a chronic medical condition.

Other types of specialty units include:

- Memory care units provide care for residents with Alzheimer's disease, dementia, and other cognitive disorders. Residents in these units have problems with their memory. Because they may wander about, safety is a major concern. These facilities are structured to ensure their safety.
- Traumatic brain injury units provide care for people who have had traumatic head injuries. The focus in this type of unit is on rehabilitation.
- Rehabilitation units have the primary goal of restoring residents to their optimal level of physical functioning. Residents are usually admitted directly from a hospital.

Why Are People Admitted to Long Term Care Facilities?

There are many reasons that drive the need for long term care. A short-term illness or injury such as a stroke may result in the need for recovery or rehabilitation for a designated period of time, with the ultimate goal of returning home. Patients with chronic diseases or terminal conditions may need care the rest of their lives.

Each resident is a special person with a unique history, and his or her individual situation determines the type of facility and support they need to support overall quality of life. The reasons for living in a long term care facility can change as a person's health care needs change. But the goal of long term care is always the same: to maintain or restore each resident's level of optimal functioning — to help all residents be the best they can be.

Residents in long term care receive one or more of the following types of care:

- **Rehabilitation.** Residents who need rehabilitation may stay several weeks to several months. They usually have an illness or injury and need help to get back to their previous level of abilities before going home. This may involve various types of therapy and restorative nursing services. Restorative nursing care is an individualized program designed to promote a resident's ability to achieve their highest level of function and to live as independently as possible.
- **Skilled nursing care.** This care is provided by or under the supervision of skilled or licensed staff that is medically necessary. Examples of skilled nursing care include physical therapy, occupational therapy, intravenous injections, or wound care.
- **Custodial care.** Most residents need ongoing help with ADL's. This care is usually provided by nonmedical staff, like nurse assistants.
- **Respite care.** Individuals may come to a facility for a temporary stay when family members or their usual caregivers are away from home or otherwise not available.
- **Hospice care.** Hospice care is special care given to individuals who are dying. Hospice services may also be provided by an outside organization.
- **Palliative care.** The focus of palliative care is to provide comfort and emotional support to those residents living with a serious illness.

complicated cancers

Some residents are active and largely independent, while others need more help. Within the facility, units are often organized based on how much care residents need. The level of care needed determines how a unit is staffed, including the number of nurses and nurse assistants. When possible, residents work with staff to develop their care plan. The resident care plan is an individualized document created after the resident is assessed. It outlines the goals of care, nursing interventions (what care is to be provided), and the time frame for accomplishment and evaluation. The care plan is a working document that is updated with any change in the resident's condition.

Who Provides Care in a Long Term Care Facility?

An interdisciplinary team cares for residents in long term care facilities. This means that staff members from many departments are involved in each resident's care (Figure 1-2).

As with all teams, the players should respect each other and work together well. As a nurse assistant, you will be in contact with people from every service area. You will talk to them casually in the hallway and more formally in team meetings. The team approach gives residents the highest quality of care because information is shared,

care is coordinated, and the plan of care is based on each resident's unique needs.

Following are the team members and their general responsibilities.

- **Resident.** The resident is always the most important person on the team. A resident's family members and significant others support the resident in care decisions (Figure 1-3).

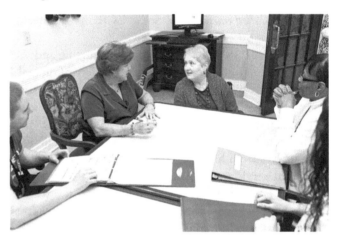

Figure 1-3 The resident and his or her family participate in decisions about the resident's care.

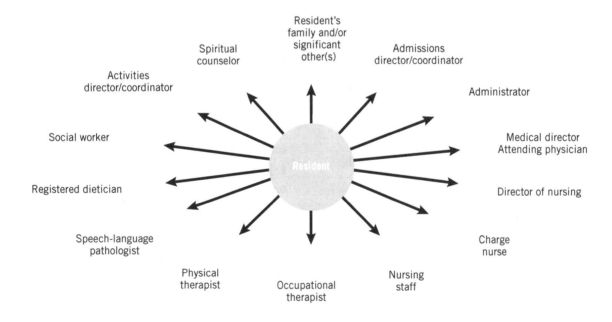

Figure 1-2 All members of the interdisciplinary team work to help the resident achieve optimal health. The resident is always the central focus.

- **Director of nursing.** The director of nursing supervises the nursing staff and establishes the philosophy and approach for caregiving.
- **Charge nurse.** This person has the day-to-day responsibility for supervising resident care. Charge nurses give the specific care assignments to nursing staff.
- **Nursing staff.** The nursing staff make up the largest department. They help residents with activities of daily living, medical treatments, medications, and health promotion. The nursing staff includes registered nurses, licensed practical nurses (known as licensed vocational nurses in some states), and nurse assistants.
- **Medical director.** This staff physician is in charge of general medical care and may provide direct care to residents.
- **Attending physician.** The attending physician directs and provides the primary care of individual residents.
- **Nurse practitioner (NP).** The NP can provide primary care for residents. They work with the interdisciplinary team to direct resident care.
- **Physical therapist (PT).** Physical therapists are highly trained professionals who help residents maintain or improve their physical abilities, such as posture, walking, and range of movement. They provide rehabilitation services following surgical procedures that affect movement to help residents return to normal function as soon as possible.
- **Occupational therapist (OT).** Occupational therapists focus on improving residents' abilities to perform everyday tasks. They assist those recovering from illness or injury and those who are dealing with a disability.
- **Speech-Language Pathologist (SLP).** These professionals, also known as speech therapists, work with residents who have difficulty speaking or swallowing. They identify communication problems and assist residents in improving speech and language abilities.
- **Admissions director or coordinator.** This person helps residents through the admission process.
- **Licensed social worker (LSW).** Social workers counsel residents and their families. They might also arrange home care services for residents who are being discharged.
- **Activities director or coordinator.** The activities director/coordinator plans and directs activities that residents enjoy and that help improve quality of life (Figure 1-4).

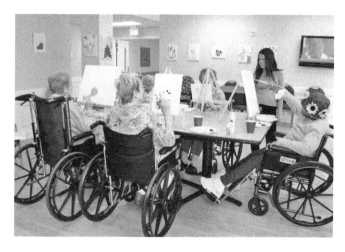

Figure 1-4 The activities director or coordinator plans a wide range of activities for residents to enjoy.

- **Registered dietitian (RD)** or registered dietician nutritionist (RDN). RDs and RDNs plan meals and design special diets to ensure good nutrition for residents.
- **Spiritual counselor.** The spiritual counselor coordinates religious services and provides counseling for residents and family members.
- **Administrator.** The administrator manages the facility and directs all staff. The administrator's goal is to make sure that each resident's quality of life and care needs are met.

Other people have important functions in the following departments:

- *Building Maintenance* maintains the physical structures (buildings) and the grounds.
- *Housekeeping* keeps the inside of the facility clean.
- *Food Services* prepares residents' meals.
- *Human Resources* hires all staff and coordinates the performance review process.
- *Financial Services* manages accounting, payroll, and purchasing.
- The *Laundry* cleans and maintains the facility's linens and residents' clothing.

Each staff member in the facility has specific skills and knowledge. All departments work together to help meet each resident's needs. As a team member, you play a very important role. You spend more time with residents than anyone else. You will learn about individual residents and develop relationships with them that no other team member may have, so effective communication with the other members of the team is vitally important to ensure individualized care.

Who Pays for Long Term Care?

Paying for long term care is often a challenge for residents and their families. Depending on the resident's age, financial status, and insurance coverage, payment may come from one or more sources. These include state and federal aid, private insurance, and personal funds.

- **Medicare.** A federal health insurance program that provides coverage for adults age 65 and older or those younger with disabilities, Medicare is a program that provides limited coverage for skilled nursing facilities (SNF), covering a specific number of days in a SNF facility after a hospital stay of at least three days. Medicare utilizes the Patient-Driven Payment Model (PDPM) to reimburse skilled nursing facilities for care. This payment model focuses on the individual needs and goals of each resident.

- **Medicaid.** A state and federal program that covers the cost of a nursing home stay for people with limited assets and income. Eligibility varies by state.

- **Managed care health insurance plan.** A type of private insurance, some managed care plans include LTC coverage in facilities that are part of the plan's provider network. Managed care plans monitor the care provided to ensure proper care and control costs. Examples of managed care plans are Health Maintenance Organization (HMO), Preferred Provider Organization (PPO), and Point of Service (POS).

- **Long term care insurance plans.** These are additional insurance policies that some people purchase in addition to their health insurance coverage. They usually help cover the costs of care when you have a chronic medical condition. Covered benefits and costs vary widely. This type of insurance is becoming more popular as people anticipate living longer and needing care.

- **Personal resources.** Residents may pay for care from their own savings or investment resources. Once a resident's personal funds are spent paying for care over a period of time, he or she may become eligible for Medicaid.

Federal rules and regulations ensure that every resident receives the same high quality of care. This does not depend on how they pay for these services or whether they can request these services themselves.

Who Oversees Long Term Care?

The **Centers for Medicare and Medicaid Services (CMS)** is part of the U.S. Department of Health and Human Services (HHS). The agency is responsible for administering a number of federal programs, including Medicare, Medicaid, the Children's Health Insurance Program (CHIP) and the federal Health Insurance Marketplace (see www.cms.gov). CMS surveys and certifies long term care facilities as approved to receive federal funding. Most facilities receive Medicare and Medicaid funds. Facilities must follow CMS regulations to continue to receive government payment.

These rules and regulations are the minimum requirements for a facility. They set service requirements for the facility, define staffing needs, and outline the rights of all residents in long term care facilities. These regulations specify how a facility determines a resident's level of care and how staff work with each new resident to develop a care plan.

Facilities must provide the services residents need to maintain at least the level of ability they had when they were admitted. Federal rules and regulations state that a long term care facility must have or provide the following:

- **Healthy and safe physical environment.** The facility must be designed, constructed, equipped, and maintained to protect health and safety. This protection is for residents, staff, and the public.

- **Physician services.** Residents are admitted to a facility by written order from the physician. While in the facility, the resident remains under their care. In some states physicians may delegate care to a nurse practitioner, physician assistant, or clinical nurse specialist.

- **Nursing services.** The facility must have enough staff to make sure the resident's assessment and care plan are effective. The resident must attain or maintain the highest practicable health. This includes their physical, mental, and psychosocial care. They should focus on all areas of health care, including health promotion, independence, and health maintenance.

- **Specialized rehabilitative services.** Special services include physical therapy, speech or language therapy, occupational therapy, and health rehabilitative services for mental health. These services can be located on site or at a nearby location.

- **Dental services.** The facility must provide each resident with routine dental care.

- **Pharmacy services.** Facilities must follow safe procedures to accurately obtain, receive, dispense, and administer medications and biologicals to meet each resident's needs.
- **Dietary/food services.** Each resident must receive a nutritious, well-balanced, and good-tasting meal. Their meals must meet their daily nutritional and special dietary needs. The food choices available are based on their preferences, always considering taste.
- **Social services.** This department coordinates admissions, discharges, and transfers of residents.
- **Recreational therapy and planned activities.** These activities encourage residents to stay involved and active. Activities provided must be based on the residents' preferences.
- **Infection control program.** This program is designed to provide a safe, sanitary, and comfortable environment. Infection control procedures must help prevent the development and transmission of disease and infection.
- **Facility administration.** A facility must use its resources effectively for each resident to attain or maintain their highest practicable physical, mental, and psychosocial well-being.

The Joint Commission is an independent, nonprofit organization that evaluates and accredits health care organizations and programs in the United States (see www.jointcommission.org). Long term care facilities often seek this accreditation, which indicates their compliance with certain quality and performance standards, in order to receive managed care contracts. To earn and keep accreditation, an organization must have an on-site survey by a Joint Commission survey team at least every three years.

Each state has a licensing organization (usually the state health department) that surveys all LTC facilities on an annual basis to ensure that they comply with state and federal rules and regulations.

What Is the Nurse Assistant's Role in Long Term Care?

In long term care, residents rely primarily on nurse assistants. As you work through this book, you will develop a clear understanding of the importance of your role. There are three main roles for the nurse assistant in long term care:

- Understanding job functions of the nurse assistant

- Working with the interdisciplinary team
- Providing care

What does it mean to provide care? Everyone has their own style of caregiving. As a nurse assistant, you will learn the standards of your profession and develop your personal caregiving style. Nurse assistants help with about 80% of all residents' care. Other team members guide this care, but you are the one with ongoing opportunities to make the everyday life of each resident better through the care and attention you provide. Your relationship with residents can make a huge difference in how they view their quality of life and the care they receive (Figure 1-5).

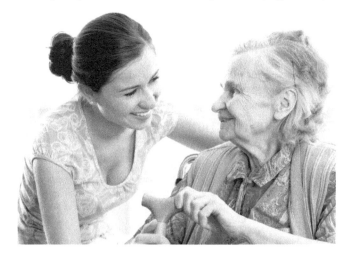

Figure 1-5 Taking the time to ask residents questions allows you to learn about their likes and dislikes.

Understanding Job Functions

When you are hired, the facility will provide you with its written *personnel policies,* along with your complete *job description.* (You may have seen some or all of the job descriptions during the interview process.) The job description typically includes this information:

- The department or unit to which the position is assigned
- Job title
- Overview of the position
- Specific list of job responsibilities and functions
- Experience and/or qualifications required to perform the job

A sample job description is shown on the following page in Figure 1-6. Carefully read your facility's nurse assistant job description. You can talk with the charge

SAMPLE NURSE ASSISTANT JOB DESCRIPTION

Department: _____

Name: _____

GENERAL PURPOSE

To perform direct care duties under the supervision of nursing personnel and to assist in maintaining a positive physical, social, and psychological environment for the residents.

QUALIFICATIONS

- Pass the state competency evaluation.
- Be a state registered nurse assistant (certified or licensed) in good standing according to all applicable federal and state certification requirements, or be in training to become a state registered nurse assistant.
- Be at least 16 years of age.
- Be able to read, write, and follow oral and written directions, and have successfully completed elementary education.
- Speak and understand English.
- Have a positive attitude toward the elderly.

ESSENTIAL JOB FUNCTIONS

A. PERSONAL CARE FUNCTIONS
Duties:

Assist residents with: daily bath, dressing, grooming, dental care, and bowel and bladder functions; preparation for medical tests and exams; ear and eye care; and transferring into and out of beds, chairs, bathtubs, etc.

Physical and sensory requirements:

Walking; reaching; bending; lifting; grasping; fine hand coordination; pushing and pulling; and ability to distinguish smells, tastes, and temperatures.

B. NURSING CARE FUNCTIONS
Duties:

Provide nursing functions as directed by supervisor, including daily perineal care and catheter care; change dressings; turn residents in bed; give sponge baths; measure and record temperature, pulse, and respirations; weigh and measure residents; perform restorative and rehabilitative procedures; observe and report presence of skin breakdowns; review care plans daily; report changes in resident conditions to supervisor; record all necessary charting entries; and report all accidents and incidents.

Physical and sensory requirements:

Bending; lifting; grasping; fine hand coordination; ability to communicate with residents; ability to distinguish smells, tastes, and temperatures; and ability to hear and respond to resident requests.

C. FOOD SERVICE FUNCTIONS
Duties:

Prepare residents for meals and snacks; identify food arrangement, and assist in feeding residents as needed; record food and fluid intake; and perform after-meal resident care.

Physical and sensory requirements:

Lifting; grasping; fine hand coordination; ability to distinguish smells, tastes, and temperatures; and ability to write or otherwise record intake.

D. RESIDENTS' RIGHTS FUNCTIONS
Duties:

Maintain resident confidentiality; treat residents with kindness, dignity, and respect; know and comply with Residents' Bill of Rights; and promptly report all resident complaints, accidents, and incidents to supervisor.

Physical and sensory requirements:

Ability to communicate with residents and to remain calm under stress.

OTHER JOB FUNCTIONS

A. SUPPORT FUNCTIONS
Duties:

Assist as directed in proper admission, transfer, and discharge of residents; inventory residents' possessions and report food articles and medications found in residents' rooms; and report defective equipment to administration.

Physical and sensory requirements:

Ability to communicate with residents and to read and write in English.

B. SAFETY AND SANITATION FUNCTIONS
Duties:

Understand and use Centers for Disease Control and Prevention (CDC) Standard Precautions, OSHA's Occupational Exposure to Bloodborne Pathogens standard, and follow established infection control, hazardous communication, and other safety rules; ensure cleanliness of assigned residents' rooms; properly maintain and record residents' restraints; and promptly report all violations of safety and sanitation rules to supervisor.

Physical and sensory requirements:

Walking; bending; lifting; grasping; fine hand coordination; ability to read and write in English; and ability to distinguish smells.

C. STAFF DEVELOPMENT FUNCTIONS
Duties:

Attend and participate in orientation, training, educational activities, and staff meetings.

Physical and sensory requirements:

Ability to understand and apply training and in-service education.

D. ALL OTHER DUTIES AS ASSIGNED

Figure 1-6 While nurse assistant job descriptions vary by facility, this sample job description lists typical qualifications, responsibilities, and job duties.

nurse about any questions in regard to your duties. Once you are on the job, you will learn your specific job responsibilities and become familiar with the facility's 24-hour routine and what happens during each shift. Each state designates what tasks nurse assistants are allowed to perform. Make sure you are aware of the scope of practice for a nurse assistant in your state.

Your general responsibilities and guidelines for success include the following:

Recognize residents as individuals.

- Find out residents' likes and dislikes.
- Ask how they want things done. Get to know their routine.
- Learn about their culture if it is different from your own (Figure 1-7).
- Find out if they have cultural preferences regarding their care, and follow their preferences.

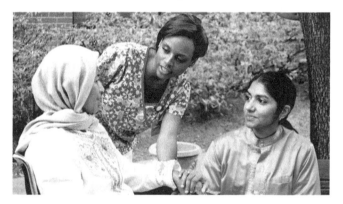

Figure 1-7 Learning about residents' cultural background helps you better understand their needs and customize care to meet those needs.

Promote residents' autonomy (making decisions for oneself).

- Understand residents' rights.
- Respect their rights when giving care.
- Encourage residents to maintain their highest level of functioning.
- Support their choices in personal care.
- Involve residents in all decisions about their care.
- Maintain their privacy.

Be aware and care.

- Balance the skills and the heart of caregiving. Observe residents closely, and watch for any changes in attitude or behavior.
- Report any changes to the charge nurse.

Be a good employee.

- Be honest and reliable.
- Be considerate of others.
- Cooperate with other team members.
- Be professional.
- Use appropriate language.
- Do not gossip.
- Be efficient with your time and supplies.
- Follow all personnel policies.
- Dress appropriately: neat and clean.
- Pay attention to personal hygiene.
- Stay healthy: Don't smoke, get enough sleep, eat a nutrient-dense diet, and exercise regularly.
- Do not use drugs or drink alcohol during work hours or before coming to work.
- Do not let personal issues interfere with your work.

Being a good employee also requires staff to be responsible and accountable for their actions. This means that when your supervisor delegates a task, you will do this to the best of your ability and take responsibility for your actions.

Working With the Nursing Team

Earlier in this chapter you learned that many different people provide services for residents. The largest department is the nursing department, led by the director of nursing. You will spend more time with nursing team members than anyone else on the interdisciplinary team, so maintaining good communication within the team is a key part in providing the best care to residents. Figure 1-8 shows a typical organizational chart for a nursing department. This is sometimes referred to as the chain of command.

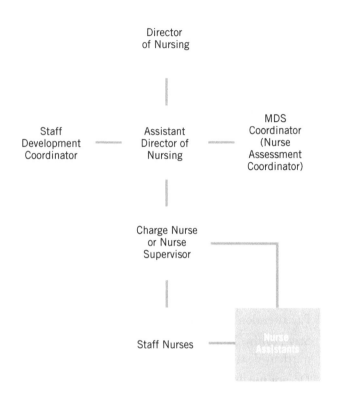

Figure 1-8 Typical organizational chart for long term care nursing services.

The **director of nursing** develops the philosophy (a belief about quality care) and approach for care. The nursing staff follows this approach. The director also determines staffing requirements. The **assistant director of nursing** helps the director of nursing put into action the philosophy and approach to care.

The **MDS coordinator** (sometimes called a nurse assessment coordinator) assesses the functional capabilities of residents and uses the data to determine the proper level of care for each resident. (MDS stands for "minimum data set," a tool used as part of the assessment process.) The **director of staff development** usually reports to the director of nursing. This nursing professional oversees nursing staff education.

Charge nurses report to either the director or assistant director of nursing, depending on the facility. They have the day-to-day responsibility for supervising resident care.

Charge nurses give the specific care assignments to the nursing team. They are a resource for problem solving and teaching, and they can help you with **in-service education**.

The number of staff nurses depends on the facility's staffing needs. Staff nurses are responsible for administering treatments and medications. A staff nurse may be a **registered nurse (RN)** or a **licensed practical nurse (LPN)**. In some states, an LPN is known as a **licensed vocational nurse (LVN)**. A staff nurse may act as a charge nurse on some shifts.

Nurse assistants report to charge nurses or staff nurses. Nurse assistants provide 80% of all resident care.

Your relationship with the charge nurse and the staff nurses is important. You need to feel that you are partners in working to achieve the caregiving goals for all residents. Follow these guidelines to develop a good relationship with the charge nurse:

- Be on time for work every day (Figure 1-9).
- Be reliable, trustworthy, accountable, and honest.
- Communicate openly.
- Make sure you understand what the charge nurse expects of you.
- Ask questions about things you do not understand.
- Be open minded and flexible in accepting your assignment.
- Be patient when you need the charge nurse's help. They have many other responsibilities, too.
- Report any resident changes immediately to the charge nurse.
- Talk about any problems or concerns you may have.
- Be ready to work at the start of your shift.
- Adhere to scheduled breaks.

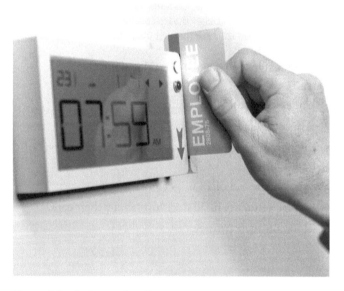

Figure 1-9 Being on time for work demonstrates that you are a reliable team member.

Establishing and maintaining a positive relationship with your co-workers is also important (Figure 1-10). A supportive work environment is a more pleasant one. Every nurse assistant has their own assignment, but you should help each other and work together. You can perform many tasks on your own, but some will require help from your co-workers, and they will need your help, as well. Remember that working well as a team improves your ability to give residents good care. Here are some actions that help in developing positive relationships:

- Offer to help co-workers when they need assistance.
- Be supportive and available to help when needed, as long as it doesn't interfere with immediate care that you are giving to another resident.
- Go to lunch together (if staff scheduling allows).
- Share ideas about caregiving (but remember, respect the residents' rights to privacy).
- Call in sick only when you are ill.
- Attend in-service education classes together.
- Be honest and reliable.
- Respect others' opinions and beliefs.
- Welcome new staff members.

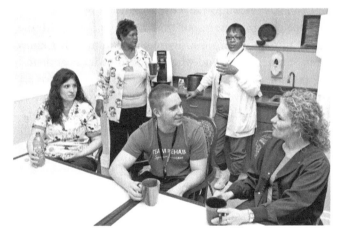

Figure 1-10   It is important to have a positive, respectful relationship with your coworkers.

Factors That Influence Care

There are many factors that influence how care is delivered:

- **The resident's needs.** A resident's needs are always the primary focus of care. Always ask yourself, "Is this what this resident wants or needs?"

- **Philosophy of caring.** The director of nursing sets the direction for care activities. Different directors have different ideas about how to do things. With time, you will become familiar with your director's approach to care.
- **New treatments and equipment.** Facilities are always looking for better ways to provide services. Your facility may try new things, such as new products or equipment.
- **Federal and state regulations.** Federal and state regulations provide a framework for caregiving. These include the Code of Federal Regulations (CFR) and Occupational Safety and Health Administration (OSHA) standards. These rules and regulations influence how much care you give, the method of providing care, and how often. This helps ensure that residents receive quality care. For example, many facilities display posters in bathrooms to remind staff to wash their hands.
- **Staffing.** The reliability of staff is a major influence on caregiving. If staff members often call in sick or there is a lot of turnover, the team does not function as well and residents' care may suffer. The attitude of the nursing staff influences all of the above factors.

These factors sometimes lead to changes in caregiving. You may not always know the reason for a change. But if you keep an open mind, ask questions, and keep residents' well-being your highest priority, you will find it easier to adapt to changes.

A Typical Day in a Long Term Care Facility

Nursing care is continuous: 24 hours a day, seven days a week, 365 days a year. Care in a long term care facility is typically organized into shifts. These shifts are scheduled based on facility staffing needs and the model of care. Shifts can overlap to allow staff ending a shift to have time to communicate with those who are coming on duty. This ensures that residents are never without someone to care for them. Most staff are assigned to one shift on a regular basis. Some may rotate between two or more shifts. Some facilities offer *flex hours* (flexible scheduling) to accommodate staff who are also in school or who must deal with childcare or other family issues.

The shift during daylight hours will often be very busy because most other team members work the day shift.

On this shift you are responsible for many of the personal care needs of residents. You will assist with two meals, scheduled appointments, recreational activities, hydration, food supplements, and snacks. Most staff meetings, care plan meetings, and physician visits occur during the day. New equipment and care procedures are first tried and evaluated on the day shift. So, it is important to manage and prioritize your time.

During the evening shift, family members and friends often visit. Fewer staff members are on duty, and there are fewer scheduled appointments. Residents relax. The evening meal is served, and p.m. care is given to prepare residents for bed. This care includes undressing, partial bathing, scheduled showers, oral hygiene, toileting, evening snacks and hydration, and comfort measures. Comfort measures may include straightening out or changing linens, providing back rubs, reading to residents, turning on soft music, and dimming the lights. On this shift you will have an opportunity to spend more time with residents and their families.

The night shift that covers residents' hours of sleep will often be considered the quiet shift, but that's not always the case. During the night most residents sleep, but some nap during the day and are awake at night. The night shift has specific duties, such as completing tasks the evening shift could not complete: helping residents with toileting, checking supplies, comforting residents who cannot sleep, and dealing with unexpected problems and emergencies. Another night shift responsibility is a.m. care. For residents who rise early in the morning, care includes helping them wash their face and hands, brush their teeth, and go to the bathroom. You may also be responsible for preparing paperwork for the upcoming day. You may make a list of residents who need showers or tub or whirlpool baths. There are important tasks to be done to prepare for the next day's activities. For example, you may have **preoperative orders** for a resident who is scheduled for a surgical procedure. The most common preoperative order is keeping a resident **NPO**. This is the abbreviation for the Latin phrase *nil per os,* which means "nothing by mouth." Residents scheduled for surgery cannot eat or drink anything after midnight.

At all times, and on all shifts, consider each resident's needs. The shifts themselves are only a framework for care, not an absolute rule for what to do or not do. Although each shift has its specific duties, never insist on doing something if a resident does not want it done at that time. Similarly, if a resident wants you to do something that is normally scheduled for the next shift, make every effort to help. With all shifts and assignments, you need to effectively manage your time, remain flexible, and prioritize care for your residents.

Nurse Assistant Assignments

Each day, at the start of your shift you will receive your **assignment** from the charge nurse. This assignment includes the residents you will care for that day. You might also meet with staff on the previous shift to hear their report about these residents, or you may get this information from the charge nurse. For example, you may learn that a resident who usually sleeps all night was awake and pacing the floor. You also learn about residents' treatments and medication status. Typical tasks performed by nurse assistants are shown in Box 1-1.

Carefully review your assignment and ask the charge nurse any questions you have to clarify your duties. Always have all the information you need before you begin giving care. This information includes the following:

- Do any residents have special needs or any special appointments today?
- Do I need help from the charge nurse at any time to give a resident a treatment?
- Does the charge nurse want any particular tasks done first?

This is a good time to ask questions if there are any tasks that you feel uncomfortable doing. Always be honest with the charge nurse about this. Talking openly with the charge nurse about your assignment lets him or her know when you need help and when you can be independent. For example, a resident needs to go to the hospital for an x-ray, but you have never done this. At this point, you do not know all the tasks involved in sending a resident to the hospital for a diagnostic exam or test, and you will need to ask for more information.

Managing Your Time

Throughout your career as a nurse assistant you will hear about the importance of being organized. You need to continually prioritize tasks to organize your day and ensure that everything gets done. **Time management** skills may not come naturally to you, so you may have to work on them. Effective time management requires an ability to prioritize tasks, organize your activities, and perform all tasks efficiently. When you use time management skills in your personal and work life, you take control and prioritize. You decide which tasks are most important and the best ways to perform those tasks. When you have mastered time management skills, you become more

BOX 1-1

COMMON TASKS OF NURSE ASSISTANTS

ASSISTING WITH PERSONAL CARE FOR RESIDENTS:

- bathing
- oral hygiene
- grooming (hair and nail care)
- dressing and undressing

ASSISTING RESIDENTS WITH MOBILITY:

- walking
- positioning
- range-of-motion exercises

ASSISTING RESIDENTS WITH MEALS:

- transporting to dining room
- preparing the environment
- preparing residents
- feeding residents
- caring for residents after meals
- recording intake and output

PROVIDING PHYSICAL COMFORT TO RESIDENTS:

- back rubs
- pillow fluffing
- hand-holding (if a resident desires)
- touching gently (if a resident desires)

PROVIDING EMOTIONAL SUPPORT FOR RESIDENTS:

- listening carefully
- working with family members
- holding a resident (if they desire)
- being with residents when they receive bad news
- sharing experiences

MAINTAINING EACH RESIDENT'S ENVIRONMENT:

- practicing infection control procedures
- cleaning residents' rooms
- making residents' beds
- preventing injuries

efficient in your job without compromising the quality of care.

In a long term care setting, there are three sets of responsibilities you need to learn to help manage your time:

- **Residents' preferences and routines.** Residents should always have a say in their own care. Residents should participate in as much of their own care as possible to maintain as much independence as possible. Allow residents to choose how they want things done. Learn about the residents' past routines and try to incorporate them into their present routine.
- **Shift responsibilities.** During each shift you will have set duties. You will learn the basics about nurse assistant tasks and responsibilities during your orientation to the job. Learn how to prioritize tasks and manage your time to complete your responsibilities during your shift. Identify which residents need baths, showers, weighing, and special turning as well as those who have medical equipment or devices such as feeding tubes, oxygen, intravenous lines, shunts, splints, or a prosthesis that will require special care.
- **Daily assignment.** As previously discussed, you receive your daily assignment from the charge nurse. It is your responsibility to make sure that you understand your assigned tasks and how to perform them.

Promoting Your Own Health

Your role as a caregiver makes it especially important to take care of yourself. Helping people as a nurse assistant is incredibly rewarding, but it does involve physical demands and may at times be stressful. You must take responsibility for your own health.

People in good health enjoy their life and their job much more than those who are tired or sick. You will give residents better care when you feel healthy and rested and have a positive attitude. In addition, you are less likely to call in sick, which causes increased workload for others on the nursing team.

To maintain or improve your health, you need to understand what it means to have a *healthy lifestyle*. Then you must evaluate what is needed to maintain this lifestyle and make a plan to achieve your goals. Actions you take to maintain or improve your health include eating a healthy, nutrient-dense diet, getting regular exercise, managing stress, and having a positive attitude. In this section, we will discuss the benefits of good health and the factors that influence health.

Part of being a good health care employee is making smart choices about your own health. You cannot provide quality care if your own health is poor. People with unhealthy lifestyles (smoking, abusing drugs or alcohol, eating a poor diet, little or no exercise, etc.) often blame their work as the cause of stress, illness, or unhappiness. They refuse to recognize that in fact it is their personal choices that are causing many of their problems. The decision to support your health is entirely up to you.

Many factors influence our health, and simple changes can sometimes make a great difference in how you feel and what you can achieve. Good health lets us lead a full, active life and reach our maximum potential. This is true for you as well as for residents. Of the factors that contribute to good health, among the most important for nurse assistants are:

- A healthy attitude
- Good nutrition
- Regular exercise
- Proper rest
- Stress management

In this section, we will focus on these five factors, although there are other factors that are very important as well. These include staying drug free, not using tobacco, and avoiding alcohol or consuming it in moderation. These substances negatively affect people's lives and job performance.

Developing a Positive Attitude

As a nurse assistant, your day-to-day attitude has a direct impact on residents' attitudes and quality of life. One of the easiest things to change is your attitude. A healthy approach to work and life begins with a positive outlook. A positive attitude influences how you live your life, how you view and perform your job, and how you treat residents and coworkers. A positive attitude can brighten your day as well as that of those around you. It is easier to have a positive outlook when you feel good about yourself and when you are well rested. Try to follow these guidelines:

- Make a difference in others' lives every day.
- Maintain a cheerful attitude — smile, it can be contagious!
- Be open to others' points of view. Avoid negative criticism.

- Stay calm when things get hectic or a crisis occurs. Breathe deeply if you start to become overwhelmed.
- Try to think through difficult situations before you react.
- Maintain a compassionate, caring attitude.
- Emphasize the positive. See the glass as half-full, not half-empty.
- Accept yourself instead of judging yourself. Be the best you can be.
- Take charge of your life. Visualize what you want for yourself and your family and work to achieve it.
- Refrain from gossiping. Refuse to participate, and remove yourself from any conversations that move in that direction.

Eating for Health

Nutrition refers to the nourishment that you take in through food and drink. The quality of your diet directly affects your quality of life. *Good nutrition* involves eating a variety of healthy foods in appropriate amounts, foods that are high in vitamins, minerals, complex carbohydrates, lean protein, and healthy fats (Figure 1-11). This promotes maintaining a healthy body weight and reduces the risk of many types of chronic disease. Many people eat a diet that is high in empty calories — those that fill you up but have little nutritional value. Some people eat compulsively or crave sweet or fatty foods when they are stressed. It is possible to consume a poor diet for years and still fulfill your daily responsibilities, but eventually the results of poor choices catch up with you and lead to poor health. You can find resources on healthy eating at www.choosemyplate.gov.

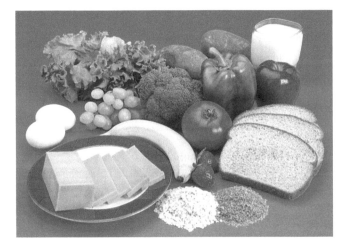

Figure 1-11 Eating nutritious foods is an important part of maintaining your health and giving you the energy you need to feel your best every day.

Exercise and Health

Physical activity and exercise are a vital part of life. Regular exercise can help you stay healthy and independent. Regardless of your current fitness status, it is always possible to improve and experience greater health. Your physician or a fitness professional can help you determine how much and what types of exercise may be best for you, and there are literally thousands of options and resources available.

The U.S. Department of Health and Human Services periodically releases *Physical Activity Guidelines for Americans*. The current guidelines state that health benefits can be obtained with a minimum of 150 minutes (2.5 hours) to 300 minutes (5 hours) of moderate-level physical activity per week. This isn't hard to do — this can be brisk walking, jogging, cycling, swimming, hiking, dancing, or any other activity or sport that you enjoy and will do regularly (Figure 1-12). You are never too young or too old to benefit from exercise! Any physical activity that gets your heart beating, your blood circulating, and your muscles working will help to improve your health and well-being. Be creative in finding ways to add physical activity into your daily routine. Keep a picture in your mind of the healthy person you would like to be.

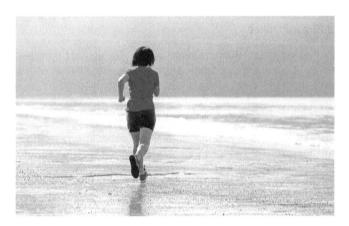

Figure 1-12 Regular exercise can help you stay healthy.

Adequate Rest

Numerous research studies show that most people function best when they get seven to eight hours of restful sleep each night. To shine at work, you have to be well rested. Make getting adequate sleep a priority in your life. The Mayo Clinic (www.mayoclinic.org) and the American Academy of Sleep Medicine (www.sleepeducation.org) offer resources and tips on improving the quality of your sleep.

Managing Stress

Managing stress is also important for good health. Chronic stress can affect your health in many ways. It contributes to high blood pressure, heart disease, and diabetes. It can also decrease your immune system's ability to fight disease or heal from injury and can contribute to the overall aging process. Poorly managed stress can increase your risk of accidents and cause you to forget important information or tasks.

No one can avoid stress, but we can learn to manage it more effectively. Some people exercise to reduce stress. An invigorating workout, yoga practice, or calming meditation class might work for you. Deep breathing and progressive relaxation exercises have been shown to have a positive effect in reducing stress. Laughter is still the best medicine, so take time to smile, spend time with friends and family (and pets!), listen to music, or participate in your favorite hobby. These activities give your body and mind a chance to calm down. If things become unmanageable, consult a licensed mental health counselor or medical professional for further advice or treatment — don't go it alone.

- In long term care, nurse assistants provide the majority (80%) of care. The focus must always be on residents' needs and providing quality care. You can make a difference in how residents feel about their lives while living in a long term care facility. Give them your best every day.

- As a nurse assistant, you are always learning. You must be willing to ask questions so that you learn tasks and procedures correctly from your first day forward.

- It is important for you to understand your role within the interdisciplinary team and work to develop positive relationships with residents and all team members.

- Remember that taking care of yourself is vital to your ability to provide the best possible care.

▷ **Key Terms**

accreditation — process of certifying that a facility meets certain quality and performance standards

activities director/coordinator — staff member who plans and directs activities for residents

activities of daily living (ADL) — tasks that are required for daily living, such as bathing, dressing, personal hygiene, and eating

administrator — general manager of a facility

admissions director/coordinator — staff member who coordinates the process of admitting new residents

Alzheimer's unit — unit that provides care for residents with Alzheimer's disease and other types of dementia

assignment — a specific set of tasks that an employee is expected to perform

assistant director of nursing — senior nursing professional who reports to the director of nursing

assisted living facilities — residential facilities that provide a limited amount of assistance with daily activities

attending physician — directs and provides the primary care of individual residents

autonomy — ability to act independently and make decisions for oneself

biologicals — medical products made from living organisms, such as vaccines or blood components

care plan — written document created after the resident assessment is completed that outlines the goals of care, nursing interventions, and the time frame for accomplishment and evaluation

Centers for Medicare and Medicaid Services (CMS) — the agency responsible for surveying and certifying long term care facilities as approved to receive federal funding

charge nurse — nursing professional with day-to-day responsibility for supervising resident care

Code of Federal Regulations (CFR) — set of rules published in the Federal Register by the departments and agencies of the U.S. government

continuing care retirement community — facility that provides several tiers of care: independent living, assisted living, and skilled nursing care

delegate — to give or entrust someone with a task or job

director of nursing — senior nursing professional who directs the approach for care and determines staffing requirements

director of staff development — staff member who develops and oversees nursing education programs

gerontology — scientific field focused on the study of aging

hospice care — care for terminally ill patients that aims to provide comfort and alleviate pain

in-service education — educational programs provided for employees while on the job

interdisciplinary team — staff members from various departments who work together to plan and implement care

intermediate care facility — provides nursing and supportive care to residents who have a variety of mental or physical disabilities

Joint Commission — nonprofit organization that accredits and certifies U.S. health-care facilities and programs; full name is The Joint Commission

level of care — classification based on the intensity of medical and nursing services provided in a health-care setting

licensed practical nurse (LPN) — health professional who provides basic nursing care under the supervision of a registered nurse or physician

licensed social worker (LSW) — licensed professional who usually has a master's degree in social work and who counsels residents and families

licensed vocational nurse (LVN) — health professional who provides basic nursing care under the supervision of a registered nurse or physician

long term care — a range of medical and nonmedical services provided for people who have a chronic illness, disability, or cognitive impairment that affects their ability to perform everyday tasks

managed care — type of health insurance coverage that monitors quality of care and is designed to contain costs

MDS coordinator — staff member who assesses residents' functional capabilities and determines the appropriate level of care; also called a nurse assessment coordinator

Medicaid — joint federal-state health insurance program for low-income individuals and families

medical director — senior staff physician who directs medical care in a facility

Medicare — federal health insurance program for individuals age 65 and older and certain people with disabilities

NPO — abbreviation for nil per os, Latin for "nothing by mouth." Used to designate a period of time during which a person cannot eat or drink before surgery or some other type of medical procedure.

nurse practitioner (NP) — works with the interdisciplinary team to direct and provide primary care for residents

nursing staff — trained members of the nursing team; includes LPNs/LVNs, registered nurses, and nurse assistants

nutrition — nourishment for the body provided by food and drink

Occupational Safety and Health Administration (OSHA) — federal agency responsible for protecting worker health and safety

occupational therapist (OT) — licensed health professional who works with residents to improve their ability to perform everyday tasks

physical therapist (PT) — licensed health professional who uses methods that include exercise, heat, massage, mobilization, and manipulation to reduce pain and improve mobility

post-acute care unit — unit that provides a high level of care for residents; may include rehabilitative services

preoperative orders — physician orders prior to surgery

registered dietician (RD) — staff member who develops food plans and special diets for residents

registered dietician nutritionist (RDN) — staff member who develops food plans and special diets for residents

registered nurse (RN) — health professional who provides an advanced level of nursing care and may supervise other nursing staff

rehabilitation unit — unit that provides specialized care designed to help residents return to a previous level of physical functioning after an illness or injury

resident — person admitted to a long term care facility

respite care — care provided for residents who enter a facility for a temporary stay until their regular caregivers become available

restorative nursing — nursing care designed to promote a resident's ability to achieve the highest level of function and to live as independently as possible

shift — scheduled period of work for a group of employees (as in day, evening, and night shifts)

skilled nursing care — care that is provided by or under the supervision of skilled or licensed staff that is medically necessary

speech-language pathologist (SLP) — highly trained professional who works with residents who have swallowing, speech, language, or other communication problems

spiritual counselor — staff member who coordinates religious services and provides counseling for residents and families

terminal conditions — illnesses from which a patient is not expected to recover; death will likely occur within a short period of time

The Joint Commission — nonprofit organization that accredits and certifies U.S. health-care facilities and programs

time management — the ability to plan and prioritize tasks and perform activities efficiently to make the best use of available time

traumatic brain injury unit — unit that specializes in rehabilitative care for residents with traumatic head injuries

1. **Long term care includes health care or personal care services provided:**
   a. During infancy and childhood
   b. Over an extended period of time
   c. In the acute care hospital
   d. In doctors' offices

2. **Settings for long term care include all of the following, except:**
   a. Assisted living communities
   b. Rehabilitation centers
   c. Adult day care centers
   d. Health and fitness clubs

3. **There are many reasons a resident may require long term care including rehabilitation, hospice care, and:**
   a. Health spa services
   b. Skilled nursing care
   c. Job training
   d. Holistic retreats

4. **The interdisciplinary team member who helps residents maintain or improve their physical abilities is the:**
   a. Licensed Social Worker
   b. Physical Therapist
   c. Activities Coordinator
   d. Spiritual Counselor

5. **The most important person on the interdisciplinary team is the:**
   a. Charge Nurse
   b. Resident
   c. Physician
   d. Admissions Director

6. **The government agency that surveys and certifies long term care facilities approved to receive federal funding is the:**
   a. Health Insurance Association of America (HIAA)
   b. Office of Management and Budget (OMB)
   c. Centers for Medicare and Medicaid Services (CMS)
   d. American Association of Retired Persons (AARP)

7. **Nurse Assistants report directly to:**
   a. The physician
   b. The family
   c. The charge nurse
   d. The Dietician

8. **One way for the CNA to develop a good relationship with the charge nurse is to:**
   a. Be on time for work every day
   b. Keep your thoughts to yourself
   c. Don't ask questions
   d. Only accept assignments you want

9. **There are many factors that influence how care is delivered including the resident's needs and:**
   a. Federal and state regulations
   b. The personal beliefs of the CNA
   c. The World Health Organization
   d. None of these

10. **In a long term care setting, there are three sets of responsibilities that a nurse assistant needs to learn to help manage time:**
    a. Residents' preferences and routines, shift responsibilities, and daily assignment
    b. What time breakfast, lunch, and dinner are served
    c. What needs to be done now, what can be held over for the next shift, and what can be omitted altogether
    d. When your coworker is available and what they can help with and when the patient can go to physical therapy

2

Communication and Customer Service

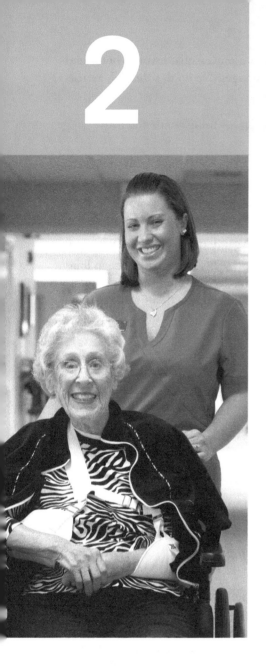

Communication is a skill we use in every interaction in life. All people need to feel that they are being heard. In this chapter, we will discuss the skills you need for effective communication with others. These skills are essential in providing excellent customer service to residents and their families.

You will learn how to communicate in various ways to meet the resident's special needs and how to use communication skills to resolve conflicts, should they arise.

OBJECTIVES:

- Define communication.

- Differentiate between verbal and nonverbal communication.

- Explain how touch is a form of communication.

- List some general guidelines for active listening and promoting effective communication.

- Describe how to successfully interact with residents with various special communication needs.

- Describe ways to communicate with residents who are behaving inappropriately.

- List the steps involved in conflict resolution.

- Define customer service and explain how poor customer service affects residents' quality of life and families' level of satisfaction with residents' care.

- Explain why providing excellent customer service is an integral part of resident care.

- List some strategies for ensuring good customer service in your daily caregiving.

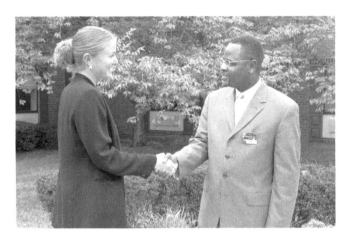

Figure 2-1 A handshake and facial expressions such as smiling are some of the ways we communicate nonverbally.

How We Communicate Counts

Moving into a long term care facility can leave residents feeling isolated and lonely. They are surrounded by strangers whom they depend on to help them meet their most basic needs. Talking with a caring person can help alleviate feelings of sadness, loneliness, or abandonment.

When you show residents that you understand their feelings, they begin to trust you. Residents who feel heard and understood are more likely to share their feelings and needs. A trusting relationship can develop when they feel cared for and know what to expect. Effective **communication** is the key to creating a trusting relationship.

It is important because it:

- Improves residents' quality of life
- Helps you gain residents' cooperation and build trust
- Adds to residents' and families' satisfaction, as well as your own
- Shares information about any changes you observe about residents
- Assists the health care team in planning individualized care for each resident
- Makes your job easier and more enjoyable.

A big part of your job as a nurse assistant involves communicating with residents. Our culture emphasizes words in many forms: print and digital newspapers, magazines, and books; radio, television, and movies; lectures, conversations, and text messages, and of course the massive amount of information available online. But communication is more than just words.

Communication is a process that involves both sending and receiving messages. We do this through a variety of methods such as:

- **Verbal communication** — using words and active listening
- **Nonverbal communication** — through body language, expressions, and touch (Figure 2-1)
- **Visual communication** — using symbols, such as traffic lights, road signs, memes, and emojis (Figure 2-2).

Words, actions, and symbols help give our lives structure, safety, and comfort. This is especially true in long term care facilities. Effective communication can improve the quality of your relationships with residents and your ability to provide the best care. All of these aspects of communication are very important in your role as a nurse assistant.

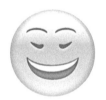  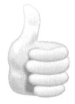

Figure 2-2 Emojis are commonly used in digital communication to express a wide range of feelings and opinions.

Verbal Communication

Verbal communication involves spoken or written words. That sounds simple enough, doesn't it? But words can have many different meanings, depending on one's background, **culture**, and education. You don't always automatically know exactly what someone means, even when they use familiar words. You have to understand the **context** of their words. This can be achieved by considering the entire situation, background, or environment that provides meaning to a person's words. As a nurse assistant, you must communicate in a manner that the resident understands, and you must pay attention to signs that show when they do not.

Your tone of voice, the speed at which you speak, and the **clarity** of your spoken message tell the listener much more than just what the words mean. You can make it easier for others to understand what you are saying if you make use of the tips shown in Box 2-1.

In an environment where residents and staff may represent many cultures, languages, and **customs**, there are some important points to remember when caring for residents:

- If you do not speak a resident's primary language, you must find someone to translate for you, such as a family member or another staff member. You can demonstrate that you really care by making an effort to learn some words in the resident's native language.
- If your primary language is not English, you must speak only English with English-speaking residents and also when you are around them. Staff members who speak to each other in a language that residents do not understand are indirectly violating these residents' rights. Some residents may feel that staff are talking about them and feel intimidated or threatened. This is particularly true with confused residents who may be having difficulty understanding what is going on around them. Speaking in another language creates the impression that you do not want them to understand what you are saying.
- Avoid using medical terms with residents, or if you must use them, clearly explain their meaning.

Box 2-1

THE DO'S AND DON'TS OF COMMUNICATION

DO

- Do use words that you know are familiar to the resident to be sure they understand.
- Do speak clearly and slowly.
- Do look directly at the person you are talking to.
- Do try to be at the person's eye level.
- Do use a pleasant tone.
- Do reduce or eliminate other sounds such as radio, TV, and housekeeping equipment. Turn down the volume or close the door to the room.

DON'T

- Don't use medical terms or slang, which many residents do not understand.
- Don't use profanity.
- Don't put your hands near your mouth while speaking.
- Don't talk with food or chewing gum in your mouth.

Nonverbal Communication

Nonverbal communication, is any type of communication that does not involve words. **Body language** includes facial expressions and eye movements, your posture and the position of your body, and your movements. Here are some examples:

- Standing with your hands on your hips or with your arms crossed may be interpreted as signs of anger or defensiveness.
- In many cultures, maintaining eye contact while speaking conveys attention and caring, but in some cultures this is regarded as a sign of disrespect.
- Moving quickly communicates that you are in a hurry and may not have time for conversation.
- Sitting down to talk with someone communicates that you are interested in them and care enough to take the time to talk (Figure 2-3).

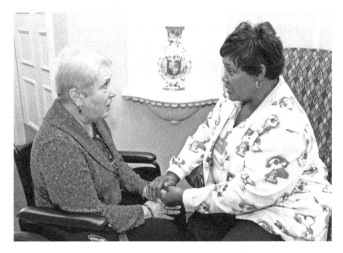

Figure 2-3 Empathetic body language communicates that you are interested in what residents have to say.

Facial expressions can convey many feelings, including happiness, humor, concern, pain, anger, frustration, and sadness. If you are experiencing negative feelings, your face will usually show it. Many times we are unaware of the nonverbal messages that our body language and expressions are sending to others. While at times we may use words to hide our true feelings, our body language usually reveals the truth. Examples of body language to avoid are:

- Rolling your eyes
- Sighing
- Smirking or using disrespectful gestures
- Turning your back on the resident
- Crossing your arms across your chest or standing with your hands on your hips

Pay close attention to the verbal and nonverbal messages that you send to residents and coworkers. For example, if a resident asks you to do a task that you cannot easily do immediately, pause to discuss alternatives instead of expressing frustration or a sense of being rushed. Together you can create a plan that works for both of you. And when caring for residents, watch for their nonverbal messages as you listen to their verbal communication.

Touch

Touch is an important form of nonverbal communication. It can be comforting, neutral, or intimidating. Some people use their hands when talking and naturally reach out to touch others. Others are not comfortable being touched — to them, touch is an invasion of their personal space. Learn about each resident's comfort level with touch (Figure 2-4). Be aware of your own feelings about touching others and being touched. Some find it easier to touch someone else than to accept being touched themselves.

Ensure that professional boundaries are maintained during all forms of communication.

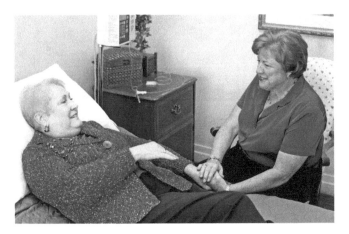

Figure 2-4 Touch can be a reassuring form of communication with residents who are comfortable with it.

Active Listening

The more you know about another person, the better you can communicate with them. You have many chances to learn about residents through your daily contact with them. The skill you need most is listening. *Active listening* is a way of listening to another person that improves mutual understanding. It means paying attention to more than just the spoken words. Active listening includes observing body language and doing your best to understand the feelings behind the words. Listening with empathy means that you make an effort to "put yourself in the other person's shoes" to understand what he or she is feeling and experiencing.

There are several important skills that you will need to practice to become a better listener. First, understand that effective listening takes time. You can learn quite a bit about residents' likes and dislikes, activities they participated in before entering the facility, and their family relationships. Take time to sit and talk, and listen to whatever is on their mind. This demonstrates that you are interested in them and that they matter to you. Other key elements of good listening are:

- Avoid distractions such as cell phones.
- Be relaxed and unhurried when you talk with residents; this helps to put them at ease.
- Make eye contact (with those who are comfortable with it), lean toward them, and nod occasionally as they speak.
- Try to keep your face at the same height as theirs by sitting, squatting, or kneeling close to the bed or chair.
- Let silence happen when residents talk; do not try to hurry them.
- If you do not understand something a resident says, ask them to repeat it.
- If you still do not understand, ask someone else for help. Do not pretend to understand when you don't, because a trusting relationship depends on honest and clear communication.

Be aware of your body language when you are listening. Maintain an *open posture,* with your arms comfortable at your sides or in your lap. Avoid crossing your arms in front of you or placing your hands on your hips. If the resident is comfortable with touch, you can touch him or her on the shoulder or arm from time to time while you talk. Sit close enough for residents to see you clearly but not so close that you invade their sense of personal space.

Validating Communication

To ensure that residents receive the precise message you mean to send, you need to *validate,* or confirm, whether or not he or she understands your intended message. Sometimes you know the communication was effective because the person does what you requested. In other cases, you know how the message was received by observing the person's body language and facial expressions (Figure 2-5).

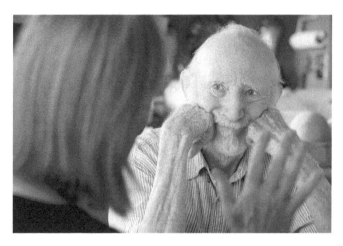

Figure 2-5 Observing the listener's body language and facial expressions tells you if your message was heard correctly.

Another way to validate communication is a technique called reflection. This means that you restate in your own words what the other person said. You also can use this technique to encourage a resident to continue talking. If your interpretation is correct, this shows that you understand the speaker's feelings and intentions. If your interpretation is not correct, this gives the speaker a chance to clarify what they were saying.

Promoting Effective Communication

In addition to the techniques you have already learned, keep in mind the following guidelines for promoting effective communication:

- Show respect for residents by calling them by their title and surname (Mrs. Jones) unless they request otherwise.
- Do not use nicknames such as "dear," "sugar," or "honey."
- Explain new procedures before you carry them out. Plan activities with residents ahead of time, and always keep your word. If something prevents you from keeping a promise, explain why.
- Respect a resident's feelings. Do not dismiss their feelings with comments such as: "Things aren't all that bad," or "Don't talk like that. It's going to be fine."
- Give hope, but not false reassurances.
- Always assume that a resident can hear you. Even if the person seems unresponsive, continue to explain who you are and what you are doing.
- Offer residents choices in all their daily activities.

- Look for ways to encourage residents to keep control over their lives. Always ask first if it is okay to do something related to their care. Ask them what they want to wear, when they want to take a bath, and when they want care.
- When possible, teach residents or family members how to do some of the resident's grooming, if they wish.
- Ask an open-ended question that encourages residents to talk, rather than asking questions with yes or no answers. Say, "How do you feel about this?" or "Tell me about that."
- Respect residents' privacy by not sharing personal information about them except with staff members who need to know.

Ending a Conversation

Communication is important, but so is getting your daily work done. How do you politely end a conversation when you must leave a resident to do something else? Try to end the conversation so that the resident feels good.

You can simply say, "I've really enjoyed talking to you. Can we continue this conversation after dinner? I have to check on some other residents now."

When you start a conversation, you can say, "I have about 10 minutes before I have to do something else. Could we talk for a few minutes?" When the time is up, you can say, "I have to go now, but I'd like to talk more later." Set a time for this if you can and be sure you come back. Never make a promise you cannot keep.

If you are not communicating effectively with a resident, will it affect their care? A resident or family member who is not comfortable talking with you may complain, withdraw, or feel that no one is interested in them. Poor communication also poses the risk of residents missing opportunities for positive relationships with other residents. Effective communication enhances residents' quality of life and keeps you engaged in your work as you continue to have a helping relationship with the residents you care for.

Special Communication Needs

Some residents have physical, mental, or emotional problems that make communication difficult. These include:

- Hearing or vision loss
- Difficulty speaking due to an illness, stroke, or improperly fitting dentures

- Depression, anxiety, or memory loss
- Behavior problems

When you are dealing with residents with special communication needs, you will need to use certain techniques that help promote effective communication.

Hearing-Impaired Residents

When communicating with residents with a hearing impairment, follow these guidelines:

- Eliminate or reduce background noise as much as possible. *don't do*
- Face the resident when you are speaking so they can see your lips. This may be helpful to residents who have developed some lip-reading ability. Speak clearly, and don't slur your words.
- Be sure you have the person's attention and maintain eye contact.
- Use gestures or point to objects as you speak and encourage the resident to use his or her hands to point to things they want.
- If the person's hearing is better on one side, position yourself so that you speak toward that side.
- You may touch a resident gently to get their attention.
- If a resident has a hearing aid, encourage its use. Be sure the hearing aid is clean and working properly (Figure 2-6).
- Repeat what you said if a resident asks you to. If necessary, say it again using different words.
- In some cases, you may need to write down on paper what you are saying.
- Always be patient.

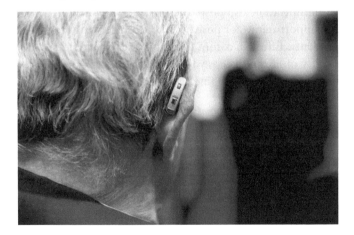

Figure 2-6 Many residents wear hearing aids, and it is important to ensure that they are in working order.

Visually Impaired Residents

When communicating with a resident who is blind or has impaired vision, follow these guidelines:

- Be sure the room has good lighting and sit where the person can best see and hear you. If a resident has glasses, make sure they are wearing them and that the glasses are clean (Figure 2-7).
- If a resident has another vision aid, such as a magnifying glass, encourage its use.
- Be sure to introduce yourself when you start talking to the resident. Continue talking so they know what you are doing and where you are.
- When appropriate, touch a resident to let them know where you are. Encourage the resident to use touch to find things in the immediate environment.
- Try to keep things in the same place (a place the resident prefers), so that the resident becomes familiar with their location. This helps residents be more independent in self-care.
- If a resident asks you to read mail or other personal documents to them, of course do so, but only when asked.
- Describe items the resident will be using, including their location. For example, describe the food on the resident's plate using the location of the items.

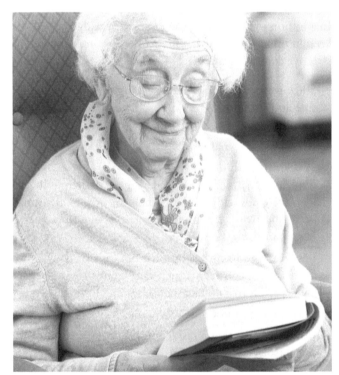

Figure 2-7 Older adults commonly need glasses to read or for other activities.

Speech-Impaired Residents

Communicating with residents with impaired speech is a necessary skill in most long term care facilities. Strokes and other brain injuries can often cause a condition called aphasia, which is characterized by a partial or total loss of the ability to communicate verbally or in writing.

Residents with aphasia may have difficulty expressing themselves and understanding what you are saying to them. A resident with expressive aphasia may have difficulty communicating but can usually comprehend what is being said to them. Some residents cannot speak but can read. Others may not be able to read, speak, or write. The specific limitation depends on the underlying reason for the loss of speech. Talk with the charge nurse to learn more about a resident's condition and how to best communicate with the resident.

Residents who have difficulty being understood may give up and become depressed or frustrated. They may withdraw and no longer try to communicate. Your time and patience can make a big difference in these instances. Try these ways to promote communication:

- Encourage the resident to use his or her hands to point or to touch things to help communicate their message.

- Ask questions they can answer with a yes or no.

- Since it is understandably frustrating for these residents to make themselves understood, let them express their anger and frustration if it occurs. If needed, simply sit quietly with them and continue your efforts to understand what they are saying.

- When you have developed an understanding of what a resident's particular sounds or symbols mean, share this information with other staff so they can communicate better with the resident. A communication board can be developed that includes signs, pictures, or symbols the person uses. The communication board can also list common phrases a resident might use; this allows him or her to point to what they need or the question they want to ask.

Cognitively Impaired Residents

Cognitive impairments include a range of conditions that affect memory, thinking, and decision-making skills. Communicating with a resident who is cognitively impaired is not only more challenging for you as the caregiver, it is frustrating for the resident as well. Some residents may have significant memory loss. Many residents cannot remember recent events (short-term memory) but clearly remember people and events from their childhood (long-term memory). Encourage them to talk about things they can remember. Follow these guidelines:

- Keep your questions and directions short and simple. Repeat information if needed.

- Try to understand the resident's feelings and their perceptions of the world, and use words appropriate for them.

- Use helpful visual reminders, such as referring to calendars and clocks throughout the facility. A wall chart in the room can help a resident remember daily routines, such as the steps in getting dressed or the times that meals are served.

- Due to memory loss, sometimes what residents say may not make sense to you. Never laugh at them or make fun of anything they say. (Figure 2-8)

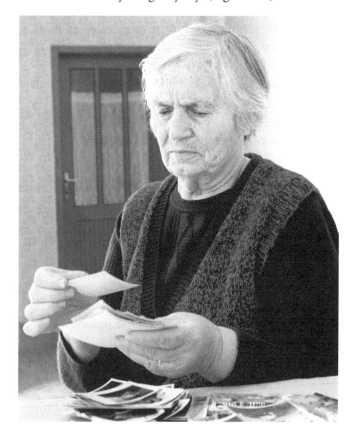

Figure 2-8   Although some residents may struggle to remember recent events, they may clearly remember events from long ago and enjoy talking to you about them.

Residents Who Are Depressed, Anxious, or Discouraged

When communicating with a resident who is depressed or feeling anxious or discouraged, there are some key things to remember. Some residents become depressed when they are having trouble adjusting to the facility. They may have experienced many losses and moving to a facility is a huge life change. Your most important guideline is to be patient, understanding, and consistent. The following additional tips may be helpful:

- Spend extra time sitting with the resident, even if they are not talking to you.

- Invite them to participate in their own care. For example, you might say, "I'll get a basin of water. While I'm doing that, why don't you get out your shaving cream and razor?"

- Set goals for the resident. Make suggestions such as, "Today we'll walk just to the nurses' station and back. Tomorrow, I'd like you to walk with me to the dining room."

- Ask family members and friends about the resident's past interests and hobbies. Then try to engage them in conversation about these interests.

- Invite them to participate in social activities when they feel ready.

- No matter what, be patient and keep trying. When you show you care, the resident may eventually respond.

The following tips are helpful in dealing with residents who need support and encouragement:

- Encourage physical activity; this helps to maintain muscle tone and flexibility of joints.

- If residents ask you to do something for them that they can do themselves, you can suggest, "You do as much as you can, and I'll help you with what you can't do." Being independent to the degree possible helps residents feel better about themselves.

- The caregiving team should use a consistent approach for residents who need more encouragement. When they begin to participate more in their care, give encouragement and praise, such as:

"You did a good job. You should be proud of your accomplishment." or "I'm glad to see you out of your room. I hope we'll see you out more." or "I'm glad you tried that. Tomorrow maybe you can do a little bit more."

Residents with Behavioral Problems

Special communication needs arise with residents who have behavioral problems or who may act out in inappropriate ways. A resident may make sexual advances or inappropriate comments. In such cases you need to communicate clearly that you do not like the behavior and that you would like for it to stop. You might say, "That makes me very uncomfortable. Please don't do it again."

Due to cognitive issues, however, some residents cannot control their behavior. In these situations, the best thing you can do is to distract them with another topic or activity. Behaviors, such as sexual advances or inappropriate remarks or jokes, may make other residents uncomfortable. It is important that residents who are not mentally competent be protected from unwanted sexual advances. Some precautions you can take include:

- Watch mentally impaired and vulnerable residents closely.

- Protect other residents from unwanted sexual advances by a behaviorally challenged resident. This often requires moving the person with the problematic behavior into a separate area to keep them from annoying or threatening other residents.

- Try to spend time with those with behavior issues and look for activities they might enjoy. Focusing their attention on a pleasant activity can help replace the inappropriate behavior with positive social interaction (Figure 2-9).

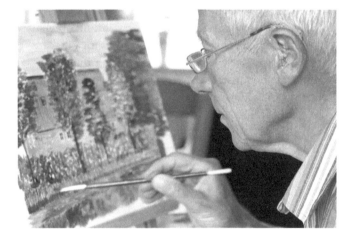

Figure 2-9 Participation in an enjoyable activity can distract a resident who is agitated or behaving inappropriately.

Aggressive Residents

Aggression is defined as hostile or violent behavior toward others. Some residents may be verbally or physically aggressive with you or with other residents. You must protect residents from harm, but you also must protect the rights of the abusing resident.

In cases of **verbal abuse**, you can acknowledge the resident's feelings. Often the person is making negative or nasty statements as a way of venting anger or frustration, as we all do occasionally. In cases of physical abuse, you must act to prevent harm to others. It is important that you do not allow an aggressive resident to injure another resident or staff member. A resident may express anger or distress by yelling or cursing, hitting, kicking, head-butting, biting, spitting, or throwing things. Residents who witness a conflict between others may become anxious and need your support and reassurance that you and other staff members will keep them safe.

The following are ways to prevent aggression and protect residents from injury:

- Get to know your residents — what they are feeling and thinking and why they act as they do.
- Constantly monitor their moods, which can change without any reason you can see.
- Try to understand what they are feeling and adjust your words and actions to meet their needs.

Understanding an aggressive resident is not always easy, especially if they are on medication, or are depressed, ill, overly tired, or in pain. Still, you can learn what the person is feeling by talking with him or her, observing facial expressions, and paying attention to what the prior shift reports about the resident's attitude or actions.

The following guidelines will help you remain calm and protect both yourself and your residents:

- Never surprise a resident or let them surprise you.
- Never approach a resident from behind and touch or startle them. When you do approach residents, smile and speak in a soft, friendly voice.
- Never give a resident a direct order or command. Always phrase your wishes as a request.
- Use short sentences and ask simple yes-or-no questions.
- When appropriate and when it will not surprise the resident, gently touch them. This can be reassuring and communicates that you care.

- Don't rush. Determine if the resident is willing to listen to you and then allow plenty of time for them to hear and understand you.
- Evaluate the situation as unemotionally as you can, and do not take a resident's actions personally or consider yourself to be the cause of negative behavior. An aggressive resident may have a brain disease or another type of mental impairment and not mean to hurt or annoy you. They are struggling with feelings or pain that may be difficult to understand or express, and you just happen to be there when they could not cope any longer.
- Never argue with a resident, no matter what they say to upset you. Always stay calm and be patient and understanding (Figure 2-10).

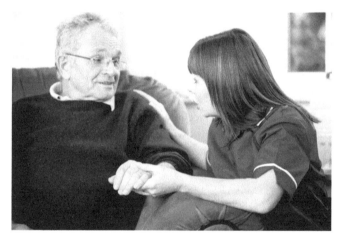

Figure 2-10   It is important to always stay calm when dealing with residents who are upset, frustrated, or angry.

Conflict Resolution

Conflict resolution is the process of finding a peaceful solution to a disagreement. Resolving conflicts can be a very rewarding experience. Successfully resolving conflicts is a key part of respecting residents' dignity and valuing their rights; it also contributes to a positive work environment.

Understanding the causes of conflict and how people react is very important. With this understanding, you can learn to resolve conflicts in a productive and rewarding way. Conflict is often a very personal thing. What you perceive as a conflict may not be viewed that way by someone else. Conflict can be defined as a situation in which:

- One side or person tries to gain something at the expense of another

- People have differing or seemingly incompatible ideas, interests, or values
- A disagreement arises among two or more people (Figure 2-11)
- People are trying to meet a goal in different ways

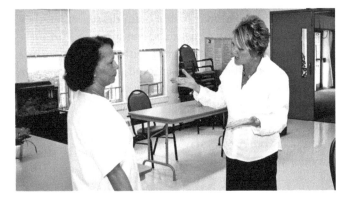

Figure 2-11 Sometimes family members become angry with staff. You should actively listen to their concerns and ask your supervisor for assistance in resolving problems if necessary.

Before you can practice effective conflict resolution, you must recognize your own reaction to conflict. When you find yourself in a situation that involves conflict, step back and look at your own motives and actions. Take stock of your emotional response and judge whether it is appropriate. Ask yourself, "What is going on? Why am I so upset?" Step back to observe the situation and yourself, and take time to understand what is going on. Ask yourself, "Am I reacting to this situation or to something else?" This process of self-discovery helps you focus your emotional energy so you can find a productive solution.

People react to conflict in different ways. Typical reactions include the following:

- **Avoidance** is trying to escape from, rather than deal with, an issue. With this approach, the conflict is not dealt with and usually continues.
- **Competition** is the opposite of avoidance. One of the parties in the conflict takes action against the other person in an attempt to "beat" that person, as in a competition. The action taken may not have anything to do with the original conflict.
- **Accommodation** is giving in to the other person. In doing so, your own needs are not being met, and you may be agreeing to something that goes against your better judgment simply to end a disagreement.
- **Compromise** means that both people give up something in order to resolve the problem. Neither one "wins" or is

completely satisfied. Most often, both parties settle for something less than or different from what they wanted, but both agree to the terms and to letting the issue go.

- **Collaboration** is the best reaction to conflict. When both sides collaborate to resolve a problem, they work together to come up with a reasonable solution. Often both parties feel they win when they make an effort to understand the other's position and work together on the solution.

People tend to react defensively when they feel another person is attacking their integrity or questioning their competence, ethics, or values. When both parties become defensive, it is very difficult to resolve the conflict. There are four common defensive reactions to conflict. Have you ever reacted in any of the following ways? Taking things personally? Running for cover? Creating a diversion or distraction? Or attacking the other person? None of these reactions are helpful, and all are likely to make it more difficult to resolve the conflict.

Effective Communication When Conflict Occurs

Understanding other people can be very challenging. Misunderstandings happen because two people may experience the same event or situation differently. Communication sometimes breaks down when people view conflict as a personal attack.

There are several common barriers to communication: defensiveness (reacting to a perceived threat), denial (ignoring or blocking true feelings or the truth about a situation), and feeling helpless or powerless in a situation. Understanding these barriers and how to deal with them will make you a better communicator:

- Understand your role in the conflict and the potential barriers to clear communication.
- Consider the timing and place of your communication. It is best to discuss problems or issues when both parties are not rushed and have time to pay attention. Try to talk in a private place. Never discuss personal issues in front of others, especially residents.
- Make sure that your nonverbal communication indicates openness and a willingness to talk.
- Always address the issue, not the person, to prevent him or her from becoming defensive.
- Be courteous, understanding, and honest. Use "I" statements, not "you" statements. With "I" statements, you take responsibility for your feelings.

- Make an effort to be clear and ask appropriate questions to ensure that the other person understands your point and you understand his or hers.

Successful Conflict Resolution

Successfully resolving conflicts requires that both parties understand the problem, discuss it, and agree to a solution. Learning to resolve conflicts is an important part of your job training because an unresolved problem can affect your ability to provide proper care and to work well with other staff. When conflict occurs, it is best to deal with it right away to prevent it from becoming a larger problem. Following are conflict resolution steps that work in many situations:

Step 1 — *Listen carefully* and try to understand the other person's position and feelings.

Step 2 — *Clearly explain* what you mean and why you feel the way you do. Both parties need the opportunity to vent their emotions and clear up any misconceptions. Making an effort to communicate clearly helps calm strong emotions, and each person has the chance to be heard. Sometimes Steps 1 and 2 are enough to resolve the conflict. When they do not, use the third step.

Step 3 — *Collaborate.* Once you both agree that you understand each other's position, you then work together to come up with a solution.

Customer Service

Customer service is the act of taking care of a customer's needs. Serving a customer—the resident—defines your job as a nurse assistant. People enter health care professions because they want to help people. Most of the people that you will serve are dealing with failing health or are in the process of recovering from an illness or injury. Everything that you do is centered on the principle of *service*.

Customer service is not just a collection of tasks; it has to be part of who you are. You will use this skill with residents, families, supervisors, peers, and guests. It is important that you think about what customer service means to you as a nurse assistant as you begin your health care career. You will learn what it takes to provide positive customer experiences through the use of communication skills, understanding customers' expectations, and being attentive to their needs. You will understand the effect of customer service on the quality of care for residents and the impact that it will have with your coworkers.

Customer service begins with the first contact that you have with someone. Research shows that a first

impression is frequently made within the first 60 seconds of meeting someone for the first time. We only have one opportunity to make a first impression, and it sets the tone for anything that follows. When a negative impression is made, we must try harder to get our customers to trust us. If we manage our first impressions well, we set a positive tone for future interactions.

Greeting residents, visitors, and co-workers is key to providing good customer service. Everyone that enters the facility should be greeted by staff members, and especially from nurse assistants caring for residents. If you ignore or fail to speak to family members or visitors, this can send a nonverbal message that they are not important to you.

When you see a new visitor in the facility, be friendly. This person may be touring the facility looking for placement for themselves or a family member. Make eye contact, introduce yourself and smile. When greeting a visitor that you are familiar with, address them by their name. The impression that facility staff members make on visitors contributes to the facility's overall reputation.

Telephone Etiquette

Impressions are not only based on face-to-face interactions but over the telephone as well. Telephone conversations are just as important as in person interactions. There are some family members that are unable to visit in person, so they rely on calling the facility for updates. A positive telephone conversation can build a strong connection with our customers and result in better customer satisfaction.

Whenever you answer the phone, you should:

- State the facility's name, the unit, and your name.
- Answer the telephone in a courteous manner and speak clearly.
- Ask the caller how you can help.
- Try to meet the caller's request. You might need to bring a resident to the phone or find the appropriate staff member to answer their question(s). If you have to get someone else to help, let the caller know that you will need to go and get them.
- Never put a caller on hold for more than 2 to 3 minutes.
- If you cannot assist with the caller's request, take a phone number, and let them know you will give the message to the right person so they can call you back.
- Thank the caller for calling.

Make sure to follow through on anything that you said you would do.

Customers

There are two types of customers. **External customers** are those who seek services from your organization (facility). External customers include residents, families, guests, vendors, medical facilities, and health care providers outside of the facility. You will also serve **internal customers** within the organization. Those include supervisors, peers, and people in other departments. Good internal customer service has a positive effect on care and can enhance your facility's image within the community. Organizations in which everyone provides good customer service to both internal and external customers report greater job satisfaction, lower absenteeism, higher morale, and less turnover.

Serving customers is a key part of every job and has a definite impact on the overall success of every type of organization. Successful facilities have fewer complaints from residents and family members and more satisfied employees. You must be willing to respond to the needs of not only residents but also their families and guests. How you treat them and respond to their concerns will affect how they feel about the facility and what they say about it to members of the community. You need to make sure that you have satisfied customers. You can do this by developing a **service mentality**. Key aspects of a service mentality are summarized in Table 2-1.

Table 2-1   Components of a Service Mentality

Service Mentality	Definition	Explanation
Empathy	The ability to understand, be aware of, and be sensitive to the feelings, thoughts, and experiences of others	▪ Customers need to know that we care ▪ A caring tone lets customers hear your concern ▪ Customers need to know they are heard and understood
Enthusiasm	Bringing a strong interest and energy to a project or service situation	▪ The enthusiasm people show affects how the world perceives their willingness to help ▪ Enthusiasm influences effectiveness ▪ Enthusiastic people enjoy thinking ahead and going the extra mile
Ownership	Being committed to solve a problem or take it to someone who will	▪ It only takes one person to provide a good customer experience ▪ Ownership is partnering with the customer to address their need and solve their problems ▪ When we own the problem, we are more committed to solving it
Responsibility	Living up to the responsibilities one accepts	▪ Important to internal customer service ▪ Important to be as considerate and responsible to our co-workers as to our customers
Adaptability	Being flexible to effectively deal with different customers and situations	▪ Adapters can handle all types of customers and situations positively ▪ Adaptability is changing your approach with each customer's needs ▪ Serving each customer respectfully and effectively
Balance	Being able to satisfy the customer while considering the resources and needs of the organization	▪ Finding a balanced solution to meet the challenge of the customer and also meet the needs of the organization ▪ Helping customers feel they are heard and treated fairly ▪ Acknowledging the feelings of the customer even if you disagree
Resiliency	Being able to bounce back from adversity	▪ Remaining calm in adverse situations, recovering quickly, and not showing signs of discouragement ▪ Speaking in a controlled, unemotional manner ▪ Handling life's setbacks by bouncing back emotionally and professionally ▪ Never taking it out on the next customer or co-worker

When you fully understand and embrace the service mentality, you can balance many different needs and make good decisions (Figure 2-12).

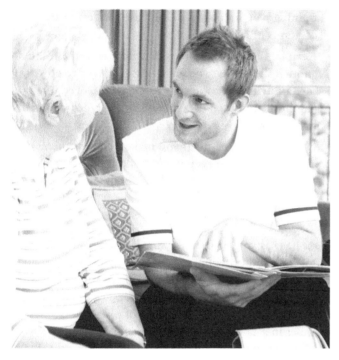

Figure 2-12 Employees who develop a service mentality are a valuable asset to the organization.

In recent years long term care services have increased to include a wide range of facility types and home and community-based programs. Customers can select the long term care environment that best suits their needs and financial resources. For your organization to be the top choice for residents and families, you must deliver good customer service. Great customer service by nurse assistants:

- Improves the quality of care for residents
- Enhances the overall quality and reputation of the organization
- Increases opportunities for the professional growth of employees within the organization

What Customers Expect

What residents expect today is not the same as even 10 years ago. People are better informed and have more choices available to them. They know how to use the Internet to research their options. Residents are more independent and want more input into their care. Excellent customer service means giving your residents both the care they need and the care they want.

To provide the best service possible, you must know the expectations customers have for your work. These expectations go beyond providing just basic service. "Average" is no longer good enough. Residents and their families want excellent care, and this has become the new minimum standard. Residents expect nurse assistants to:

- Be confident and friendly
- Smile when you greet them and talk with them
- Build relationships and rapport
- Be accountable for your actions
- Provide all necessary care and find solutions for problems quickly
- Be consistent in what you say, do, and how you provide care

Providing Excellent Customer Service

Customer service begins with the first contact. A positive first impression sets the tone for everything that happens from that point on. Greeting staff members, visitors, and residents is a key part of good customer service. Everyone who enters the facility deserves a hello from staff members (Figure 2-13). If you ignore or fail to greet or speak to family members, this sends the message that they are not important to you. It is important to treat our residents and families the way we would want to be treated. This means we have to be flexible and do all we can to make the resident and family happy. We need a "whatever it takes" attitude.

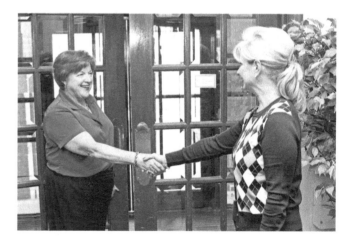

Figure 2-13 The first impression is made when the customer enters the facility.

Awareness is being conscious of what is going on in your environment. It is an important skill to develop in everything you do, especially as you observe and attend to residents' needs. You need to understand what the resident and the family want, need, and expect, so that you can respond appropriately. As you give care to residents, observe what they say and be aware of any changes in their physical appearance, speech, and behavior. Always report your observations to your supervisor. Often you are the first to notice even the slightest change in a resident's appearance or behavior. Sometimes these small changes are very important because there may be a serious underlying reason for the change. You play a major role in their care by observing and reporting all changes you see. Maintaining a keen sense of awareness is essential in maintaining great customer service skills.

The Family as Customer

While you primarily serve the resident, his or her family is also your customer. How you greet family members, how you talk with them about the resident, and how you address their concerns all affect their view of their loved one's care. It is important to have a positive relationship with the resident's family, friends, and significant others. They can provide valuable feedback and guidance and should be considered part of the resident's care team.

Think of the family as your partner (Figure 2-14). With a partner, you share common goals and decision making. Family members who are well informed will support the resident's goals for care. Keep them informed, treat them with respect, and they will usually support your efforts.

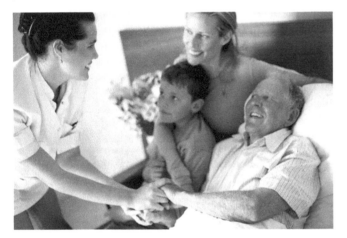

Figure 2-14 How you relate to family members and address their concerns affects their perception of the quality of care their loved one is receiving.

Trust is needed for good customer service. Customers who trust the caregiver are happier and spread positive feelings in the community. To gain the trust of residents'

families, you need a consistent approach, which includes the following:

- Use common language that people without medical training will understand. Don't use medical or technical terms or abbreviations.
- Keep family members informed. Talk with them often and tell them what you are doing and why. Keeping family members updated about their loved one's condition and progress makes them feel included and helps to build trust.
- Honor commitments. If you make a commitment, do all that you can to keep it and to do it on time. If you cannot carry out a promised task right away, then it is important to let the family know that you will complete it as soon as you can.

As hard as you try to make sure you are communicating well and providing excellent customer service, occasionally concerns or conflicts will arise. This can occur if family members have unrealistic expectations. It can also happen due to the stress of placing a family member in a care facility. Family members may express hostility toward staff and be critical of the care provided. They may request that a physician be called in more frequently than necessary or demand special treatment for their loved one. They may overreact to situations or make numerous complaints. They may even threaten legal action against the facility.

There are often reasons we are unaware of behind negative or critical behaviors. Family members may be experiencing emotional and/or financial stress. Their loved one's need for care may be a reminder that they won't have them forever. Be sure to keep in close communication with the health care team about any situation that arises. If you inform your supervisor about family members' actions and inquiries, they can take appropriate measures and, if needed, set up a meeting to address any concerns.

How Residents Perceive Their Care

For residents, customer satisfaction involves how they perceive the quality of their care and the services they receive. In all daily tasks, you must always consider how the resident feels about their care. Remember that residents should direct their care to the degree that they are able.

We have all had experiences with customer service. Think about a situation where you are the customer, such as eating out or purchasing something new. What makes the experience positive for you? Is it when some-one smiles, and asks, if they can help you and then allows time for you to ask other questions without feeling rushed?

Nurse assistants who understand and implement the following steps provide the best customer service:

- Always ask for the residents' permission before providing care
- Always ask the residents what they want.
- Provide high-quality care and services with a smile (Figure 2-15).
- Do whatever it takes to make the answer "Yes," within facility policies and procedures
- Adopt the attitude that you will always try to do the job right the first time.
- Always keep your promises.
- Ask for and encourage input from family members.
- Go out of your way for all your residents.
- Over-deliver — strive to make "extra effort" your standard effort.

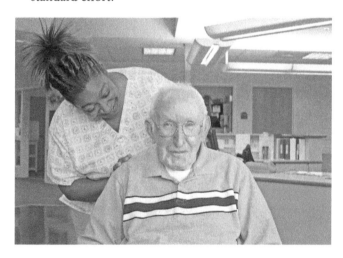

Figure 2-15 You must create an environment that gives the customer more than they expect.

Customer Service in Difficult Situations

Sometimes, no matter how hard we try, problems occur. When people are upset, they get emotional (Figure 2-16). Your ability to respond to the emotional needs of your residents and their family members is one of the best skills for dealing with difficult situations. The customer needs to know that you understand what he or she is trying to tell you about their needs. There are three key things to remember in dealing with problems or conflict:

listen, don't take anything personally, and be aware of your responses.

Listening is an essential skill for nurse assistants. The first step in identifying residents' needs is listening to what they say. Let them present the issue, and actively listen to what is on their mind. Be sure not to interrupt before they are finished. Residents, families, and your team all make requests, and it is important that you understand what is being said (and sometimes what is not being said). As you learned earlier, people communicate both verbally and nonverbally.

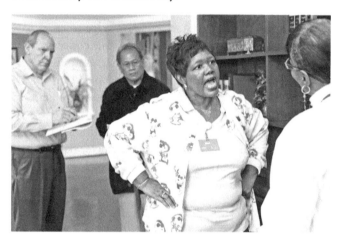

Figure 2-16 While it's easy to become emotional if you are challenged, excellent customer service means listening to others' concerns, not taking things personally, and responding appropriately so you are part of the solution.

When you are attentive and aware, you will be able to:

- Determine what the resident (customer) wants and needs
- Prevent misunderstandings and errors
- Gather clues about ways you can improve the service you provide
- Build long-term trusting relationships

Becoming defensive is a natural response in any difficult or emotional situation, especially if you feel that you are being attacked or wrongly accused. But it is important to *not take things personally* and to stay focused on the resident's needs and well-being. When you respond with empathy, you remain calm and in control. Only then are you at your absolute best. You can then be ready, willing, and able to help your customer.

Successfully managing difficult situations depends on good communication skills and *responding appropriately*. You need to understand how your own behavior and language affect other people. You must be careful to avoid *trigger words,* which are words or phrases that can make a situation worse by provoking the other person. Examples of trigger words are "Calm down!" "Be quiet!" "You need to listen!" or "You don't understand." Phrases such as these give the impression that you are being disrespectful and talking down to someone. This type of response only makes the situation worse by keeping everyone angry or frustrated.

How you physically react is also important. Do not roll your eyes or turn away while others are talking. Pay attention to what is being said and keep an empathetic attitude. Maintain eye contact. Acknowledge what is being said with phrases such as "I hear your concern" or "I see that this is very upsetting to you." Responses such as these show compassion. When people know that they are heard, this goes a long way in defusing tense situations.

At times you may need help managing difficult conversations or situations with family members, visitors, or staff members. Always keep your supervisor informed if any of these situations arise.

Your Role with Supervisors, Peers, and Others

Customer service also involves how you interact with your supervisors, peers, other members of the health care team, visitors, and guests. Working as a team requires respect for all individuals who make up the team. You can show respect on a daily basis by following these guidelines:

- Do not gossip. Gossip hurts people. While it may seem harmless, it can be insulting and abusive. Avoid sharing negative information about other people. You should also refuse to listen to gossip. If someone takes a conversation in that direction you can simply say that gossip is not something you are comfortable with.

- Start each interaction with a greeting. A simple smile and a warm greeting are important in developing positive relationships with your peers and creating a more positive work environment. Other people recognize a genuine response and a service-oriented attitude.

- Be courteous and personable with others at work. Ask people how they would like to be addressed. Everyone feels honored when they are called by the name they prefer and appreciates when others remember it.

- Always show respect for your peers and supervisors. This is vital in the long term care environment.

Quality of care can suffer as a result of a poor working relationship among team members. Even when you are in a hurry, remember to speak kindly to your fellow workers. Always treat your coworkers with the same respect that you want for yourself. It is very important for the organization to have an honest and respectful work environment at all levels. Maintain professionalism at all times.

Blending Customer Service into Daily Care

As you incorporate customer service into your caregiving, you must understand your role in meeting residents' needs and helping to solve residents' problems (see Table 2-2). If you do not know how to handle a specific problem, discuss it with a supervisor or coworker who does. Tell the resident what you are doing to solve the problem, and then make your best effort. While not every issue has a solution, customer satisfaction depends on the effort you make to solve the problem and meet the resident's needs.

Table 2-2 Golden Rules of Customer Service

Principles of Customer Service	How to Act
People come first	▪ Give the resident your complete attention
Don't rush	▪ Take time to get information ▪ Remember speed is not success
Be friendly always	▪ Treat everyone equally ▪ Remember their behavior mirrors how they are treated
Don't be too busy to be nice	▪ Don't give short answers ▪ Keep your sense of humor
Don't use technical language	▪ Use easy, understandable words ▪ Explain unfamiliar words
Remember your manners	▪ Don't slip into slang ▪ Good manners never go out of style ▪ "There ya go" is not "Thank you" ▪ "Uh huh" is not "You're welcome"

When you have a customer service focus, you use active listening skills when talking with residents. You never make excuses for poor service. You work to solve problems by taking a positive approach. You remain thoughtful and never let caregiving tasks become routine. Balancing your technical skills with the art of caregiving shows residents that they are important to you.

Good customer service during daily care includes making residents feel more comfortable and maintaining their dignity. Residents may feel embarrassed about having to rely on others to care for their basic needs, which they have done for themselves for most of their lives. Asking about their preferences, offering choices, and making accommodations to meet their requests help establish a good relationship. Often it is simple things that make a difference for residents. Always give residents a choice in their care. They need to be involved in choosing how and when they are bathed or showered and dressed, and you can make sure that their hair is combed or styled the way they prefer.

There are aspects of customer service related to meals. Is the food presented in a way that you would want to eat it? Is this when, where, and what the resident likes to eat? Who do they want to eat with, or do they prefer to eat in their room while watching a favorite show? A *mindful caregiver* considers what the resident likes and wants. Some individuals have specific requests for meals based on cultural and dietary preferences. Individual choice and resident-centered care are not only expected in long term care facilities, but they are also required.

Customer service also relates to residents' participation in activities. Asking and honoring each resident's requests for their activities is very important. Learning about activities and hobbies they participated in before coming to the facility and working to re-create those can provide hours of enjoyment for residents (Figure 2-17). This type of socialization can play a significant role in maintaining residents' overall well-being and enhancing their quality of life.

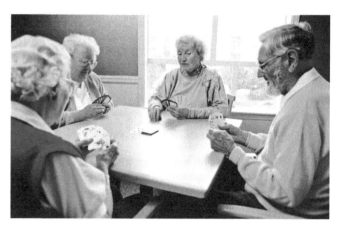

Figure 2-17 When residents have the opportunity to participate in their favorite activities, this enhances their overall quality of life.

- Verbal communication involves using words to express oneself and active listening to understand what others are saying.

- Nonverbal communication is communication that occurs through body language, expressions, gestures, and touch.

- Touch is a form of nonverbal communication that can be pleasant, reassuring, neutral, or intimidating. It is important to learn residents' comfort level with touch and to respect their boundaries.

- Active listening improves mutual understanding. It involves paying attention to spoken words and nonverbal cues.

- Effective communication is based on respect for each resident and developing an understanding of each resident's unique needs and capabilities. Effective communication is also an essential part of building positive working relationships with supervisors and coworkers.

- You will care for residents with special communication needs. You'll need to learn and use techniques that promote effective communication with people who have problems with hearing, vision, and speech, and those who are cognitively impaired.

- Residents with mental impairments and other conditions may behave inappropriately or aggressively. You must remain calm at all times and help guide the resident toward more appropriate behaviors to ensure their safety and the safety of other residents.

- Successful conflict resolution involves three steps: 1) Listen carefully to the other person's concerns and viewpoint; 2) clearly explain your perspective on the issue; and 3) collaborate to find a mutually acceptable solution to the issue or problem.

- Customer service is the act of taking care of a customer's needs. The resident is your primary customer, and a key focus of your job is to effectively meet residents' needs and help improve their quality of life. Residents' families are also important customers you will serve.

- Excellent customer service by nurse assistants improves residents' quality of care, enhances the quality and reputation of the facility, and increases your opportunities for professional growth within the organization.

- High-level customer service during daily care includes making residents feel more comfortable and maintaining their dignity at all times.

Key Terms

accommodation — resolving conflict by giving in to the wishes of another person

aggression — hostile, threatening, or violent behavior toward others

aphasia — communication disorder that results from damage to parts of the brain responsible for language; affects ability to speak and understand speech and ability to read and/or write

avoidance — staying away from a person or issue instead of dealing with a conflict

awareness — consciousness of one's environment

body language — nonverbal communication that includes posture, gestures, and facial expressions

clarity — clearness of communication

collaboration — working together to accomplish a task or resolve a conflict

communication — sending and receiving messages verbally, nonverbally, in writing, or through symbols

communication board — a device used for those who have difficulty communicating verbally, it is customized with signs, symbols or pictures that help the resident communicate their needs

compassion — sympathetic understanding of another person's suffering or situation coupled with a sincere desire to help

competition — challenge or contest in which there is a winner and a loser

compromise — resolving conflict by both parties agreeing to something less or different than they originally wanted to achieve a peaceful resolution

conflict resolution — process for settling a dispute or disagreement

context — the entire situation, background, or environment that provides meaning to a person's words

culture — the collective customs, attitudes, and beliefs of a particular group of people; may relate to ethnic or religious background and/or social groups

customer service — the actions involved in serving a customer's needs

customs — traditional practices of a particular group of people

defensiveness — being overly sensitive to perceived criticism from others

denial — ignoring or blocking true feelings or the truth about a situation

dignity — a sense of pride and self-respect; being worthy of honor and respect

empathy — ability to understand and share the feelings or perspective of another person

expressive aphasia — communication disorder that involves difficulty communicating but the person can usually comprehend what is being said to them

external customer — residents, families, and customers who are outside of the long term care facility

internal customer — customers who are part of the same organization; supervisors and coworkers

mentally competent — capable of rational decision making and being responsible for one's actions

nonverbal communication — sending and receiving messages without using words

open-ended question — question that requires a more complex answer than a simple "yes" or "no."

physical abuse — any action that causes physical harm

reflection — restating in your own words what another person has said to be sure that you understand the speaker's meaning and feelings

service mentality — dedication to making sure that customers' needs are satisfied

verbal abuse — using profanity or other words that attack, insult, threaten, bully, or humiliate another person

verbal communication — sending and receiving messages using spoken or written words

visual communication — using symbols, such as traffic lights, road signs, memes, and emojis

1. **Body language such as facial expressions and eye movements are examples of:**
   a. Verbal communication
   b. Open communication
   c. Nonverbal communication
   d. Poor communication

2. **Touch is an important form of nonverbal communication. Before using touch, the nurse assistant needs to:**
   a. Put on protective gloves and gown
   b. Find out if the resident is comfortable with it
   c. Obtain signed permission from the resident
   d. Ask the charge nurse if it is okay

3. **Verbal communication uses spoken or written words which can have different meanings depending on one's:**
   a. Background
   b. Culture
   c. Education
   d. All of these

4. **Reducing background noise and facing the resident when speaking are useful guidelines for communicating with residents who have:**
   a. Impaired memory
   b. Impaired hearing
   c. Impaired sight
   d. Impaired smell

5. **Cognitive impairments include conditions that affect the resident's decision-making skills, and, for effective communication, the nurse assistant needs to:**
   a. Keep questions and directions short and simple
   b. Be very detailed and lengthy when giving directions
   c. Complete the residents' sentences for them
   d. Laugh if what the resident says doesn't make sense

6. **Aggression is defined as hostile or violent behavior toward others. When a resident becomes aggressive, you must:**
   a. Rush to get out of there
   b. Stay calm and never argue
   c. Yell as loudly as possible to stop it
   d. Take it personally

7. **Steps for conflict resolution include all of the following, except:**
   a. Listen carefully
   b. Clearly explain
   c. Compromise
   d. Ignore

8. **Customer service is the act of taking care of a customer's needs; in this case, the resident. Customer service is not just a collection of tasks; it has to be:**
   a. Part of who you are
   b. Written down
   c. Optional
   d. Mandatory

9. **Great customer service by nurse assistants enhances the organization's reputation, increases opportunities for professional growth of employees, and, most importantly:**
   a. Increases satisfaction of families
   b. Improves quality of care for residents
   c. Neither of these
   d. Both of these

10. **Strategies for good customer service include:**
    a. Not being flexible
    b. Being a mindful caregiver
    c. Always deciding what is best for the resident
    d. Always doing what is best for you

3

Maintaining Quality of Life

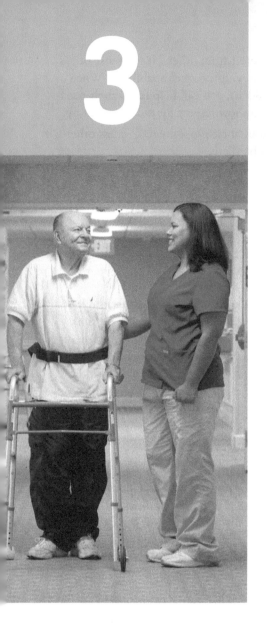

Residents often think that moving into a long term care facility will be a negative experience. Despite any fears or concerns they may have about this major life change, residents still value their lives. It is important for them to know that they are valued and respected for who they are. By demonstrating this on a daily basis, you can better support them and help them find meaning while in your care.

How do you want your residents and families to answer the question: "What is it like to live in this facility?" Do you want them to say that they feel they are well cared for, that they are treated with respect, and that their permission is always asked before something is done to them? Do you want them to say they feel well informed about what is happening in the facility? That staff members are pleasant and truly doing the best they can to help residents maintain as much dignity and independence as possible?

It is important to have a positive relationship with residents' family members, friends, and significant others. Most often, they know the resident best and can give you valuable information and guidance. You will come to understand the important role that residents' family members play in maintaining quality of life. We focus on how to ensure that the resident's quality of life is the best it can be and how to support the resident and family through this phase of their lives.

OBJECTIVES:

- Explain Maslow's hierarchy of human needs and how they relate to a person's quality of life.

- List Erikson's eight stages of psychosocial development.

- Define family and explain why residents' family members are important to quality of life.

- Describe ways that nurse assistants can include the resident's family as part of the care team.

- Explain why it is important to develop a positive relationship with residents' families and provide examples of effective communication with family members.

- Explain why treating a resident with dignity and respect is an important part of caregiving.

- Describe how activities contribute to a resident's quality of life.

- Define themes of care, name the eight themes, and give examples of how to use themes to enhance residents' quality of life.

- Describe the key principles of alternative care models.

Understanding the Resident

Every person that you meet throughout your life has unique qualities that make them who they are. While people have widely differing preferences, backgrounds, and experiences, we all have the same basic human needs. We need to keep our physical bodies safe and functioning well. We need to nurture our social, intellectual, sexual, and spiritual selves. Through our unique life experiences, we have developed ways to meet those needs. Abraham Maslow was an American psychologist and researcher who studied human behavior. He developed a theory known as *Maslow's hierarchy of needs* that ranks basic human needs in order of importance (Figure 3-1):

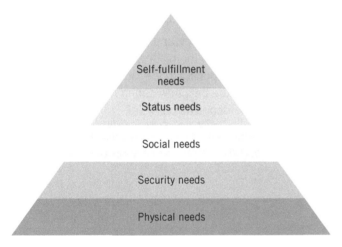

Figure 3-1 Maslow's hierarchy of needs. The most basic human needs must be met before a person focuses on addressing higher-level needs.

- *Physical needs* such as oxygen, food, and water are essential to maintain life. Everyone wants to meet their physical needs independently, but that may change as we grow older. Because of physical changes that occur as we age, we may need help meeting our physical needs. These needs must be met before addressing the next level of need.

- *Security and safety* — feeling safe and free from bodily harm. These needs are met after physical needs are met. For example, if you were starving, you might risk your safety to get food. Once you meet your need for food, you behave more cautiously to protect yourself from danger.

- *Social needs* include feelings of approval, acceptance, love, and belonging. Everyone wants to feel wanted and cared for. Social needs also include interaction with others and being recognized.

- *Status* involves respect from others. It is a sense of valuing oneself and your unique capabilities. When you care for a resident, you can help fulfill their need for status. You can show respect for each resident by:
  - Calling them by their proper name, unless otherwise directed by them.
  - Always asking their permission before acting.
  - Explaining all tasks and procedures.
  - Knocking on their door and waiting for permission to enter.
  - Respecting their belongings.
  - Recognizing their achievements.

- *Self-fulfillment,* also known as self-actualization, is at the highest level on the hierarchy. This is a person's need for a sense of satisfaction that comes from living in a way that maximizes one's full potential. Encourage residents to be as independent as possible and set goals. As a nurse assistant you can help residents reach their goals.

Psychosocial Development and Quality of Life

Erik Erikson was a developmental psychologist who established the stages of psychosocial development throughout the lifespan. His theory outlines the milestones that are commonly mastered during each life stage and the types of conflict that can develop if they were not (Table 3-1). Most of the individuals you will care for will be adults, but it is important to remember that previous stages of their life still influence their current feelings and behavior.

Providing psychosocial care meets the resident's social, spiritual, and emotional needs, not just their medical needs. Mental health disorders have a strong tie to psychosocial needs, which can have an impact on a resident's overall physical health.

How a Resident's History Affects Quality of Life

Prior to entering a long term care facility, every resident had a life with many experiences and relationships. To successfully care for your residents, you must understand their history and become aware of any cultural, sexual, religious, or spiritual preferences they may have. It will be important for you to respect all residents' beliefs and practices, regardless of your own views. Residents should never be judged for their beliefs or opinions, and nurse assistants should never attempt to push their personal beliefs on a resident.

Table 3-1   Erikson's Eight Stages of Psychosocial Development

Age	Success/Conflict	Task	What the Nurse Assistant Can Do
Infant	Trust vs. mistrust	The infant must form a loving, trusting relationship with the caregiver.	In this phase the nurse assistant should hold the infant and be consistent and reliable to encourage trust. Feeding is the primary means to achieve success. Holding the infant during feeding supports this development.
Toddler	Autonomy vs. shame/doubt	The child develops physical skills, including walking, grasping, and bowel and bladder control. The child learns control at this stage.	The nurse assistant must support the toddler's physical development in walking and independent eating. Playing ball and other games is critical to develop gross motor skills. Helping with toilet training is critical for success. Praising the child and never scolding will help support their development.
Preschool child	Initiative vs. guilt	The child continues to become more assertive and independent and starts to take more initiative.	The nurse assistant must support the preschool child's need to develop independence. The child will use their imagination in play. The child needs to be encouraged in their game playing.
School-age child	Industry vs. inferiority	The school-age child deals with demands to learn new skills and knowledge.	Helping the child be successful in learning is critical in this stage. This child needs to feel they are productive and can succeed. The child should be praised for completing their tasks.
Adolescence	Identity vs. role confusion	A teenager must achieve a clear sense of identity in sex roles at home, at school, and at work.	Talking with teenagers about their goals and friends is critical at this stage. Supporting them in decision making or even teaching decision making is important as teenagers sort through who they are and what they will do.
Young adulthood	Intimacy vs. isolation	The young adult learns to develop intimate relationships.	The ability to make a commitment is critical for the young adult's success. Discussing the person's relationships and supporting their commitments will help the person achieve success.
Middle adulthood	Generativity vs. stagnation	Adults need to feel they have accomplished something or supported the next generation.	A resident in this stage needs to feel they have accomplished something good. They must feel they have shared a part of themselves with people who are close to them. Talking with the resident will help them identify their successes.
Maturity	Ego integrity vs. despair	An older adult must have a sense of feeling fulfilled, that they have lived successfully.	In this stage the resident has to accept both the good and bad of their life. Allowing and encouraging the resident to discuss issues will help them in this stage.

Religious and spiritual practices can be influenced by a person's culture and personal history. These practices and rituals play an important role in many residents' lives as they move closer to the end of life.

Spirituality involves much more than religion. Spirituality can help a resident meet their security, social and self-fulfillment needs. It involves a meaning of life and feeling related to something greater than ourselves. A resident may express spirituality through prayer, mediation, reading, and religious rituals.

It is important that all staff members are accepting of each resident's culture and beliefs and interacts with each person without prejudice (Figure 3-2). It is important to never impose your beliefs on a resident.

Religious practices often give residents spiritual comfort. This is especially true when residents are coping with major life changes like the loss of a loved one or their own approaching death. If a resident requests a visit from their spiritual counselor, such as a priest, rabbi or minister, let your charge nurse know so a visit can be scheduled. Provide privacy when the spiritual counselor visits.

Many religious and ethnic groups observe special religious holidays. These could involve ceremonies and traditional foods. Find out what special holidays your residents observe. Facilities often plan special activities for religious holidays.

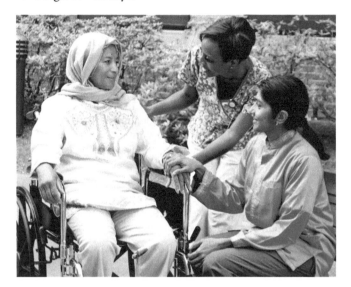

Figure 3-2 Nurse assistants care for people representing a wide range of cultural, ethnic, and religious backgrounds.

How a resident meets their needs is influenced by their culture and values along with the resident's family structure, education, and financial status. Culture represents the customary beliefs, social forms, and traits of a particular nation, religion, or social group. Every culture has what is considered cultural norms, which are standards that a particular culture or social group live by. Take touch or hugging, for example. There are some cultures that it is the norm to give your friend a hug when you see them, but in other cultures this may be considered unacceptable. Understanding the cultural background of your residents will better equip you to meet their needs and deliver quality care.

Sexuality

Sexual expression is both a physical and social need. Sexual needs are not limited to sexual acts; they can also be met through close physical contact. Older individuals have sexual needs and desires, just like younger people. The desire for intimacy does not decrease as we age, but, due to physical changes and life situations, the older adult may need to make adjustments to meet their needs.

Sexuality is the sexual habits and preferences of individuals. Sexuality includes gender identity or sexual orientation. Gender identity is how an individual perceives their gender. One may associate with being male, female, both, or neither. Sexual orientation differs from

gender identity as it relates to those in which an individual is attracted.

There are many different terms associated with sexual orientation or gender identity. Heterosexual refers to an individual that is attracted to the opposite sex. Those attracted to the same sex are known as homosexual. A bisexual is someone who is attracted to both sexes. Transgender refers to an individual whose gender identity is different than the sex that they were assigned at birth.

A resident's lifestyle or sexual preferences may be very different from your own, but regardless of your personal beliefs, his or her rights and preferences must be respected (Figure 3-3).

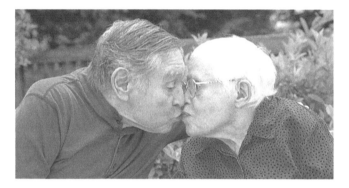

Figure 3-3 Residents' lifestyle and relationship choices must be respected.

Remember to maintain confidentiality at all times and to avoid gossip. Every resident is a human being, and their beliefs and lifestyle choices are to be respected. As you get to know residents, their personal history, and their families, you will be developing relationships based on trust. These relationships are essential in helping residents maintain their quality of life.

Understanding the Role of the Family

Think about the people who matter the most to you: your family, friends, and your romantic partner, if you have one. These are your significant others. Family members affect us emotionally because of their personalities and actions. They bring meaning into our lives as we share experiences. Residents may have just a few or many significant others in their lives. Their family may include a spouse, partner, brothers and sisters, nieces and nephews, children and grandchildren. Their significant others may include friends, neighbors, and former coworkers. Because of their special bond with residents, family and significant others are very important. Going forward, we will use the term "family" to refer to all significant others in a resident's life.

Why Is Family Important?

Think of family members as an extension of the resident. They share many experiences and special memories.

Often these relationships have lasted many years. Family members usually know a resident better than anyone else. Family members are reassuringly familiar to residents when everything else in the facility is at first unfamiliar. Family members can provide comfort and help care for a resident. They can share their knowledge about the resident, and they may provide financial support. Residents who have been close to family all their lives want to keep these relationships after entering a facility.

Not all families are the same. Each resident has a unique relationship with his or her family. Some have strong family relationships (Figure 3-4). Others are more distanced. Some have difficult or stressful relationships. Be careful not to impose your own family values when interacting with residents and their families. Support each resident and their family, whatever form their relationship takes, even if you don't agree with what you see or find it hard to understand.

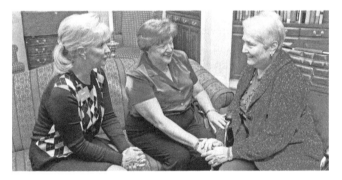

Figure 3-4 Many residents have close relationships with family members.

What Happens to Families When Residents Are Admitted?

When a resident is admitted to a facility, it is usually stressful for their family, as well, because many changes happen at once. The resident is physically and emotionally affected by this move, and these changes also affect the family. Family members may have a range of feelings when their loved one enters the facility. Many find it hard to accept that they can no longer care for their loved one or that the person is no longer independent. They may have difficulty accepting that the resident may never come home.

New residents must redefine their life when they leave their home and enter the facility. Your assistance with the transition will also help the resident's family. For the first time, sons and daughters may be in the uncomfortable position of having to make major decisions for their parents. Often, they have to take a more active role in their loved one's financial and property matters. Now they are turning the day-to-day caregiving responsibility over to you and other team members who are strangers to them. They may feel as if they will have only a secondary role because you have become their loved one's primary caregiver. With all these changes and stresses, family members may disagree or argue at times as everyone adjusts to new roles.

It is often stressful for family members to care for elderly or ill relatives at home. Caring for one's parents is especially challenging for adults whose children also live at home. They may feel torn between the needs of their children and the needs of their parents. Families can feel burned out — physically and mentally exhausted — after caring for their loved one for a long time. You will encounter many families suffering from this type of chronic stress. Communicating understanding as you talk with family members can help them cope. Sometimes it helps just to tell the family that you understand that the changes must be difficult. If you see that further help may be needed, ask the charge nurse to arrange for a social worker to talk with them.

The Adjustment Process

Like residents, families must adjust before they can feel comfortable with their loved one's new living arrangements. It also takes time for the family to develop a trusting relationship with you.

During this time, family members may have many different reactions. Be observant and try to understand their feelings. Cycling through a range of feelings is a normal part of the adjustment process, and these feelings affect how they behave toward you and their loved one. Accept that this adjustment period lasts until everyone is comfortable and a trusting relationship develops. Let's explore some of the most common reactions families may have when placing a loved one in a facility:

Guilt. Family members may feel guilt when they place their loved one in a facility. Some feel that they are abandoning the person, no matter how difficult it would be to keep caring for them at home. They may try to make up for it by visiting often and becoming very involved in care and decision making. You can build trust by helping them stay involved and feeling useful. Their attention is often very beneficial for their loved one and makes the transition easier for everyone.

Anger and Resentment. Some family members may be angry when they lose control of the care of their loved one. They may resent staff, including you, because they feel as if you are replacing them. They may also be angry because of family disagreements about placing the loved one in a facility. Angry family members may be critical and demanding of you and other staff. Sometimes a social worker or a more senior staff member can help.

Uncertainty. Some families feel uncertain or anxious about their decision. They are not sure what to expect from the facility. They may worry whether they made the right decision. These families can be very emotional when they visit the resident. By acting professionally and compassionately, you can help them feel confident that you do care about their relative and are doing your best.

Sadness. Some family members are very sad. They may have a hard time coping with being separated from their loved one if they have lived together or cared for them. They may grieve over the person's dependency or declining health. Even though they visit the resident, they may feel a tremendous sense of loss.

Loss of Control. Many family members who cared for their loved one for a long time feel a loss of control when you and other staff take over the caregiving. Sometimes a family member's main role in life was to care for the loved one. Now they may feel that they have no purpose. They may try to keep some control by becoming involved in care and decision making for their loved one.

Relief. Some family members feel relieved when their loved one enters a facility. Taking care of the person at home may have been stressful and exhausting. This is especially so when family members have other responsibilities such as jobs and children. These families are relieved by the respite from caring for their loved one.

During the adjustment process, family members often move back and forth through different emotional stages. The key is to help them recognize what is happening and to support them through the stages. Once they feel comfortable with you and other staff members, they will come to trust and rely on you.

Your Relationship with the Family

From the moment you meet them, consider the resident's family part of the caregiving team. Family members can

share information about the resident (Figure 3-5), interact with them, and help with their care. You can help families feel comfortable in this role. When a resident is admitted, take the opportunity to get to know his or her family. Help make them comfortable by welcoming them and introducing yourself. Get to know them by name. Take the time to understand their relationship with the resident, and explain how you will help with their loved one's care.

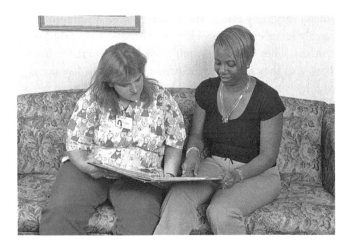

Figure 3-5 Family members are good sources of information about the resident.

Families are interested in their loved one's activities. Let them know about upcoming events. Share the calendar of events and explain the activities that are available for residents. Your facility may have special events that involve families. Encourage family members to participate as often as they are able.

Family members need to feel important and useful. Help them decide if they want to be involved in their loved one's care. If so, what would they like to do? If not, make sure they know that is okay, too, because you will make sure that all necessary care is provided. Family members can help motivate a resident who seems depressed or is upset by illness or medical treatment. They are often the best cheerleaders.

Involving the Family in Care

Family members can participate in the resident's care in many ways. They can do all or part of a resident's personal grooming at bath time. They may want to help their loved one eat and drink. They can be good companions during physical therapy sessions. They may want to join in activities such as crafts, music, or games. The family can also assist by shopping for clothes or special items for the resident.

Family members should be encouraged to participate in resident care conferences. Their knowledge is valuable. They can become involved in the family council and help shape the facility's policies for the benefit of all residents. Both care conferences and family councils are good opportunities for families to be actively involved and to make valuable contributions (Figure 3-6).

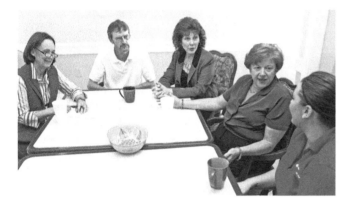

Figure 3-6 Resident care conferences and council meetings provide opportunities for family members to get involved.

You will work with the family as part of caring for their loved one. How the family feels about the care being provided affects their attitude toward you and other staff. If the family feels that their loved one is receiving good care, they will have positive feelings for you and other staff. They will trust you. But if they feel that their loved one is unhappy or not well cared for, they will react negatively, which is understandable. Because you spend so much time with each resident, you have the opportunity to get to know the family, to understand their feelings, and to help them adjust to their loved one's new circumstances.

Communicating Effectively with Family Members

Good communication begins when the family knows you and you know them. Be available to talk with the family during their visits or via phone. Let them see how you interact with their loved one. Show your support by really listening to their comments and concerns. If a family member asks to speak to you when you are busy, agree on another time in the near future when you will have time to focus on them. Find a quiet spot so you can both relax and talk. This helps develop a positive relationship (Figure 3-7).

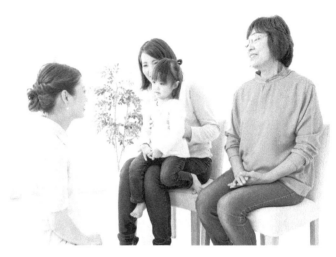

Figure 3-7 You can support family members by taking the time to listen to their questions and concerns.

In speaking with family members, be courteous and remain objective. Do not agree or disagree with their opinions, especially if they are angry or frustrated. If family members disagree with each other or with their loved one, do not take sides. You can paraphrase the feelings, questions, and concerns they have expressed to ensure that you understand exactly what they are saying. When you communicate that you understand their feelings, they are reassured that you have been listening. If you are uncomfortable discussing an issue raised by a family member or if you cannot answer a specific question, ask them to speak to the charge nurse or social worker. The charge nurse is the person who should report any change in a resident's condition to the family.

Family members need to feel connected to their loved one, and most families stay in contact through visits, telephone calls, cards and letters, online communication, and outings. If you become aware of any barriers to communication, work to remove them. Be sure that residents have access to a telephone, paper, or computer so that they can contact family members. By encouraging family members to visit, making their visits comfortable, and involving them in care, you enhance a resident's relationship with their family.

Often, you will have more contact with residents than their own family members do. Some residents may come to rely on you and even trust you more than their own family. You may be the most consistent and caring person in their life and may develop a close, caring relationship with them (Figure 3-8). You may come to feel like a family member yourself. Enjoy this special relationship and treasure their trust. You and the family are an important part of the residents' ability to maintain their quality of life.

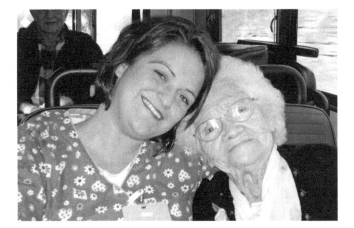

Figure 3-8 Getting to know the residents you care for can lead to close, caring relationships.

Family Visits

Most residents look forward to interactions with their families, and regular contact should be encouraged (Figure 3-9). If a resident cannot communicate or is in failing health, visits can be difficult. In these situations, continue to offer your support to the resident's family.

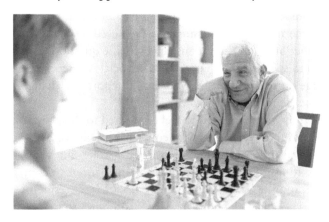

Figure 3-9 If the resident wishes, family members should be encouraged to visit as often as possible.

Sometimes family members express their distress in ways that make you uncomfortable. They may become emotional and may not have adjusted well to their loved one being in the facility. Remember that they may have other stresses in their life, as well. These may cause them to be demanding, critical, or to speak unkindly to you and other staff. Do not take their comments personally. Be supportive. Try not to judge the situation but report it to the charge nurse.

A family support group or family council can be a great help to family members who are feeling distressed. They will get emotional support from others who are dealing with similar circumstances. Encourage the family's participation. Tell them when these groups meet and how to obtain more information. Sometimes the social worker can help. Families need to know about all available resources and where to find them. You are a necessary and important link.

Dignity and Quality of Life

What does *dignity* mean to you? If you ask different people what dignity means to them, you will get many different answers. Dignity is generally described as a sense of feeling worthy and deserving of respect. If we grew up in a healthy environment, our parents and teachers showed us that we were valuable and deserved respect. Our sense of self-worth must be reinforced throughout our lives, particularly if we become impaired or vulnerable in some way.

When you consider a resident's quality of life, you should think about dignity and respect. Why is it important to promote a resident's dignity, and how can you ensure it?

Treating residents with dignity and respect means that you are meeting their needs and supporting their quality of life. In addition, you enhance residents' quality of life when you support their existing relationships and help them create new ones both inside and outside of the facility.

Nurse assistants can maintain residents' dignity by:

- Always showing respect and demonstrating that they are important
- Treating them as you want to be treated
- Calling residents by their preferred name
- Asking permission before giving care
- Providing individualized care in a pleasant and comfortable manner
- Maintaining privacy during personal care
- Remaining sensitive to their needs, wants, likes, dislikes, and preferences
- Being careful with their belongings

You can promote the dignity of residents by getting to know them as the important people they are. When residents are treated with respect, they feel better about themselves. When their self-esteem improves, they play a more active role in their own care. Their health may improve, and they may regain physical capabilities that they seemed to have lost. They engage in more social activities. They eat and sleep better and reach their optimum level of wellness.

Honoring a Resident's Life

How can you best understand each resident in your care? Ask the resident or his or her family or friends what the person likes and dislikes. Ask about where they grew up, what traditions they follow, their job or volunteer experiences, and what they like to do to relax. You can also learn more about a resident's background from nurses, therapists, and social workers. Remember that your initial perceptions about a resident may not always be accurate. Learning about residents' values, culture, religion, home environment, travels, and professional and personal experiences will help you promote their dignity by honoring who they are as individuals (Figure 3-10).

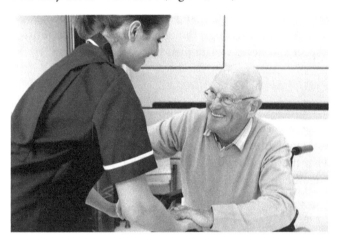

Figure 3-10 Residents have had many interesting life experiences. You will enjoy getting to know them.

It is important to make an effort to understand who the residents are when they enter your facility. And, equally important is what you can do to help residents transition from their past lives to their new life in the facility. You can encourage them to bring personal items for their rooms and to talk about their past while getting used to their present situation. For example, you can learn about past habits and preferences and help them find new ways to do the same or similar things now. Although the setting may be different, they need to know that their quality of life can still be good.

Activities and Quality of Life

In a long term care facility, activities are an important part of residents' lives. Activities help residents maintain their independence, sense of purpose, and feeling that they are contributing members of society. The facility activity program is a critical part of the resident's care plan. Activities must be meaningful to the resident. Once you have gotten to know a resident, you and the care team will have a better idea of what type of activities to offer or suggest. You can help the activities director by sharing your knowledge of the residents. In thinking about activities, consider the resident's former job or profession and his or her hobbies and interests. Encourage residents to select activities that will provide positive experiences. Try not to involve them in an activity that involves skills they may not have. As a nurse assistant, you will assist residents in going to and from their activities of choice.

The facility should offer both structured group activities and unstructured activities. The goal of both types of activities is to help residents become actively engaged — not sitting passively in front of the television or napping. Activities should not be childish. They should stimulate residents and help them feel involved (Figure 3-11). Most facilities post a schedule of events. Talk with residents about upcoming events so they can choose to participate in those that appeal to them. If a resident says that none of the activities interests them, tell the activities director and talk with the resident about what they would like to do.

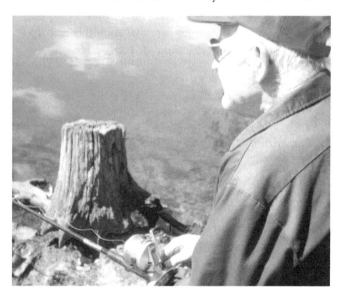

Figure 3-11 It is important that residents are able to continue to engage in activities they enjoy after entering long term care.

As the person who spends the most time with the resident, you can give the charge nurse and the rest of the care team useful information about how the resident responds to activities. Then adjustments can be made to the resident's care plan, if necessary. Just remember that not all residents like to do the same thing.

Resident-Centered Care

By this point you may be wondering how you are going to meet the needs of the residents you will care for. As you are beginning to see, the key to success involves combining skillful and caring service with effective and respectful communication. The **resident-centered care** model focuses on the resident's individual preferences and needs with each resident being an active participant in their care. Using a resident-centered care approach allows the resident to make choices about their care and increases their independence, which will increase resident outcomes and satisfaction.

To give excellent care while promoting residents' quality of life, you have to incorporate **themes of care** into all your activities.

A *theme* is a central idea or an underlying meaning.

Themes of care are the basis for all that you do. Your specific tasks will vary throughout the day, or they may be different for every resident because of their preferences, but the themes of care should always stay the same. In every interaction with a resident, these themes must be part of what you do. This is how you balance the art of caregiving with the essential skills of your job.

There are eight themes of care that should be incorporated into every aspect of caring for your residents:

- Communication
- Autonomy
- Respect
- Maximizing capabilities
- Safety
- Observation
- Infection control
- Time management

Communication

You communicate with residents throughout the day. If you did not communicate with a resident, or if you failed to notice the resident's nonverbal messages, how would you know if they were unhappy or in pain? Residents have the right to know what is happening to them and around them. Communication is an important component for developing a trusting relationship with residents and other staff on the care team.

Autonomy

Autonomy means making decisions for oneself and being independent. You must help each resident be as independent as possible. Encourage residents to take responsibility for their care by making their own choices. Then support them in the choices they make, even when it means you have to change how you do a task. Residents are entitled to make their own decisions about how care will be given.

Respect

Everyone deserves to be treated with dignity and respect. Simple courtesies show that you are respectful. Treating each resident with respect must be part of everything you do. Remember that all residents are human beings with their own feelings, thoughts, and beliefs. You must respect and never violate their basic human rights.

Maximizing Capabilities

Maximizing capabilities means that you work with the resident's capabilities and support them to their fullest. You emphasize what the resident is still able to do, not what they cannot do. You work with the resident to help them be the best they can be (Figure 3-12).

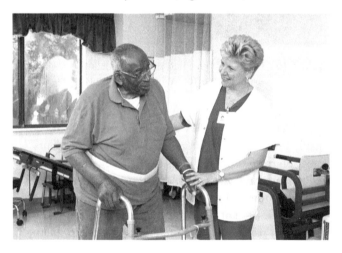

Figure 3-12 Always work with residents to help them achieve their goals.

Safety

Safety means being free from harm or risk and secure from threats or danger. The facility's environment is designed to be a safe place where the staff can focus on giving care in a home-like setting. But if care becomes a quick and careless routine, injuries and accidents are likely. Both residents' safety and your own always depend on acting thoughtfully and carefully (Figure 3-13).

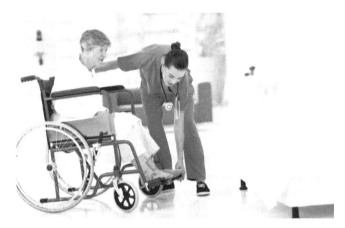

Figure 3-13   Locking the wheels on the wheelchair helps to ensure safety.

Observation

Observation means to watch and pay attention to details. You must pay close attention to your residents every day and look for any changes in their physical, mental, or emotional condition. Report any changes immediately.

Since you spend the most time with residents, it is very likely that you will observe changes before anyone else on the care team does.

Infection Control

The infection control procedures you will learn in later chapters will help prevent the transmission of harmful germs (Figure 3-14). The transmission of microorganisms can be kept to a minimum if everyone follows the proper hygiene protocols. You will learn to incorporate this theme in all your caregiving tasks. This is extremely important to protect the resident, you, and other staff.

Time Management

Time management is the skill of organizing and prioritizing your activities and performing them efficiently. You will learn to prioritize your work by deciding which tasks are most important in providing the highest quality of care while completing all your assigned tasks for a given shift.

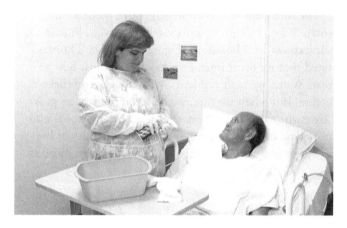

Figure 3-14   Using proper infection control procedures minimizes the spread of bacteria and other microbes.

How to Use Themes in Your Work

Remember to think about the themes of care as you complete each task. How you perform each step is as important as finishing the task. It is a good practice to ask yourself these questions every time you begin a new task:

- What do I need to know or consider about the resident?
- Did I get permission to do the task?
- How should I do this task?
- What do I need to do before I get started?
- What supplies or equipment do I need to complete the task?
- How can I incorporate the themes of care in this task?

In Chapter 5, you will learn important preparation and completion steps and specific strategies for integrating the themes of care in your daily work.

Alternative Ways to Provide Care

Professionals who work in long term care want residents to feel that their life is still worth living. Based on this, Dr. William Thomas created a different type of long term care environment known as the Eden Alternative®. To use this approach, staff in long term care facilities must understand three basic principles of care:

- Every resident can grow as a person.
- A resident's needs and capabilities must determine how we care for them.
- Care must be continuous and long-lasting, unlike treatment, which typically is intermittent and brief.

The idea behind this approach is that to make life worth living, caregivers must work to prevent loneliness, helplessness, and boredom (Figure 3-15). Dr. Thomas stated that we must learn how to care, not just how to treat. When we treat residents, we manage only their disease. But when we care, we help the resident to grow. Currently, the Eden Alternative® is an international non-profit organization dedicated to creating quality of life for elders and their care partners. You can learn more at www.edenalt.org.

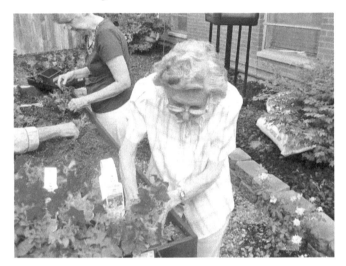

Figure 3-15 The Eden Alternative® program encourages residents to plant their own flower and vegetable gardens.

A variety of alternative care models have emerged in recent decades. Some new facilities are built in a home-like cottage design. Residents share common living areas, and meals are served family-style. A primary caregiver model is used to staff these units of 6 to 10 individuals per cottage. Using innovative care models is a growing trend. In many of these models, the goal is to make the facility less of an institution and more of an environment that welcomes residents into a home and meets their needs for companionship, variety, and for connection to others (Figure 3-16).

Long term care facilities that implement the homelike models include pets and vegetable gardens in the environment. Residents have the opportunity to care for the home, their plants and animals, gardens, and even enjoy meals made with vegetables they grow. Some programs include children. Daycare centers and after-school programs may be part of the facility, and children interact with the residents on a regular basis. In such an environment, residents grow and feel that they are still a valuable part of their community. It is a process that transforms the entire facility, the staff, and the residents.

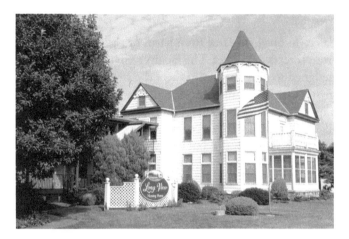

Figure 3-16 Long term care facilities include homes that have been converted into facilities.

Remember that regardless of the type of facility in which you work, everything you do to make residents feel more at home in their new environment contributes significantly to their quality of life.

Quality of Life Requirements

The Centers for Medicare and Medicaid Services (CMS) requires facilities to care for residents in a manner and environment that promote enhancement of every resident's quality of life. This includes:

- Treating the resident with dignity and recognizing their individuality.
- Encouraging self-determination and participation. This means giving residents choices about all aspects of their life in the facility, including activities, schedules, personal care, and health care. Encouraging the organization of and participation in resident and family groups.
- Encouraging participation in social, religious, and community activities as long as they do not interfere with the rights of other residents.
- Accommodating the individual's needs and preferences, within reason.
- Providing a program of activities to meet the residents' interests and promote their physical, mental, and psychosocial well-being.
- Maslow's hierarchy of human needs is a psychological model that ranks human needs from the most basic to the most complex.

Points to Remember

- Psychologist Erik Erikson outlined eight stages of psychosocial development that all humans experience and described the challenges that must be faced at each stage.

- Residents' family members play a significant role in helping the resident achieve the best quality of life possible. The resident's family is an important part of the care team.

- The nurse assistant's role involves working to develop a positive relationship with residents' families based on respectful and effective communication with the resident and family members.

- Residents must be treated with respect and kindness at all times.

- Participation in activities to the level that a resident is able is an important part of maintaining quality of life.

- The themes of care are the basis for everything that a nurse assistant does. The eight themes are: communication, autonomy, respect, maximizing capabilities, safety, observation, infection control, and time management.

Key Terms

psychosocial — relating to the psychological and social aspects of mental health

resident-centered care — focuses on the resident's individual preferences and needs with the resident being an active participant in their care

themes of care — core principles that form the basis for all care provided to residents

1. **What is our highest level of needs in Maslow's hierarchy?**
   a. Social needs
   b. Sexual needs
   c. Self-fulfillment needs
   d. Safety and security needs

2. **What is the task for the older adult in Erickson's theory of psychosocial development?**
   a. The must feel fulfilled with their life.
   b. They must learn to develop intimate relationships.
   c. They must learn to be assertive and to take the initiative.
   d. They must achieve a clear sense of identity in sex roles.

3. **Ways to enhance a resident's relationship with their family include all of the following EXCEPT:**
   a. Ask family members to only visit once a month
   b. Encourage family members to visit
   c. Make their visit comfortable
   d. Involve them in the resident's care

4. **Who is considered part of a resident's family?**
   a. All significant others
   b. Only relatives of common ancestry
   c. Only people related to the resident
   d. Everyone the resident knows

5. **It is important to develop a positive relationship with residents' families because they:**
   a. May influence the resident to not like you
   b. Will complain if you are not nice
   c. Are a part of the caregiving team
   d. Really want to be your friend

6. **It is important to treat a resident with dignity and respect because when residents have dignity:**
   a. They feel better about themselves
   b. Their self-esteem improves
   c. They play a more active role in their care
   d. All of these

7. **Activities are an important part of residents' lives because they help residents:**
   a. Maintain their independence and sense of purpose and feel they are a contributing member of society
   b. Feel tired, so they will nap throughout the day
   c. Feel stressed
   d. Feel helpless because it involves skills they do not have

8. **The themes of care are a basis for all you do to provide excellent care, while promoting a resident's quality of life. They include:**
   a. Communication, autonomy, and respect
   b. Maximizing capabilities, safety, and observation
   c. Infection control and time management
   d. All of the above

9. **Key principles of the Eden Alternative care model include:**
   a. Every resident has the same needs and capabilities
   b. Every resident can grow as a person
   c. Every resident shares the same interests
   d. Every resident just needs medical treatment

10. **Understanding the cultural background of your residents will better equip you to:**
    a. Meet the needs of each resident and deliver quality care
    b. Allow you to make judgements about other cultures
    c. Limit the care that you can provide
    d. Keep a closed mind about other cultures

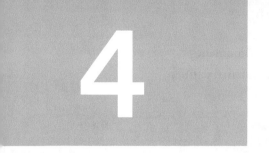

4

Resident Rights

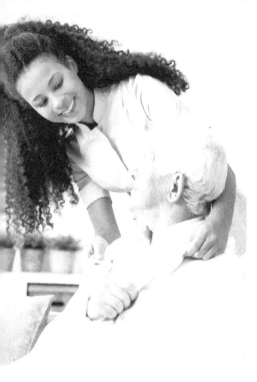

Rights are things to which a person is entitled. Residents are individuals who have the same human and legal rights as all U.S. citizens. They have a right to be treated with respect and dignity, to pursue a meaningful life, and to be free from fear. All residents have the right to high-quality care. The facility and its staff must protect and promote each resident's rights. Violating a resident's rights is breaking the law, and punishment can include being fired, fined, or sent to jail. In this chapter you will learn about residents' rights and your responsibility to protect those rights.

OBJECTIVES:

- Define resident rights.

- List and describe the rights that apply to residents of long term care facilities.

- Explain why protecting residents' rights is essential in maintaining quality of life.

- Identify signs of resident abuse, and state the guidelines for reporting suspected abuse.

- Explain the role of an ombudsman.

Legal Rights

In 1987, a federal law called the Omnibus Budget Reconciliation Act, was passed. Since then, this law, also known as OBRA '87 or the Nursing Home Reform Act, has been updated several times. This law guarantees the rights of residents in long term care facilities. Nurse assistants must understand residents' rights and know how to protect them while delivering care. In general, residents have the right to a dignified existence, to self-determination, and to communication with and access to persons and services inside and outside the facility. Facilities must care for residents in a manner that promotes maintenance or enhancement of each resident's quality of life.

The Code of Federal Regulations specifies resident rights in 42 CFR Part 483, Subpart B, requirements for Long Term Care Facilities. These regulations state:

- The resident has a right to a dignified existence, self-determination, and communication with and access to persons and services inside and outside of the facility.
- The facility must treat each resident with respect and dignity and care for each resident in a manner and in an environment that promotes maintenance or enhancement of his or her quality of life.
- The facility must promote care for residents in a manner and in an environment that maintains or enhances each resident's dignity and respect, in full recognition of their individuality.

Residents have many specific rights, listed in the Residents' Bill of Rights (Figure 4-1). Resident rights can be grouped into the following categories:

- Right to exercise one's rights
- Right to privacy and confidentiality
- Right to information
- Right to choose
- Right to notification of change
- Protection of residents' personal funds
- Grievance rights
- Admission, transfer, and discharge rights
- Right to be free from restraint and abuse

- Right to a safe environment
- Right to contact external entities

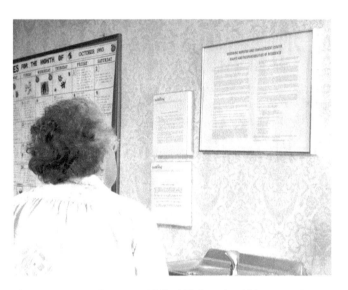

Figure 4-1 The Residents' Bill of Rights should be posted where all residents can see it.

Right to Exercise One's Rights

The facility must inform each resident about their rights both orally and in writing. Residents have the right to exercise the rights they have as a resident of the facility and as a citizen or resident of the United States. Each resident has the right to be free of interference, coercion, discrimination, and reprisal from the facility when they exercise any of their rights. If a resident is judged incompetent under the laws of a state, the person appointed by the state to act on their behalf may exercise their rights.

A person's legal rights do not change just because they enter a long term care facility. Residents may ask your permission to do something like use the phone. Always tell the resident that of course they can use the phone (Figure 4-2). Remind them that they can do the normal activities they did at home here in the facility. You should encourage residents to exercise their rights. Provide assistance and offer choices whenever possible. For example, you can help them vote using an absentee ballot if they cannot go to a polling location.

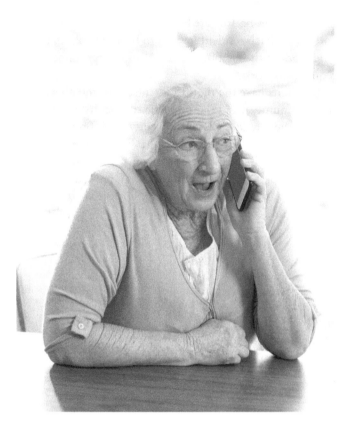

Figure 4-2 Residents should have access to a phone whenever they need it and privacy during calls.

Right to Privacy and Confidentiality

Residents have the right to confidentiality in regard to their personal and medical records. They may decide whether anyone outside the facility may see these records. An exception occurs when a resident transfers to another facility. Then, the law requires release of their records to the other facility.

There have been ongoing updates made to the Health Insurance Portability and Accountability Act (HIPAA) of 1996. These regulations determine how confidential health information should be handled and communicated. You need to be familiar with your facility's policies concerning compliance with this federal regulation.

Residents also have the right to privacy in their rooms. This includes privacy in written and telephone communications, during personal care and medical treatment, and when visiting with family members, friends, and other guests.

You can help protect residents' right to privacy by following these guidelines:

- Do not discuss residents' personal or medical information with anyone unless they have a legitimate need to know it and are legally entitled to the information.

- Do not share residents' personal information with other residents or staff members. This information should also not be shared with the resident's relatives, friends, visitors, or with the news media or your own friends. Other staff members should be told only the information they need to care for the resident, and you should share this information in private. Do not gossip.

- When you care for a resident, always provide privacy. Knock on their door and give them time to say, "Come in." Then introduce yourself and ask if this is a good time. When giving care, pull the curtain and close the door. For personal care, drape their body correctly. You may have to ask visitors or other residents to leave the room when you provide care.

- If asked, you may help a resident read or write letters. Never open their mail unless they ask you to. If there is not a private telephone in each room, allow residents to have private phone conversations in a designated area.

- Give residents time alone with visitors. Help them find a private place for visits, especially for visits with spouses or significant others. If needed, involve their roommate in some activity outside the room to give the resident privacy.

Right to Information

Residents have the right to see their personal and medical records within 24 hours after asking. If they request a written copy of their records, they must receive it within two working days. They have the right to be fully informed, in words they can understand, about their total health status.

Residents must be given a written description of their rights. This should include their eligibility status for Medicaid benefits. They also have a right to know the rules and regulations governing resident conduct and responsibilities during their stay in the facility. If needed, a translator or interpreter must be present when giving information.

Residents must be informed about services and fees and also services that they cannot be charged for. This information must be given before or at the time of admission and periodically during their stay. Residents must also be informed about any change in services. They have a right to see their financial records and to have everything explained to them.

The facility must post in an obvious place the names and addresses of resident advocacy groups and the ombudsman program (discussed later in this chapter). Residents have the right to read the facility's most recent survey report written by federal or state surveyors. They also have the right to read the facility's plan for correcting any problems noted in the surveyors' report.

You can help ensure that residents receive all appropriate information by following these guidelines:

- While residents' rights are explained during the admission process, you must know where to find this information in the event that a resident has questions after admission.

- The Residents' Bill of Rights and instructions for contacting the ombudsman and other advocacy groups must be posted where residents and their families will see them (usually in lounge or dining areas). Read the written residents' rights statement with them, or to them if needed. Go with them to read the posted information.

- A resident may see procedure manuals that contain the facility's policies if they wish. If a resident asks questions, help them find answers.

- If a resident asks to see their records, tell the charge nurse right away.

- If residents express concerns about their medical condition or treatment plan, ask the charge nurse or physician to talk with them.

Right to Choose

Residents have the right to choices regarding their living arrangements and medical care, as long as their choices do not interfere with other residents' rights. Each resident has the right to choose their personal physician and to help plan their own care. They must be informed in advance about changes in care or treatments that may affect their well-being. Residents have the right to take their medications by themselves if the health care team believes it is safe for them to do so. Residents have the right to refuse a specific treatment and to refuse to participate in research. Residents have the right to keep and use their own things as long as there is room and it is safe to do so. Married residents have the right to share a room with their spouse if both live in the facility and both give consent.

Residents have the right to choose their own activities, schedules, and health care based on their own interests and needs. Each resident has the right to do voluntary or paid work in the facility. However, residents cannot be required to work.

Residents have the right to interact with members of the community, inside and outside the facility and the right to meet with others. The facility must provide space and support staff for such meetings. Each resident has the right to have the facility reasonably meet their individual needs and preferences. For example, if a resident wants to have an annual family gathering, if space allows, the facility could help host the event (Figure 4-3).

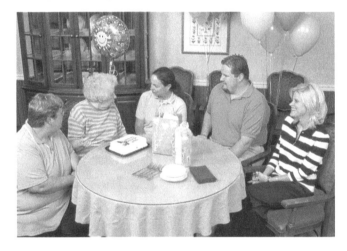

Figure 4-3 Residents have a right to hold special events like a birthday party in the facility.

You can help residents exercise their right to choose by following these guidelines:

- Make sure that residents are aware of their choices. Tell them about activities in the facility. Learn about their interests and help them keep doing things they enjoy.

- Some residents may want to help with tasks like watering plants and making their own beds. Some people feel more useful and have more self-worth if they do things for themselves and help others.

- If residents want to stay active in the community, encourage their involvement with activities that interest them. They can attend meetings and events if their health allows. Think of ways to enhance residents' independence. Encourage residents to set up their own routines as much as possible.

- A resident's choices may have to be limited if they interfere with other residents' rights. To prevent such problems, make sure you are familiar with facility rules that ensure the fair treatment of all residents.

Right to Notification of Change

Residents, family members, and physicians must be told of any change in a resident's physical, mental, or psycho-social status and any accident that causes an injury. If treatment must change because of the resident's condition or resources, the resident must be informed of this change. Residents must be told in advance of any planned change in their room or roommate and about any changes in residents' rights.

The facility must keep and update addresses and phone numbers of each resident's legal representative and family members.

Follow these guidelines when notifying residents and families of change:

- If you must change a resident's care, such as changing a treatment time, tell the resident in advance. When possible, give them a choice of times to schedule the treatment. Even with simple things like a meal delay, tell residents what time they will eat.

- Residents should be involved in decisions such as moving them to another room or assigning a different roommate. Help the resident become comfortable with the decision.

- If you see an accident in which a resident is injured, tell the charge nurse so that the physician and family are informed.

- If a family member gives you a new address or phone number, note it in the resident's record.

Protecting Residents' Personal Funds and Belongings

Residents have the right to keep and manage their own funds or have someone else do it for them. If a resident wants the facility to manage their funds, the facility must safeguard these funds. The facility must provide quarterly statements when the resident or legal representative asks. Funds over $100 ($50 for Medicaid residents) must be maintained in an interest-bearing account. The facility is required to maintain petty cash on hand to honor resident requests.

If you know a resident has a lot of money or is not managing their money appropriately, immediately tell the charge nurse, family, or legal representative so that they can protect the resident's funds. All staff must help safeguard residents' belongings. The facility must make every effort to prevent theft or mismanagement of residents' belongings and money.

Grievance Rights

A grievance is a formal complaint of some type of wrong, injustice, or unfair treatment. Each resident has the right to make complaints without fear of retaliation or discrimination, and the facility must respond promptly to resident complaints.

Federal law requires each state to have an ombudsman program. The ombudsman investigates complaints from residents and family members. The ombudsman also acts as their advocate to resolve complaints (Figure 4-4). The facility must provide information to residents and their families about this program.

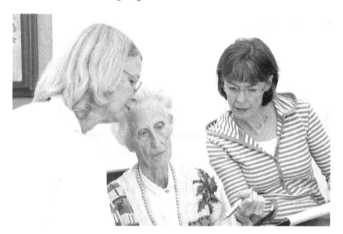

Figure 4-4 The ombudsman hears concerns voiced by residents and family members and works to investigate and resolve problems.

You can help residents exercise their grievance rights by following these guidelines:

- Encourage residents to join resident councils.
- Provide written information to residents about the procedure for filing a grievance.
- If a resident complains to you, tell the charge nurse as soon as you can. Never ignore a resident's complaint.
- If a resident or family member complains or claims that the facility has not resolved a problem, refer them to the charge nurse or social worker.

Admission, Transfer, and Discharge Rights

Transfer and discharge involve moving a resident to a different location. A resident must be told about a transfer or discharge at least 30 days in advance. A resident can be transferred or discharged against their will only with proper advance notice, when another suitable place can be found, and only in one of these situations:

- The situation threatens their life or that of others.
- The resident no longer needs the services of the facility.
- The resident has failed to pay for services after reasonable notice.
- The facility ceases to operate.

Enough advance notice must be given to ensure that the transfer or discharge process is safe and orderly. If the resident plans to return to the same room, such as after hospitalization or therapeutic leave, the same bed may be held for the resident, depending on the facility's policy.

If a resident is unhappy or frightened about a move, listen to their concerns. Do not discount their feelings. Help them understand why the change is needed. Make sure they have time to adjust.

Right to Be Free from Restraint and Abuse

Residents have the right to be free from physical or chemical (medication) restraints, and free from verbal, sexual, physical, or mental abuse and from corporal punishment or involuntary seclusion. The facility must follow written policies to prevent mistreatment, neglect, or abuse of residents and their property.

If a resident or family member complains of a violation of these rights, this complaint must be reported to the administration and other officials as required by state law. The facility must fully investigate these complaints and report the findings.

The Centers for Medicare and Medicaid Services (CMS) requires every facility to have a seven-part abuse-prevention program that includes staff education (Box 4-1). You will learn about this program as part of your employee orientation. You are required to participate in your facility's program and follow its guidelines in your caregiving.

Each facility is required to post the resident's rights, make sure that you know where it is located in your facility.

Right to a Safe Environment

Each resident has a right to a safe, clean, comfortable, and homelike environment, including but not limited to receiving treatment that supports daily living safely. The facility must provide housekeeping and maintenance services necessary to maintain a sanitary, orderly, and comfortable interior. The facility should ensure comfortable and safe temperature, sound, and lighting levels in all areas. It is the responsibility of the nurse assistant to report any environmental concerns according to facility policy.

Right to Contact External Entities

A facility cannot prohibit, prevent, or in any way discourage a resident from communications with federal, state, or local officials, including but not limited to state surveyors, or federal or state health department employees.

Elder Justice Act of 2010

In March 2010, the federal government passed guidelines regarding reporting requirements for any suspicion of a crime committed against an older adult. The guidelines state: If an individual such as a health care worker has a reasonable suspicion that a crime has occurred involving a resident or person receiving care at the facility, that individual has the responsibility to report the suspicion directly to both local law enforcement and the state survey agency without fear of retaliation. The Act also specifies serious bodily injuries that must be reported within two hours. Any other suspicion of abuse is required to be reported within 24 hours. It is important to know your facility's specific policies, guidelines, and definitions regarding elder abuse.

Defining Abuse and Neglect

Abuse is willfully injuring a resident, unreasonably confining a resident, intimidating or punishing a resident, or causing physical harm, pain, or mental anguish. There are various types of abuse:

- **Verbal abuse** includes using profanity, calling a resident names, yelling at a resident, making verbal or written threats, or teasing in an unkind manner.
- **Mental abuse** includes any action that makes a resident fearful, such as threatening them with harm or threatening to tell others something they do not want them to know. It includes actions that belittle or make fun of a resident.
- **Physical abuse** is any action that causes actual physical harm. This includes handling a resident too roughly, giving a wrong treatment, or hitting, pushing, pinching, or kicking a resident.
- **Sexual abuse** includes any sexual act where the resident doesn't or is unable to give consent. It may also include touching residents in an intimate or suggestive manner, making sexual comments, or allowing another resident to engage in unwanted sexual acts with a resident.

BOX 4-1

SEVEN COMPONENTS OF ABUSE PROHIBITION PROGRAMS

Screening Policies for Potential Hires:

- Interview applicants, keeping in mind desirable employee behaviors.
- Do criminal background checks.
- Check references.
- Conduct a screening for drug use.
- Check licensing or certification boards to be sure employees are in good standing.
- Start all employees with a probationary period.
- Screen all employees for past and present alcohol and substance abuse.

Training of Employees That Includes:

- definitions of abuse
- how to handle a difficult resident
- stress and burnout
- residents' rights
- regulations and responsibilities
- missing items, theft

Facilities Must Have Prevention Policies and Procedures That:

- identify residents at risk
- define roles during the probationary period
- set up an ongoing education plan
- recommend staffing levels
- establish a plan for reporting incidents
- describe the investigation of missing items and theft

Procedures for Investigating Incidents and Allegations That Include:

- identifying when the suspected abuse may have occurred
- identifying all staff and residents who may have had access to the resident
- interviewing staff and residents in person
- obtaining written statements from both staff and residents about what happened, including:
- the resident's behavior
- staff members' response to the resident's behavior
- unusual occurrences
- observations
- communications
- everyone's immediate response to the situation

Procedures for Identifying Possible Incidents or Allegations That Include:

- what to do about complaints
- observations of what happened
- how to investigate injuries of unknown cause

Procedures for Protecting Residents During Investigation That Include:

- securing the environment
- assessing the resident for harm and threats
- reassuring the resident

Procedures for Responding and Reporting That Include:

- reports to required agencies
- corrective actions
- analysis of the problem and solutions

- **Physical restraints** are any devices that limit a resident's movement or access to their body. Restraints may include bed rails, vest restraints that keep a resident in bed or in a chair, limb restraints that limit a resident's use of their arms or legs, tables that lock over a resident in a chair, or lap pillows that keep a resident from standing or walking. The resident must be able to remove any device or equipment used. Otherwise, it is considered a restraint. *released q2h*

- **Chemical restraints** are medications used to sedate a resident, slow their muscle activity, or change their behavior.

- **Neglect** is failing to do something you should have done. Neglect includes not giving proper hygiene care, not turning a resident over in bed to improve their

circulation, not giving food and water regularly, or not taking the resident to the bathroom when they ask. Neglect may also be considered physical abuse.

- **Negligence** is failing to act in the same way that a reasonable person with the same training would act in the same situation. Gross negligence is any action that shows no concern for the resident's well-being.

- **Corporal punishment** is physical punishment, such as spanking or slapping.

- **Involuntary seclusion** is the isolation of a resident against their will, such as locking them alone in a room.

- **Misappropriation of resident property** is the act of deliberately misplacing a resident's belongings or money or using a resident's belongings without his or her permission. It is considered theft and is a form of abuse. You can help prevent theft by marking belongings with the resident's name and helping residents keep their possessions in a safe place. List all personal belongings on the inventory record. You may suggest that family members take home expensive items.

- **Domestic violence** is when abusive behavior occurs within a relationship. It is used to gain power or control over another person. Anyone can be a victim of domestic violence regardless of age, gender, social class, race, education, sexual orientation or religion. It is important to keep in mind that this type of abuse can occur within the long term care setting as well.

In addition to the direct forms of abuse noted above, abuse can be indirect, such as talking to another nurse assistant while ignoring a resident. Indirect abuse also includes saying negative things about a resident outside their room (whether or not the resident is likely to hear it) and ignoring a resident's call light when you are about to go on break.

Use of a Restraint

You will learn your facility's policy for the use of restraints during your orientation. A restraint may be used temporarily to help give a resident a medical treatment. For example, a resident may be placed in a limb restraint if they pull out tubes needed for medical treatment. The limb restraint is used to restrict the resident's ability to move their arm and pull out the tube. A restraint may also be used in an emergency if needed for a life-saving treatment. For example, an infection can cause a resident to become confused or delirious, and if they are not treated, they could die. A resident who is uncooperative or combative cannot be evaluated properly, so there may be a need to restrain them so the nurse or physician can draw blood and do the proper assessment. The restraint would then be removed.

If a restraint is needed, the charge nurse will tell you which type of restraint to use and the proper procedure for using it. However, a physician's order is needed to use the restraint. The charge nurse must document the reasons for using the restraint according to the facility's policies. Any restraint used should be the least restrictive device that allows the most movement while still meeting the needs of the resident.

When a resident is restrained, check that the restraint is used properly. Check the resident often to make sure the restraint does not cause a circulatory problem. Release the restraint frequently (without actually removing it), following your facility's policy.

Necessary care should never be withheld when a resident is restrained. Their needs for nourishment, hydration, hygiene, and toileting must be met. Also, a resident who is restrained may be frightened, angry, resentful, or confused as to why they are being restrained. It is important that the resident's emotional needs are met as well.

A resident who is sleeping much of the time or is suddenly slurring their speech may be receiving too much medication. Tell the charge nurse about any situation like this. Make sure it is documented in the resident's chart. This situation may be considered a chemical restraint.

Signs of Abuse

As a nurse assistant you will spend more time with the residents than other staff members, so it is important to be able to recognize signs of abuse. Signs of abuse may not be limited to physical signs, such as a bruise, cut, or laceration that cannot be explained. It may be a change in the residents' emotional or social status. You could have a resident that is outgoing and attends activities but all of a sudden stops attending activities and isolates themselves in their room. Or you could be caring for a resident that is tearful or acts scared around others. These could be signs that abuse has occurred.

Your Role in Preventing Abuse

Sometimes on-the-job or personal stress leads to abuse. Recognize your own stress level and that of others around you. It may help to take breaks with coworkers and to join a stress management program offered by your facility or another health care resource.

Report any signs of abuse to the charge nurse and the administrator. If you know about abuse and do not report it, you are just as responsible as if you did it.

The law requires the facility to have procedures to protect residents, and it severely punishes anyone who abuses residents. This can include fines and imprisonment of anyone convicted of abuse. Staff can be charged with assault for threatening to harm a resident. Anyone who causes physical harm can be charged with battery. You must protect **vulnerable residents** from abuse by other residents or others outside the facility.

Whenever a resident or family alleges abuse, the facility must investigate and report its findings to state agencies. During the investigation, you may be asked about your actions. This does not mean that you have done anything wrong, but the facility must be able to document that it tried to protect its residents.

If a charge is brought against a staff member, that person has the right to a hire a lawyer. The person may not be at fault even if charged with an offense. The same rule applies to all U.S. residents: innocent until proven guilty.

A health care professional found guilty of resident abuse loses their job and is reported to the state registry. Facilities refer to the state registry when hiring because they are not allowed to hire anyone who has been found guilty of neglecting, abusing, or mistreating residents or stealing their property.

Ombudsman Program

The Long Term Care Ombudsman Program was established in 1972 under the authorization of the Older Americans Act to protect residents' rights. It was set up because of growing concern about poor care in nursing facilities. The facility must tell residents how to contact the local ombudsman program.

Each state has an Office of the State Long Term Care Ombudsman, directed by a full-time state ombudsman. There are also ombudsman programs at the local level operated by professional staff and community volunteers. Ombudsmen are charged with investigating complaints by residents or others about violations of rights. According to the U.S. Department of Health and Human Services, the ombudsman program has these responsibilities:

- Identify, investigate, and resolve complaints made by or on behalf of residents.
- Provide information to residents about long term care services.
- Represent the interests of residents before government agencies, and seek administrative, legal, and other remedies to protect residents.

- Analyze, comment on, and recommend changes in laws and regulations concerning the health, safety, welfare, and rights of residents.
- Educate and inform consumers and the general public about issues and concerns about long term care, and facilitate public comment on laws, regulations, policies, and actions.
- Promote the development of citizen organizations to participate in the program.
- Provide technical support for the development of resident and family councils to protect the well-being and rights of residents.
- Advocate for changes to improve residents' quality of life and care.

The state ombudsman has authority to solve problems for a resident. If the ombudsman cannot resolve the problem, they may represent a resident, negotiate a solution, or file a lawsuit.

Ombudsmen also monitor state regulations and help strengthen laws that protect residents' rights. Ombudsmen help educate the public and train volunteers to help residents and their families. Since 1995, the National Ombudsman Reporting System (NORS) has collected information about complaints that are investigated. This information is helping families, facilities, and government agencies improve the quality of long term care.

Facilities are required to post information about all relevant state client advocacy groups, including:

- The state's survey and certification agency
- The state's licensure office
- The state's ombudsman program
- The protection and advocacy network
- The Medicaid fraud control unit

Points to Remember

- Residents in long term care facilities have the same rights as all U.S. citizens. They have a right to be treated with respect and dignity. All staff members must be aware of and protect each resident's rights.

- It is the responsibility of all staff members to report any suspected abuse.

- Any restraint used should be the least restrictive device that allows the most movement while still meeting the needs of the resident.

Key Terms

abuse — cruel or inhumane treatment that causes physical and/or psychological harm; threats made to a person

advocate — someone who takes the side of another person and speaks for them

allegation — a person's statement that someone has done something wrong or illegal

chemical restraints — medications used to sedate a resident, slow their muscle activity, or change their behavior

corporal punishment — physical punishment, such as spanking or slapping

discrimination — an unfair or unjust treatment of people or groups of people

grievance — formal complaint of a wrong, injury, or injustice

involuntary seclusion — the isolation of a resident against their will, such as locking them alone in a room

mental abuse — any action that makes a resident fearful, such as threatening them with harm or threatening to tell others something they do not want them to know

misappropriation of resident property — includes deliberately misplacing a resident's belongings or money, or using a resident's belongings without his or her permission or theft

neglect — failure to provide proper care

negligence — failure to act in the same way that a reasonable person with the same training would act in the same situation

ombudsman — official or designated person who investigates and resolves complaints; advocate for resident rights

physical abuse — any action that causes actual physical harm

physical restraints — any devices that limit a resident's movement or access to their body

retaliation — the act of getting revenge or punishing a person for doing something

self-determination — freedom to make your own choices and choose your own activities

sexual abuse — any sexual act where the resident does not or cannot give consent

verbal abuse — includes using profanity, calling a resident names, yelling at a resident, making verbal or written threats, or teasing in an unkind manner

vulnerable resident — someone in need of special care, support, or protection because of age, disability, or risk of abuse or neglect

1. **What federal law guarantees the rights of residents in long term care facilities?**
   a. Omnibus Budget Reconciliation Act, also known as OBRA '87
   b. The Elder Justice Law
   c. The Older American Act
   d. The Nursing Facility Act of 1900

2. **In the chain of command, to whom do you report any suspected abuse?**
   a. The activity director
   b. The director of housekeeping
   c. The staff development coordinator
   d. The charge nurse

3. **What is the Elder Justice Act?**
   a. Guidelines for reporting facility revenue
   b. Guidelines for reporting resident grievances
   c. Guidelines regarding reporting requirements for any suspicion of a crime committed against an older adult
   d. Guidelines for reporting the facility census

4. **Abuse is defined as:**
   a. Cruel or inhumane treatment that causes physical and/or psychological harm or threats made to a person
   b. As only physical abuse
   c. An accident that was not intentional
   d. An act that does not need to be reported

5. **What type of abuse occurs when a staff member steals money from a resident?**
   a. Physical abuse
   b. Misappropriation of resident property
   c. Sexual abuse
   d. Theft is not considered a type of abuse.

6. **The failure to notify a resident that they will be moving is a violation of which of the resident's rights?**
   a. The right of protection of personal funds
   b. The right to choose
   c. The right to privacy
   d. The right to notification of change

7. **If suspected abuse is reported, the facility must:**
   a. Investigate the allegation and report the findings to the appropriate state agency
   b. Investigate the allegation and only report the findings to the charge nurse
   c. Wait a week to investigate the allegation
   d. Only interview the roommate of the resident involved in the allegation

8. **Which of the following is a violation of resident rights?**
   a. Delivering mail unopened to the resident
   b. Allowing privacy for family visits
   c. Talking about a resident's medical condition in the breakroom
   d. Allowing the resident to choose their own physician

9. **Not taking a resident to the bathroom would be considered:**
   a. Misappropriation of resident property
   b. Neglect
   c. Improper use of physical restraints
   d. This would not be considered abuse

10. **Using a medication to make a resident sleep so they will not bother staff would be considered:**
    a. A physical restraint
    b. A chemical restraint
    c. An acceptable method to ensure that a resident gets the sleep they need
    d. A violation of the resident's right to have a private phone conversation

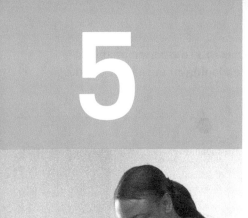

5

Preventing Infections While Providing Personal Care

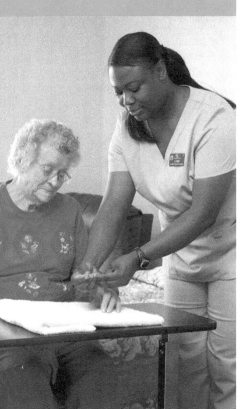

Residents in long term care facilities are at risk of exposure to bacteria that have become resistant to antibiotics. Unfortunately, people die every day from these serious bacterial infections. Residents who are elderly, frail, or already weakened by another illness are most at risk for contracting some type of infection. Many of these infections can be prevented. The challenge is to provide personal care in a way that protects both residents and staff.

Infections spread because of careless infection control practices. Adherence to established protocols while caring for the resident can often prevent these tragedies.

You have a very important role in preventing and controlling infections in your facility. In this chapter, you will learn how microorganisms are transmitted and what you can do to prevent the spread of infection. You will learn how to incorporate infection control practices into the personal care routines you will use every day.

OBJECTIVES:

- Explain how microorganisms are transmitted from one person to another.

- Name and describe each link in the chain of infection.

- Define standard precautions and explain how these measures prevent the spread of infection.

- Demonstrate proper hand hygiene techniques.

- Demonstrate the proper way to put on and remove gowns, gloves, masks, and other personal protective equipment.

- Explain how soiled linen and wastes in the resident's environment must be handled.

- Explain when and why isolation precautions are used.

- Name and describe the different types of transmission-based precautions.

- Differentiate between cleaning, disinfection, and sterilization.

- Explain why observation is an important part of providing personal care.

- Explain how completing the preparation steps can help perform procedures efficiently.

- State the common completion steps in providing personal care and describe each step.

- Demonstrate the proper way to carry out the following procedures: complete bed bath, tub bath, shower, whirlpool bath, shampooing, brushing and flossing, cleaning dentures, providing mouth care for comatose residents, shaving a male's face, shaving a female's legs and underarms, trimming facial hair, brushing/combing/styling hair, caring for fingernails and foot care, dressing and undressing a dependent resident.

What Are Microorganisms and How Do They Cause Infection?

Microorganisms are organisms so small that they can be seen only with a microscope. They are usually single cells or infectious particles and include **bacteria**, **viruses**, **fungi**, and **parasites**. The commonly used term for these microorganisms is "germs." *Pathogens*

Many microorganisms live naturally on the skin. They also live in the intestines, vagina, mouth, and other parts of the body. These bacteria are called **natural flora**. In a healthy person, these bacteria are in balance and do not cause problems. However, if the natural balance is disrupted due to illness, poor nutrition, stress, fatigue, or certain drugs, these microorganisms may cause **infection**. Infection occurs when there is an invasion and multiplication of microorganisms, such as bacteria and viruses that are not normally present in the body, that may or may not produce symptoms.

Microorganisms that live in one part of the body without causing problems can cause a serious infection if they reach another part. For example, *Escherichia coli* bacteria (abbreviated as *E. coli*) normally live in the gastrointestinal tract. If these bacteria reach the bladder, they can cause a urinary tract infection. You may have heard of *E. coli* infections reported in the news related to food contamination caused by improper food handling, contaminated water, or food products such as meat and produce.

The Chain of Infection

Microorganisms are transmitted from one organism (person or animal) to another in a process called the **chain of infection** (Figure 5-1). Six elements or conditions must be present for the infection to be transmitted:

1. The microorganism is capable of causing an infectious disease.

2. The microorganism resides in a **reservoir** (person, animal, or environment). *where germs live*

3. It leaves the reservoir via a **portal of exit** (route of transmission) *sneeze/cough*

4. It travels via a **mode of transmission** (the means by which it is transferred).

5. It reaches a **portal of entry** (the place where it enters the second organism)

6. It enters a **susceptible host** (the person or animal who is at risk of developing an infection from the microorganism).

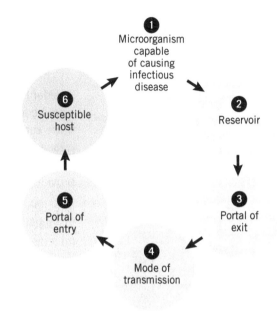

Figure 5-1 The chain of infection. Transmission of microorganisms involves six links.

The Microorganism

The first link in the chain is the microorganism that causes the infection. Many types of viruses, bacteria, and fungi cause infections. Microorganisms that cause infections are called **pathogens**; those that do not are called **nonpathogenic**. Without a pathogenic microorganism, there can be no infection.

The Reservoir

The second link is the reservoir. This is where the microorganisms live. The human body is a reservoir for many different types of microorganisms. They also live in animals, plants, soil, food, and water as well as on surfaces in the environment.

Human reservoirs may not show any signs of the disease but can pass the infection on to others without knowing.

Portal of Exit

The portal of exit is the route by which the microorganism leaves the reservoir. Microorganisms must exit from an infected person or another reservoir to be transmitted to another person. Portals of exit include all natural body openings and breaks in the skin such as tears or wounds.

They also include openings made during medical, dental, and surgical procedures. For example, microorganisms in the lungs can exit the body when a person coughs or sneezes. Microorganisms in the bladder exit in urine, and those in the intestinal tract exit in stool.

Modes of Transmission

Organisms are transmitted from the portal of exit of one person to the portal of entry of a susceptible person. This can happen in several way (modes), including direct, indirect, and airborne transmission:

- **Direct transmission** of microorganisms from one person to another can occur via physical contact such as kissing, skin-to-skin contact, and sexual intercourse. Direct transmission also occurs through **droplet spread**. This occurs when a direct spray of mucus from coughing, sneezing, or talking comes in contact with another person's eyes, nose, or mouth when people are within three to six feet of each other. Droplet-transmitted diseases such as chicken pox and measles spread quickly among children. Direct transmission also occurs when one person's infected blood or other body fluids come in direct contact with another person's broken skin or mucous membranes.

- **Indirect transmission** occurs when a microorganism is transferred from one person to another via a **vehicle** (some type of inanimate object) or a **vector** (living agent that transmits infection) such as a tick or mosquito. Infectious organisms may be transmitted via soiled linen or dressings and contaminated surfaces, water, and food.

- **Airborne transmission** occurs when microorganisms are carried in aerosols (tiny particles suspended in air) and a susceptible host inhales the particles. The bacteria that cause tuberculosis (TB) are transmitted in this way. TB microorganisms can live in the air, but airborne transmission can be prevented if the facility has proper ventilation and air exchange systems. The measles virus can also be spread this way; it can live up to two hours suspended in air. Some viruses, such as COVID-19 can be transmitted by indirect, droplet and airborne transmission. According to the CDC, the principal mode by which people are infected with COVID-19 is through exposure to respiratory fluids containing the virus.

Portal of Entry into Host

Most often, the portal of entry is a natural opening in the body. For example, a susceptible host may breathe in microorganisms through the nose and mouth when a nearby person coughs or sneezes. The portal of entry may also be an open wound. This includes skin tears and pressure ulcers. Microorganisms that cause diarrhea can enter a susceptible host's digestive system when a person preparing or handling food did not wash their hands after using the bathroom. Bacteria and viruses that cause sexually transmitted disease can enter through the mouth, vagina, penis, or anus.

Susceptible Host

We are all susceptible to infections caused by viruses, bacteria, fungi, and other pathogens. A resident can become more susceptible to infection due to existing diseases or health conditions. For example, a person with respiratory disease may be more susceptible to inhaled pathogens.

Other reasons for increased risk of infection include treatment with steroids or chemotherapeutic agents that weaken the immune system, breaks in the skin, use of invasive devices such as catheters, an unclean environment, or simply advanced age.

Strategies for Breaking the Chain of Infection

If even one link in the chain of infection is broken, disease cannot be transmitted. Many different infection prevention and control measures can be used to break various links in the chain (Figure 5-2 and Table 5-1).

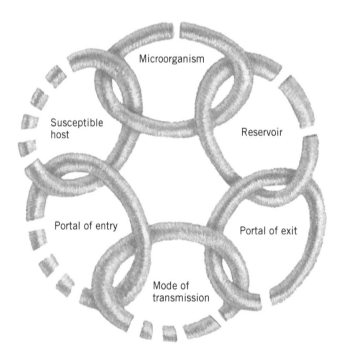

Figure 5-2 The chain of transmission can be broken by using proper infection control procedures.

Table 5-1 Breaking Links in the Chain of Infection

Link	How the Chain is Broken
Microorganism	▪ Facility cleaning procedures ▪ Handwashing
Reservoir	▪ Environmental sanitation ▪ Identification and treatment of infections with antibiotics ▪ Food sanitation procedures such as cleaning equipment and adequate refrigeration ▪ Handwashing
Portal of exit	▪ Use of barriers such as gloves, masks, and face shields ▪ Handwashing
Mode of transmission	▪ Use of barriers such as gloves, masks, and face shields ▪ Handwashing
Portal of entry	▪ Use of barriers such as gloves, masks, goggles, and face shields ▪ Proper disinfection of equipment ▪ Handwashing
Susceptible host	▪ Immunization against disease ▪ Use of barriers such as gloves, masks, and face shields ▪ Handwashing

Standard Precautions

Standard precautions are evidence-based practices designed to prevent the transmission of infectious disease. According to the Centers for Disease Control and Prevention (CDC), standard precautions represent the minimum infection prevention measures that apply to all patient care, regardless of the infection status of the patient, in any health care setting.

The goal of standard precautions is to reduce the risk of transmission of microorganisms from both recognized and unrecognized sources. This means that you use the same precautions around someone you think is healthy as you would use around someone who is known to have a virus or other infectious disease. You should assume that all blood, body fluids, wounds, and mucous membranes may be infected.

Standard precautions include many work practices that minimize or eliminate your exposure to pathogens. Key elements are:

▪ Proper hand hygiene
▪ Proper use of gloves, gowns, and facial protection

▪ Proper handling of linens
▪ Proper environmental cleaning and waste disposal
▪ Proper use and disposal of patient care equipment
▪ Prevention of needle sticks and injuries from other sharp instruments
▪ Respiratory hygiene and cough etiquette

Hand Hygiene

Hand hygiene is the process of cleaning your hands by using either handwashing or using an alcohol-based hand rub.

Proper hand hygiene is essential to making sure that the skin is free of contamination by potentially infectious microorganisms. Hand hygiene is the most effective way to prevent the spread of germs and infections. According to the CDC, the use of alcohol-based hand rubs is the preferred method for cleaning your hand in most clinical settings. Alcohol-based hand rub should contain at least 60% alcohol and must be used according to the manufacturer's guidelines to be effective.

Handwashing is recommended when your hands are visibly soiled, after caring for a resident with diarrhea, or after coming in contact or suspected exposure to a spore (Procedure 5-1). Your facility will have guidelines in place for when specific hand hygiene methods should be used.

Alcohol-based hand rub can be used:

▪ Before and after each shift
▪ Before and after contact with a resident or their environment
▪ Between care activities (after helping the resident toilet and before helping with the bath)
▪ After contact with blood or body fluids
▪ Before and after cleaning an area
▪ Before and after handling body fluids collected for testing
▪ Before putting on gloves
▪ After removing gloves
▪ After a cough, sneeze, or blowing your nose

There are certain situations in which handwashing MUST be done. You must wash your hands:

▪ When hands are visibly soiled
▪ Before and after handling food
▪ Before and after using the bathroom
▪ When caring for a resident with diarrhea

1 Before you begin, check that the sink is clean and the soap dispenser is within reach. Paper towels must be within reach without touching the dispenser to avoid contaminating your hands.

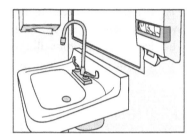

2 Remove your watch and roll up your sleeves.

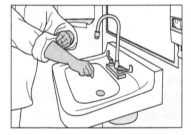

3 Turn on the water and adjust to a comfortable temperature. Wet your hands and wrists.

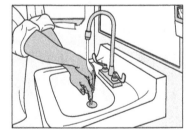

4 Apply soap to your hands.

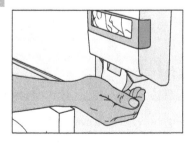

5 Rub your hands together in a circular motion with friction for a minimum of 20 seconds.

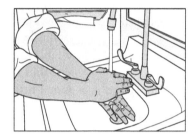

6 Clean all surfaces of your hands, including your wrists. Lace your fingers together to wash in between them. Clean under your fingernails using a nail brush or orange stick, or rub your nails briskly in your palm to clean them.

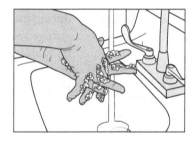

7 Rinse your hands with warm water, keeping them downward, allowing the water to run from the wrist to the fingers.

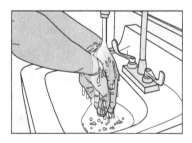

8 Get paper towels from the dispenser. Touch only the clean towels, not the dispenser.

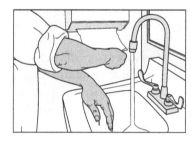

9 Dry your hands with paper towels. Start at the top of the fingers and work downward toward the wrists.

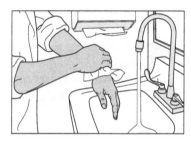

10 Turn off the faucet(s) using a clean paper towel.

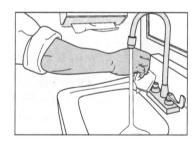

11 Discard paper towels in appropriate receptacle.

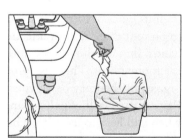

- After coming in contact or suspected exposure to *clostridium difficile* (*C difficile*) or anthrax

Studies have shown that even after proper hand hygiene, pathogens can be present under longer fingernails. The CDC recommends that nails should be no longer than one fourth of an inch. Artificial nails harbor bacteria and should not be worn in a health care setting. It is also recommended to wear as little jewelry as possible, since rings and bracelets can also become contaminated with microorganisms.

Remember to perform hand hygiene before putting on gloves and immediately after removing gloves or other personal protective equipment. If you come in contact with blood or other potentially infectious materials, immediately wash your hands and the affected skin areas with soap and water. If your mucous membranes (such as your eyes or inside your nose or mouth) are splashed with blood or fluid, flush the area with water immediately and report the incident according to facility policy. Such contact may occur from the splattering of fluids, such as when emptying a urinary drainage bag or rinsing a bedpan.

Procedure for Using Alcohol-based Hand Rub:

- Apply the hand sanitizer to the palm of your hand. Make sure to follow the manufacture guidelines on how much product to use.

- Rub your hands together.

- Rub the hand sanitizer to all surfaces of your hands, making sure to get in between fingers and under nails until your hands are dry. This process should take about 20 seconds.

Gloves and Other Personal Protective Equipment

According to the Occupational Safety and Health Administration (OSHA), **personal protective equipment (PPE)** is equipment worn to minimize exposure to hazards that cause serious workplace injuries and illnesses. PPE provides a barrier between you and microorganisms that can cause diseases. These include gloves, gowns or plastic aprons, masks, face shields, and eye protection. Various types of PPE are used, along with hand hygiene, to prevent the spread of infection. PPE protect your hands, skin, clothing, eyes, and mucous membranes from microorganisms. They also protect residents from microorganisms that may be on your hands, skin, or clothing. Review your facility policies and procedures related to when and how to use PPE. There are different methods that can be used to put on and remove PPE. This chapter will cover one method that can be used.

Standard precautions require that gloves be worn in the following situations:

- When touching blood, body fluids, **secretions**, excretions, or contaminated items.

- When touching mucous membranes or broken (nonintact) skin.

Most often, you will need single-use disposable gloves. Gloves are made from different materials. Most are made of nitrile, vinyl, or latex. These gloves are packaged as clean, not sterile. Some types of gloves fit better than others. Your facility will have various sizes of gloves on hand. Good-fitting gloves are needed for fine motor skills. Most of the time, you do not need sterile gloves or tight-fitting gloves.

Gloves must be changed between tasks, before giving care to another resident, and before touching noncontaminated items and environmental surfaces. Change your gloves and perform hand hygiene before caring for each resident and anytime the gloves become visibly contaminated. You must perform hand hygiene after removing gloves because they may become contaminated from small defects, from tears in the gloves that occurred during use, or when removing the gloves. You must also change your gloves when moving from a contaminated body site to a clean one. There are several different methods used for putting on and removing gloves. One method is shown in Procedure 5-2.

When you clean equipment or surfaces like a bedside table, you should wear heavy utility gloves (Figure 5-3) rather than single-use disposable gloves. The chemicals in cleaning solutions can irritate your hands, and heavy utility gloves offer better protection. You can reuse utility gloves unless they are cracked, torn, or worn out, just as you reuse similar gloves at home.

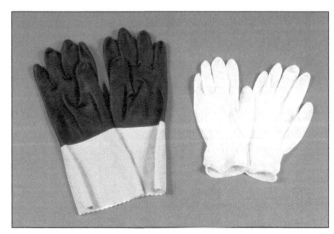

Figure 5-3 When cleaning, heavy utility gloves (left) should be worn rather than single-use gloves (right).

PUTTING ON GLOVES:

1. Perform hand hygiene

2. Slip gloves on, covering your entire hand and wrist.

3. If you are putting on gloves along with a gown and mask, put the gown on first, then the mask, and then the gloves. Pull the gloves up over the gown's cuffs.

REMOVING GLOVES:

Gloves are removed after you complete a task. Use the steps shown below if you are right-handed. If you are left-handed, use the opposite hand.

1. Using your right hand, grasp the outside of the glove on the left hand at the inside of the wrist, turning the glove inside out as you pull it down over your left hand.

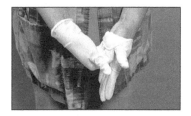

2. Hold the used left glove in a ball in your gloved right hand.

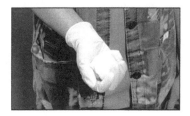

3. Grasp the inside of the right glove at the top of the wrist with your left hand.

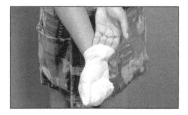

If you are wearing fitted, sterile gloves, you will not be able to grasp the inside of the top of the right glove, so you must cuff (fold over) the top of the right glove before you begin to remove the glove.

4. Pull the right glove down over your right hand and over the used glove held in that hand. The right glove is now inside out, with the left glove enclosed in it.

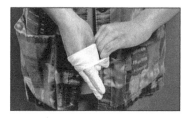

5. Place the gloves in the trash receptacle. Follow your facility's infection control policies to dispose of soiled waste.

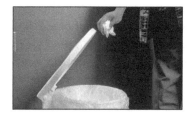

6. Perform hand hygiene by washing hands or using an alcohol-based hand rub.

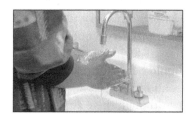

Gowns

Gowns are made of cloth, paper, or plastic. A clean, nonsterile gown should be worn to protect your skin and prevent soiling of your clothing when you perform tasks that may splash or spray you with blood, body fluids, secretions, or excretions. Wear a gown when a resident has diarrhea, is **vomiting**, or has large amounts of drainage from a wound. A soiled gown should be removed as soon as possible after completing your task. If you are using gloves and a gown, put the gown on first and then the gloves. Remove the gown after completing your task with the resident. The correct steps are shown in Procedure 5-3.

Plastic aprons are barriers that cover the front of your clothing. They are particularly useful in situations in which your clothing may get wet, such as when you are helping a resident to bathe. Plastic aprons are also useful when changing soiled linen that cannot easily be folded in on itself to contain the soiled area. Disposable plastic aprons usually have a neck strap and ties at the waist. They do not protect your arms. When you need to wear gloves and a plastic apron, put the apron on first, then the gloves. Remove the gloves first, then the apron. Be sure to wash your hands after removing the apron.

Face Protection

Surgical/procedure masks, visors, goggles, and face shields are used to protect the mucous membranes of your eyes, nose, and mouth during tasks that are likely to involve splashes or sprays of blood, body fluids, secretions, or excretions. For example, face protection is used when emptying a Foley catheter drainage bag or assisting a nurse with suctioning a resident.

Masks. Masks are an effective barrier to splashes or splatters, and they also protect against inhaling droplets in the air. The mask must fit tightly so that you do not inhale air easily around the sides of the mask. If you will be spending a long time with a resident with an infectious disease, change your mask every 20 minutes, sooner if it becomes moist or this is the policy at your facility. Some situations may require you to wear a N95 respirator mask. Respirators should have a tight fit, and a seal check should be performed to make sure air is not escaping around the edges.

Although there are different kinds of masks, all have a metal bar on the bridge of the nose and ties, straps, or elastic to secure the mask. If you need to wear a mask, gloves, face shield or goggles, and a gown or apron, put on the gown or apron first. Then put on the mask, then the face shield or goggles, and put on the gloves last.

Remove the gloves first, then the face shield or goggles, and finally the mask. Perform hand hygiene after removing PPE and at any point your hands become contaminated during the process. If you are wearing a N95 mask, do not remove until after you have let the resident's room and closed the door. The correct steps for removing a mask are shown in Procedure 5-4.

Eye and face protection. Goggles or face shields protect the eyes and face from splashes and splatters (Figure 5-4). You will rarely be in a situation that requires eye protection, but you must know how to use it. If you wear eyeglasses that you want to use for splash protection, they must have side shields, which are add-on devices. The infection control practitioner in your facility can help you locate the correct side shields for your glasses.

If you do not wear glasses and need eye protection, you can use goggles or a face shield. Goggles can be washed, dried, and reused, as can most face shields. Some manufacturers make a single-use combination mask and eye protection shield. These shields can be worn over corrective eyeglasses and protect against splashes from the front and sides.

If you are using eye protection and a mask along with a gown or plastic apron and gloves, put on the eye protection after you put on the mask. As always, wash your hands after you remove all barriers.

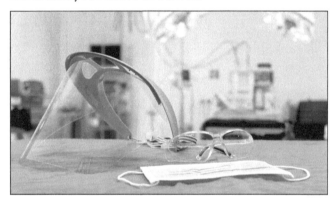

Figure 5-4 Goggles and face shields protect the eyes from splashes or splatters.

HOW TO APPLY AND REMOVE PPE

There are different methods for applying and removing PPE. This procedure demonstrates one method. Review your facility policies and procedures related to when and how to use PPE.

To Apply PPE

- Remove jewelry.
- Perform hand hygiene.

- Put on gown:
  - Gently open the gown without shaking.
  - Insert your arms in the sleeves, with the opening in the back.
  - Tie the gown at the neck and waist. The gown should cover your uniform from you neck to your knees.
- Put on mask or respirator:
  - Put mask or respirator over your nose and mouth.
  - Extend under your chin.
  - Tie or secure the straps around the back of your head so that the mask fits tightly.
  - Pinch the metal piece on the bridge of the nose to make a tight seal. If a N95 respirator is used, perform a seal check/fit-check.
- Put on goggles and face shield:
  - If a N95 respirator is used, make sure that it does not interfere with proper position of your goggles.
- Put on gloves:
  - Gloves should extend and cover the cuffs of the gown.

To Remove PPE

Remove the respirator after leaving the resident's room and closing the door.

The outside surface of the gloves, face shield, goggles and front and sleeves of the gown, and the front surfaces of the mask are considered contaminated. If at any time your hand become contaminated while touching the outside of these surfaces, stop and perform hand hygiene before continuing.

- Remove Gloves: Use the steps shown below if you are right-handed. If you are left-handed, use the opposite hand.
  - Using your right hand, grasp the outside of the glove on the left hand at the inside of the wrist, turning the glove inside out as you pull it down over your left hand.
  - Hold the used left glove in a ball in your gloved right hand.
  - Grasp the inside of the right glove at the top of the wrist with your left hand.

- If you are wearing fitted, sterile gloves, you will not be able to grasp the inside of the top of the right glove, so you must cuff (fold over) the top of the right glove before you begin to remove the glove.
- Pull the right glove down over your right hand and over the used glove held in that hand. The right glove is now inside out, with the left glove enclosed in it.
- Place the gloves in the trash receptacle. Follow your facility's infection control policies to dispose of soiled waste.
- Remove Goggles or Face Shield:
  - Remove goggles or face shield from the back by lifting head band or ear pieces.
  - If the item is reusable, follow facility policy on cleaning. Otherwise, discard in a waste container.
- Remove Gown:
  - Untie the gown at your neck and waist.
  - Pull the gown away from the neck and shoulders, touching the inside of the gown only. The gown can also be removed by, grasping the cuff of one of the sleeves and pull the sleeve down over that hand.
  - Pull the other sleeve off with your covered hand.
  - Carefully roll up the gown, keeping the soiled surface inside, making sure not to touch the outside of the gown.
  - When removing a cloth gown that will be laundered, put it in the appropriate linen hamper. Place a disposable paper gown in the appropriate trash receptacle, following your facility's policy.
- Remove Mask or Respirator:
  - Remove the mask by untying the ties or pulling the straps over your ears or head. If a respirator is worn, pull the bottom strap over your head first, then pull the top strap on over your head.
  - Fold the outside edges of the mask together, keeping the soiled sides together. Dispose of the mask or respirator in the trash, following your facility's policy.
- Perform hand hygiene.

Linens

Used linens must be handled and transported in a way that prevents exposure to pathogens and prevents the spread of microorganisms. Linens that are soiled with blood, body fluids, secretions, or excretions must be handled in a way that prevents exposure of your skin and mucous membranes or contamination of your clothing. At a minimum, wear gloves. Always carry linens by holding them away from your uniform, even if not visibly soiled. If the linens are wet, you should also wear a gown (Figure 5-5).

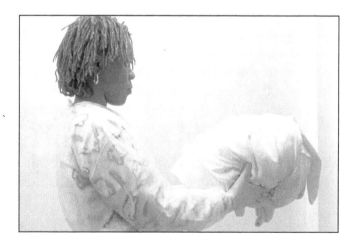

Figure 5-5 Wear gloves and a gown if linen is soiled or wet.

PUTTING ON A GOWN

1 Remove jewelry. Perform hand hygiene. Gently open the gown without shaking.

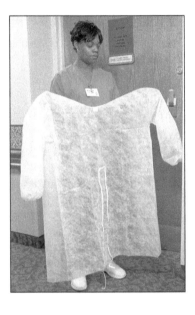

2 Insert your arms in the sleeves, with the opening in the back.

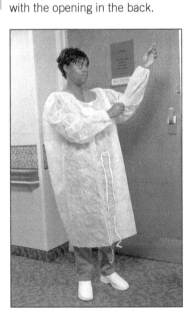

3 Tie the gown at your neck and waist. The gown should cover your uniform from your neck to knees.

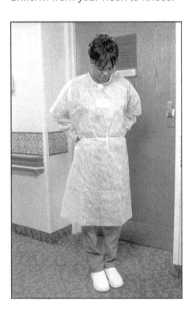

4 Put on your gloves and pull the gloves up over the gown's cuffs.

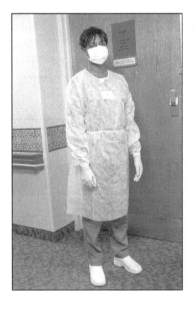

REMOVING A GOWN

1 Remove your gloves first and dispose of them properly.

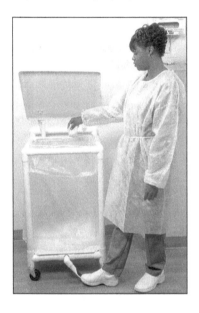

2 Untie the gown at your neck and waist.

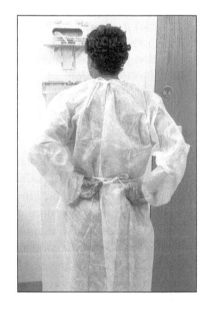

3 Grasp the cuff of one of the sleeves and pull the sleeve down over that hand. Gown can also be removed by pulling the gown away from the neck and shoulders, touching the inside of the gown only.

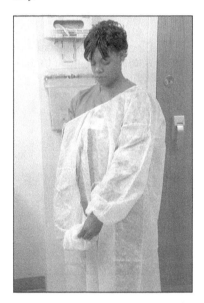

4 Pull the other sleeve off with your covered hand.

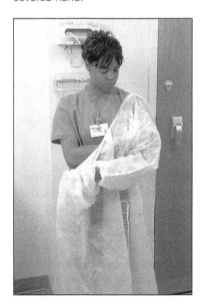

5 Carefully roll up the gown, keeping the soiled surface inside, making sure not to touch the outside of the gown

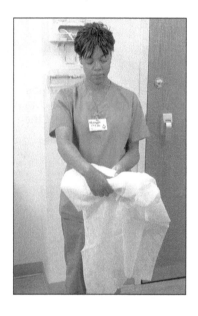

6 When removing a cloth gown that will be laundered, put it in the appropriate linen hamper. Place a disposable paper gown in the appropriate trash receptacle, following your facility's policy.

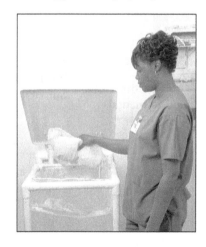

7 Perform hand hygiene by washing hands or using an alcohol-based hand rub.

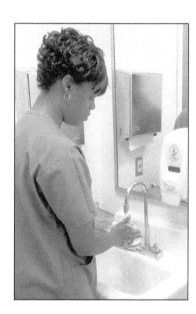

5-4: Putting on and Removing a Mask

PUTTING ON A MASK

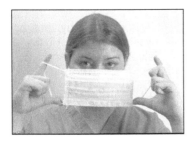
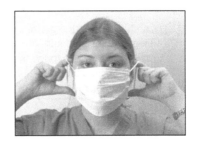
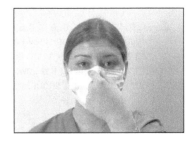

1 Put the mask over your nose and mouth.

2 Tie or secure the straps around your ears or the back of your head so that the mask fits tightly.

3 Pinch the metal piece on the bridge of the nose to make a tight seal.

REMOVING A MASK

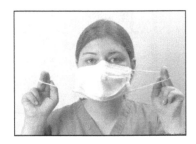
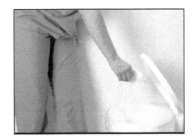
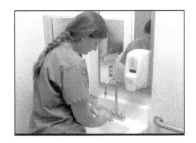

1 Remove the mask by untying the ties or pulling the straps over your ears or head.

2 Fold the outside edges of the mask together, keeping the soiled sides together. Dispose of the mask in the trash, following your facility's policy.

3 Perform hand hygiene by washing hands or using an alcohol-based hand rub.

Environmental Cleaning and Waste Management

You will need to learn your facility's procedures for the routine care, cleaning, and disinfecting of environmental surfaces, beds, bedrails, bedside equipment, and other frequently touched surfaces.

Wastes that Require Special Handling

A number of terms are used to designate wastes that require special handling. These include **biohazardous waste**, regulated waste, infectious or infective waste, and special waste. All states have regulations regarding the handling and disposal of waste material that is contaminated with blood or secretions and excretions. Waste regulations vary from state to state and from city to city. Your infection control practitioner will inform you about your facility's procedures for waste handling and disposal.

Equipment Used for Resident Care

Equipment used as part of daily resident care must be handled and transported in a way that prevents the spread of microorganisms. Equipment that has been soiled with blood, body fluids, secretions, or excretions must be handled so that contact with your skin and mucous membranes or contamination of your clothing does not occur. At a minimum, wear gloves and a gown. You must ensure that reusable equipment is not used for

- dedicate a set for vitals

the care of another resident until it has been properly cleaned and disinfected and that disposable (single-use) items are disposed of according to local and facility waste management guidelines.

If a resident frequently contaminates the environment or does not (or cannot) help maintain appropriate hygiene or environmental cleanliness, you should discuss this with the charge nurse. Alternate rooms or additional precautions may be needed.

Preventing Transmission of Bloodborne Pathogens

Needles and other sharp objects such as razors can spread infection if not handled or disposed of properly. An injury may occur when handling sharp instruments after procedures, when cleaning used instruments, or when disposing of used needles. The following guidelines will help protect you and your residents:

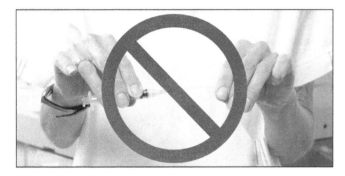

Figure 5-6 Never recap a needle.

- Never recap (put a cap back on) used needles (Figure 5-6).
- Use needles with attached safety devices.
- Place used disposable syringes and needles and other sharp items in designated puncture-resistant sharps containers (Figure 5-7).

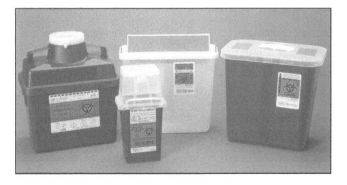

Figure 5-7 Discard needles and other sharps in a designated puncture-resistant container.

Breaking the Chain at the Reservoir Link

Some microorganisms, such as certain bacteria, are susceptible to the effects of antibiotics, which may be used as a treatment for these infections. This treatment reduces the number of microorganisms and the severity of the infection, allowing the person to get well so he or she is no longer a reservoir.

Proper food handling practices prevent food from becoming a reservoir for microorganisms. This includes using clean equipment for preparation, adequate refrigeration for storage, and proper hand hygiene, especially after using the bathroom, coughing, or sneezing. If food sanitation is not maintained, many people can become ill from eating contaminated food.

Breaking the Chain at the Mode of Transmission Link

Diseases such as gonorrhea, syphilis, and human immunodeficiency virus (HIV) are transmitted by direct contact during sexual activity. HIV can also be transmitted through direct contact with the blood of an infected person. There are no vaccines for these diseases. Using condoms during sex is one way to prevent the spread of sexually transmitted diseases.

The herpes simplex virus is also transmitted by direct contact. One strain of this virus causes fever blisters and cold sores, and a second type causes genital herpes. You must wear gloves when giving mouth care. A mouth care sponge with a handle can be used to avoid touching the affected area.

Airborne transmission can be reduced when the facility has appropriate ventilation and air exchange. Staff members also need to recognize when a resident's cough is a symptom of infection and to report this or other symptoms to the nurse. Recognizing and treating airborne diseases (such as measles and tuberculosis) at an early stage helps to prevent further transmission.

Breaking the Chain at the Susceptible Host Link

People develop immunity to some microorganisms after one infection, but many types of pathogens can cause repeated infections. Breaking the chain at the susceptible host link depends on the microorganisms and the individuals. If a vaccine is available, the best way to protect susceptible hosts is to vaccinate them. Immunization against certain diseases can keep you and residents from being susceptible hosts.

Annual flu shots should be given to residents and staff if not contraindicated. CMS currently recommends that all eligible residents be offered an influenza vaccine every year and a pneumococcal vaccine unless the vaccines are medically contraindicated, or the resident has already been immunized. Pneumococcal vaccines are recommended for adults 65 years of age and older, or younger populations with certain medical conditions. The best way to protect residents from becoming sick from microorganisms that are already in their bodies is to help them maintain their nutritional status and mobility. You can protect yourself from infectious diseases by keeping up with the recommended immunization schedule, staying as healthy as you can, and following established infection control procedures, especially in regard to frequent and thorough handwashing.

Table 5-2 provides an overview of the most common types of infections seen among residents of long term care facilities. To prevent the spread of these diseases, you must never let infection control activities become routine. Ask yourself these questions if you suspect an infection is present:

1. *Who or what may be infected?* The source of infection may be a resident, staff member, visitor, or something in the environment such as equipment in a resident's room or a food source.

2. *Who is at risk?* A resident may be more susceptible to infection due to advanced age or underlying disease. Risk is also increased by treatments with steroids or chemotherapeutic agents, breaks in the skin, and the use of invasive devices such as urinary catheters, intravenous catheters, and G-tubes.

3. *How can the microorganism be transmitted?* Microorganisms can be transmitted through all routes. The most common routes in a facility are direct and indirect contact, droplet, and airborne transmission.

4. *What do I need to do to protect residents and myself?* Use protective equipment, perform hand hygiene between residents and procedures, and change your gloves often. Change gloves between residents and whenever they are contaminated. Promote good nutrition and exercise. Encourage annual influenza and pneumococcal vaccinations.

Table 5-2   Most Common Infections in LTC Residents

Type of Infection	Description	Signs/Symptoms/Treatment	Vaccine Available
Urinary tract infection (UTI)	▪ Most common bacterial infection in older adults. More common in women than men ▪ Risk increases if a resident has diabetes or must use a catheter	▪ Pain or discomfort during urination ▪ New or sudden urinary incontinence ▪ Worsening confusion or dementia ▪ Treatment includes increased water intake and may require antibiotics.	No
Skin infection	▪ May be caused by bacteria, viruses, fungi, or pressure on the skin	▪ Itching or pain ▪ Lesions ▪ Various treatments depending on the cause ▪ Good hygiene is important	Vaccine available to prevent shingles caused by the varicella-zoster virus (same virus that causes chickenpox)
Bacterial pneumonia	▪ Bacterial infection in one or both lungs ▪ Air sacs in the lung become filled with fluid and other material	▪ Respiratory problems ▪ Weakness or confusion ▪ Fever, chills, cough ▪ Commonly treated with antibiotics	Some types can be prevented by the pneumococcal vaccine
Influenza (flu)	▪ Highly contagious viral infection of the respiratory passages ▪ Can lead to pneumonia	▪ Fever, chills, cough ▪ Muscular pain ▪ Weakness or confusion ▪ Antiviral medications may reduce symptoms	Some strains can be prevented by vaccines

Type of Infection	Description	Signs/Symptoms/Treatment	Vaccine Available
Gastrointestinal infection	▪ Infection of the stomach and/or GI tract ▪ Common causes are bacteria: ▪ *Helicobacter pylori* ▪ *Clostridium difficile* (often due to antibiotic treatment that kills off healthy gut flora)	▪ Nausea ▪ Abdominal pain ▪ Fever ▪ Diarrhea ▪ *H. pylori* treated with various drugs ▪ *C. difficile* treatment usually involves stopping the antibiotic	No

(Source: American Academy of Family Physicians)

Treatment-Resistant Microorganisms

Healthcare-associated infections (HAIs) are infections contracted while receiving care in some type of inpatient, outpatient, or residential facility. Multidrug-resistant organisms (MDROs) are among the most serious threats in any health care facility. MDROs cause infections that cannot be managed with usual forms of treatment, and these infections are very serious, especially in older adults and those with compromised immune function.

The most common threats to long term care residents include:

- *Clostridium difficile (C. diff)*: These bacteria cause diarrhea in patients after antibiotic use. It is classified by the Centers for Disease Control and Prevention (CDC) as a severe threat due to the number of people who are affected and the severity of the symptoms.
- Methicillin-resistant *Staphylococcus aureus* (MRSA): These bacteria cause a range of illnesses from skin and wound infections to pneumonia and potentially fatal blood infections that can cause sepsis.
- Vancomycin-resistant *Enterococcus* (VRE): These bacteria cause a range of illnesses, including surgical site infections and infections of the bloodstream and urinary tract.
- Extended spectrum beta-lactamases (ESBL): These bacteria most commonly cause an infection in the urinary tract, but can cause infections in wounds, surgical sites, body organs and in the bloodstream.

Infections caused by an MDRO are hard to treat and can be fatal. As a nurse assistant, you must make sure that you follow all isolation and infection control policies within your facility. The CDC issues guidelines for long term care facilities to prevent and control the spread of each type of (MDRO).

Isolation Precautions

Isolation precautions are actions that facilities take to keep microorganisms from spreading from one resident to others. Specific practices are usually described in the facility's infection control manual or isolation manual. You should be familiar with the isolation precautions used in your facility. The infection control practitioner will teach you how to implement the steps involved in isolation precautions. Talk to the charge nurse if you have any questions about your duties in regard to these precautions (Figure 5-8).

The CDC has specific recommendations for isolation precautions. In addition to the standard precautions previously described, the CDC recommends using transmission-based precautions for residents who are known (or suspected) to be infected with highly transmissible pathogens.

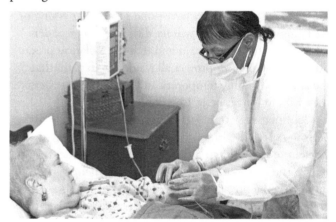

Figure 5-8 Use proper infection control procedures when caring for a resident with an infectious disease.

Transmission-Based Precautions

Three types of transmission-based precautions are used along with standard precautions: airborne, droplet, and contact precautions.

Airborne precautions are used in caring for residents who are known (or suspected) to be infected with microorganisms transmitted by airborne droplets, such as those associated with active tuberculosis. Airborne droplets remain suspended in the air and can be dispersed by air currents.

Droplet precautions are used in caring for residents who are known (or suspected) to be infected with microorganisms transmitted by droplets produced by coughing, sneezing, talking, or performing procedures. These precautions would be used if there was a flu outbreak among residents.

PPe + Mask + goggles

Contact precautions are used in caring for residents known (or suspected) to be infected with microorganisms that can be transmitted by direct or indirect contact. Transmission can occur when you perform care activities involving hand or skin contact. Microorganisms can also be spread through indirect contact, such as touching environmental surfaces or items in the resident's room that have been contaminated. These precautions are used when a resident has a draining wound or diarrhea.

- gown + gloves

Psychosocial Needs of Residents in Isolation

A resident in isolation will likely be confined to their room but in most cases can still have visitors and contact with staff. Residents who are not allowed to leave their rooms may feel that they have done something wrong or are being punished. You will need to help them understand how germs are spread and that the isolation precautions are designed to protect all residents. Explain that the situation is only temporary and when they are better, they will no longer be in isolation.

Confinement can be very disorienting for an elderly person, especially those with cognitive impairments. Explain to the resident and family why the resident must stay in the room and for how long. Help them understand that the precautions are in their best interest. Provide as much mental stimulation as possible by offering activities that the resident enjoys.

Cleaning, Disinfection, Sterilization, and Asepsis

To practice infection control, you must understand the concept of *clean* versus *dirty*. If something is considered clean, it remains clean until it is contaminated with something considered dirty. For example, if you wash your hands properly before preparing supplies for bathing a resident, your hands are considered clean. But if you answer a phone call, open the door for someone, or blow your nose, your hands are now considered dirty until you perform hand hygiene. The safest approach is to assume that everything is dirty and needs to be cleaned. This includes objects such as tables, trays, glasses and dishware, personal care items, and your hands. Keep the concept of clean versus dirty in mind at all times. This awareness will help decrease the spread of germs that could be harmful to you and to residents.

Cleaning

Cleaning is the removal of soil from objects. Water, detergent, and scrubbing are used to clean things. Cleaning helps control and prevent infection and keeps the environment pleasant and free of odors, dust, and dirt.

The facility's housekeepers regularly clean floors, carpets, walls, and large items. They also clean drapes, curtain dividers, and furniture as needed. When a resident is discharged, housekeepers should thoroughly clean the bed, chairs, over bed and bedside tables, and the entire room, so the environment is clean and ready for the next resident.

In some facilities, nurse assistants clean the resident's immediate environment during daily care activities. Be sure you know which staff member is responsible for cleaning furniture and smaller items in residents' rooms and understand your area of responsibility.

Disinfection

Disinfection is a process that kills or inhibits the growth of virtually all microorganisms on objects and surfaces using heat, special chemicals, or ultraviolet rays. Chemical disinfectants are sometimes combined with a detergent, and the solution is used to clean objects such as over bed tables, side rails, and plastic-covered mattresses. When you use a disinfectant, wear gloves to protect your hands from chemical burns or other damage. Every facility has **safety data sheets (SDS)** on file that contain information about the chemicals used in your facility. If your skin comes in contact with any disinfectant, consult the SDS for guidance on what action to take.

Sterilization

Sterilization is a process that completely eliminates all microorganisms from a surface or object. Many items used for resident care come in a sterile condition or are disposable. This includes gauze pads, surgical supplies, urinary catheters, needles, and bags of fluid used for intravenous (IV) therapy.

Asepsis

Asepsis refers to the absence of bacteria. There are two types of asepsis, medical and surgical. Medical asepsis reduces the number of microorganisms, also known as clean technique. The goal is to prevent the spread of infection. Using PPE and performing hand hygiene is an example of using medical aseptic practices. **Surgical asepsis** also known as sterile technique, is the process of eliminating all microorganisms. Surgical aseptic practices are used during sterile or surgical procedures.

Designated Clean and Dirty Areas

Most facilities have designated clean and dirty utility rooms or other areas. These are used to separate clean and dirty supplies, equipment, and operations. Clean utility rooms are used to store supplies such as bandages and tape, dressings, urinary catheters and tubing, bed pads, irrigation fluid, irrigation sets, feeding tubes and supplies, bedside kits (with wash basin, water pitcher, cup, and **emesis** basin), and other clean supplies.

All objects and supplies that have been used by a resident or caregiver are considered dirty. Some used supplies, such as soiled dressings or bed pads, are disposable. These may be discarded in an appropriate waste disposal container. Other supplies will be reused after being cleaned. Be sure to follow your facility's policy for cleaning reusable supplies.

Many dirty utility areas also have waste receptacles for the disposal of sharps containers and other regulated wastes. This may be called "red-bagged trash." Because regulations vary from state to state, you must know your facility's procedures for disposal of hazardous waste.

Providing Personal Care

Your role in preventing and controlling infection is very important. Now that you understand how microorganisms cause infection, you can apply this knowledge as you learn how to incorporate infection control practices into everyday care routines for your residents.

Personal care includes bathing, mouth care, grooming, and dressing. How much help you give a resident depends on each individual's needs. When you help residents with personal care, remember that you are assisting them with tasks they previously did on their own, in private, with no help. This includes their bathing and toileting routines and possibly incontinence care. Receiving your assistance may be difficult or embarrassing for some people. You must treat each resident with respect and dignity as you provide individualized care. Keep in mind that most people care how they look, and everyone has their own style and preferences. Helping residents keep up their grooming and appearance can help them feel better about themselves and improve their quality of life.

Residents' Personal Preferences

In long term care facilities, the term **routine care** is often used to refer to daily care activities. Keep in mind that the word "routine" does not mean that you do not pay attention to each resident or that all residents' needs are the same.

Before you assist with personal care, you need to take the time to learn each person's likes and dislikes. Residents have specific ideas about cleanliness, grooming, and dressing. Always base the care you give on each resident's personal preferences. If a resident cannot express their preferences, ask family and friends for their input. During all personal care activities, encourage the resident to participate as much as possible, and explain each step as you go.

Observation and Determination of Assistance Needs

In this chapter, you will learn how to perform the tasks involved in personal care but remember that your job involves much more than this. Before you take any action, you need to observe the resident and determine his or her capabilities related to each task. This requires that you analyze the situation to see how to best help the resident. By first determining the resident's needs, you will be better prepared and more organized. Residents also will find the experience more pleasant and will appreciate your attention.

Observation is very important when helping with personal care. Your job is to observe residents for any physical or psychological changes. Think of observation as a head-to-toe look at a resident that involves a quick check to see, hear, smell, and feel for any changes. Of all staff, you have the best opportunity to observe residents and monitor both their physical health and emotional status. Record and report any changes you observe.

Use of Gloves in Personal Care

As noted earlier in this chapter, infection prevention and control depend on implementing proper techniques as you provide personal care. You should always wear gloves when helping with tasks that involve a resident's body secretions or excretions. This includes assistance with toileting, incontinence care, oral hygiene, bathing, and caring for a resident with skin sores, a rash, or a wound. Wear gloves if you have an open sore, rash, or wound on your hands. Be sensitive to how residents may feel when you put on gloves and explain that gloves must be worn for certain tasks to protect both them and you from infection.

Common Preparation and Completion Steps

Much of your job involves preparation. Preparing in advance for all tasks reduces your workload by helping you get the job done efficiently. All nurse assistant skills involve preparation. Often you will use the same preparation steps every time you do the task. Because residents have different needs and preferences and because the environment changes, small variations are often necessary.

The exact steps of care may differ somewhat from task to task and even from moment to moment. Remember that tasks are not performed the same way for all residents at all times. Quality care involves adjusting tasks to meet the individual's needs. You must be flexible and adapt your care to each resident's preferences. Different equipment and settings may also require adjusting the preparation steps.

How you will complete procedures will be similar for most of your daily tasks. Completion steps let residents know that you are finished with a particular task and also ensure that residents are safe and comfortable. These steps also allow residents the opportunity to ask questions if they need to do so.

Become familiar with these preparation and completion steps. Use them daily with all tasks you perform. Note that in some cases, you will need to change the order of some steps because of a resident's specific needs.

Table 5-3 Common Preparations Steps

STEPS	RATIONALE	THEMES
Check the care plan.	▪ The care plan gives you information about the resident, including details about their capabilities or if any additional equipment is needed before entering the room.	Maximizing Capabilities
Knock, introduce yourself, and address resident by preferred name.	▪ Knocking respects the privacy rights of the resident. An introduction lets them know who is entering their room. Addressing the resident by their preferred name shows respect.	Communication, Autonomy, Respect
Perform hand hygiene.	▪ Hand hygiene prevents the transmission of infections.	Infection control
Gather supplies and secure assistance if needed.	▪ Give an explanation of what you are about to do and seek the resident's input so they are more comfortable and involved with their care. Make sure that safety needs are met throughout the care by locking the wheelchair, locking the bed wheels, adjusting the height of the bed, and using all equipment properly.	Autonomy, Safety, Time Management
Explain procedure and ask about resident preferences.	▪ Explaining the procedure gains the resident's cooperation and creates a more relaxed atmosphere. It helps the resident feel more involved and in charge of their care needs. Courtesy and politeness are important in your relationship with your resident.	Communication, Autonomy, and Respect
Respect privacy and rights at all times.	▪ Provide privacy by closing the door, pulling the curtain, and keeping the resident covered during care. Respect resident rights throughout the procedure.	Respect

Table 5-4 Common Completion Steps

STEPS	RATIONALE	THEMES
Determine the resident's preferred position for comfort and ask them if they need anything else.	▪ Making the resident comfortable is a part of your responsibilities.	Autonomy, Respect, and Communication
Examine the environment for safety and cleanliness.	▪ The bed should be in the lowest position. The wheelchair should be locked as appropriate and bed wheels should be in a locked position. It is your responsibility to make sure that you minimize any safety concerns. All equipment should be cleaned and stored according to facility policy. All dirty items should be removed from the room according to facility policy.	Safety and Infection Control
Secure the call light and any other needed items within reach of the resident.	▪ Residents must be able to reach you throughout your shift.	Safety
Perform hand hygiene.	▪ Hand hygiene helps prevent the spread of infection.	Infection control
Document the procedure and report any findings to the staff in charge.	▪ Detailed records help staff identify the resident's normal patterns. Documentation helps the charge nurse identify potential problems with a resident. Remember that often you are the first person to notice when something may be wrong.	Communication, Observation

Bathing

Bathing helps keep skin healthy and prevents skin problems. The three main purposes of bathing are to:

- Remove dirt, perspiration, and microorganisms from the skin
- Increase circulation to the skin
- Help the resident feel better and more comfortable

If a resident can leave the bed, help with a bath or shower. Facilities have schedules for residents who need help with bathing, based on their hygiene needs and comfort. Bathing too often may cause skin dryness, which can cause skin breakdown. Give partial baths between complete baths as needed. A partial bath involves washing only certain body parts. When giving a partial bath, you help residents wash their face, hands, and underarms, and also provide perineal care. Residents who cannot get out of bed need bed baths (Procedure 5-5).

Remember, bathing is a very personal activity, and residents may feel uncomfortable receiving assistance. Give them as much privacy as possible during bathing and encourage them to make their own choices about how to bathe. Procedure 5-6 outlines the steps for a tub bath, and Procedure 5-7 shows the steps for assisting with a shower. When bathing a resident, it is important to make

sure the water is not too hot. You can have the resident test the water prior to bathing, but you may have some residents that are unable to communicate or determine if the water is too hot. According to CMS, 100°F is a safe temperature for bathing.

Whirlpool Bath

A whirlpool bath is a special therapeutic bath that cleans, helps to relieve pain, and is used as treatment for a wound that needs daily cleaning or for poor circulation that needs stimulation. Whirlpool baths have jets that move the water in the tub. Some have a mechanical lift for use in getting residents into and out of the tub. Follow the facility's guidelines for using the whirlpool, including cleaning and infection control measures before and after use (Procedure 5-8).

Using a Resident's Personal Products

A resident or family member may want you to use certain bath or personal hygiene products for personal care. Honor their requests and become familiar with their preferred products such as shower gels, bath oils, or fragranced soaps. Most products come with directions for use. Check the directions and talk with the resident about how they like to use them.

PREPARATION STEPS

1. Check the care plan.
2. Knock, introduce yourself, and address resident by preferred name.
3. Perform hand hygiene.
4. Gather supplies and secure assistance if needed.
5. Explain procedure and ask about resident preferences.
6. Respect privacy and rights at all times.

ITEMS NEEDED

- 3 washcloths
- 2 towels
- bedpan
- basin half filled with warm water
- soap or preferred body wash
- gloves
- plastic trash bag or waste basket
- lotion
- plastic-covered pad or waterproof pad
- bath blanket
- resident's clothing

PREPARATION:

1 Before beginning the bath, remove the resident's blanket and bedspread and put them on a clean surface.

2 Place a bath blanket over the top sheet and pull down the top sheet to the foot of the bed, leaving the bath blanket covering the resident.

3 Remove the resident's clothing under the bath blanket to expose only the part of the body you are washing. This allows for privacy and prevents them from becoming cold. The best position for the resident is flat in bed, if they can tolerate it.

4 Fill the water basin halfway with water that is warm to the touch. Test the water with your bare hand. The water temperature should be 98.6°F to 100°F. Test the water temperature with the inside of your wrist. After you do this, have the resident feel the water to be sure it is comfortable.

MAKING A BATH MITT:

A bath mitt provides a soft surface for the person's skin and is easier to use than an unfolded washcloth. The edges of an unfolded washcloth may get cold and make the resident uncomfortable.

1 After wringing out the wet washcloth, put your hand in the center of the washcloth.

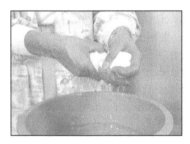

2 Fold the side of the washcloth over from your little finger, and hold the fold with your thumb.

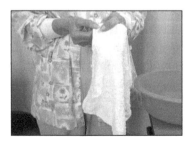

3 Fold the remaining cloth over and hold it firmly with your thumb.

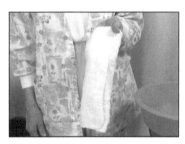

4 Fold the top edge of the cloth down and tuck it into your palm. Hold it with your thumb.

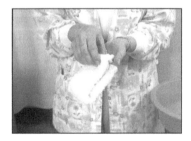

5 The mitt is now ready to use. Rinse the cloth and refold the mitt as needed during the bath.

GIVING A COMPLETE BED BATH:

1 Begin with the resident's eyes, using only water — no soap.

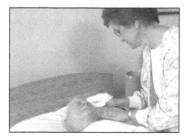

Start with the eye that is farther from you. With one corner of the washcloth, wash from the inner corner of the eye outward toward the ear. Clean away any crusting that may be stuck to the lower part of the eye. Use another corner of the washcloth to wash the eye that is closest to you. Be sure to move the washcloth from the inner corner of the eye outward.

2 Wash the resident's face.

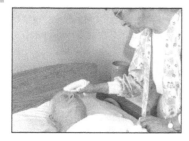

Some residents prefer not to use soap on the face. In this case, use water only or a facial cleanser that the resident prefers. To wash with soap, wet the washcloth and apply a small amount of soap. Wash the face and be sure to rinse off all the soap. When you dry the resident's skin, pat it dry, being careful not to rub too hard. Once dry, inspect the area.

3 Wash the resident's ears and neck. Be sure to wash behind the ear as well as inside (gently). Wring out the wash cloth so that excess water does not enter the ear canal. Rinse, dry, and inspect the area.

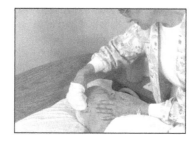

4 Wash the arms, underarms, and hands. Remember to expose only the areas to be washed and use a bath blanket to cover the rest of the body. Use soap sparingly because it dries the skin. Wash the side away from you first, then the side near you, so that you are moving from a clean area to a dirty area, unless you feel you have to stretch too far and might injure yourself. (If so, wash one side of the resident's body, then move to the other side and wash it.) Rinse, dry, and inspect the area.

5 Fold the bath blanket down and cover the resident's chest with a towel. Wash the chest and abdomen as far as the pubic area. Rinse, dry, and inspect the area. Pay particular attention to the skin under a female resident's breasts and or any skin folds on the chest and abdomen. These are common areas for skin irritation and breakdown. Note any redness, odor, or skin breakdown. Cover the chest with the bath blanket.

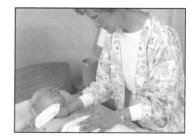

6 Expose one leg and foot. Cover the exposed leg with a towel. Wash the legs and feet. Don't forget to wash between the toes. Rinse, dry, and inspect the area. Check between the toes for any redness, irritation, or cracking of the skin. Note any swelling of the feet and legs.

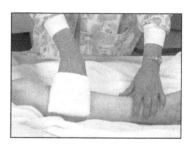

7 Change the water at this point or at any time during the bath if the water gets too cold, soapy, or dirty. (Using the same water after foot washing could potentially spread a foot fungus.) Cover the resident before leaving to change the water. Follow safety procedures when leaving the bedside.

8 Help the resident to turn to one side. Keep him or her covered with a bath blanket.

9 Expose the resident's back and buttocks. Wash the resident's back and buttocks. Rinse, dry, and inspect the area.

10 Give the resident a back rub. Rub a small amount of lotion into your palms. Rub hands together to warm the lotion. Starting at the lower back, massage with gentle motions, working your way up toward the shoulders then downward to the lower back. Give the back rub for at least three minutes. Back rubs are comforting and relaxing and stimulate circulation, helping to prevent skin breakdown.

11 Help the resident move back onto their back.

12 Before providing perineal care (washing the genital and anal areas), put on gloves and place a waterproof pad under the resident. Alternately, you can use a bedpan, which allows a good view of the perineal area because it raises the resident's pelvis and lets you use more water for washing and rinsing. Since the bedpan might be uncomfortable for a resident, ask first. Sometimes you can use a fracture pan or a folded towel under the buttocks to raise the pelvis.

REMEMBER THESE GUIDELINES:

- Always change the water before perineal care, when the water gets too cold, soapy, or dirty.
- Always change the washcloth and towel.
- Always wear gloves when giving perineal care.

PERINEAL CARE FOR FEMALES

1 Put on gloves.

2 Help the resident onto the bedpan or pad.

3 Drape the resident by folding back the bath blanket to expose only her legs and perineal area. Ask the resident to bend her knees.

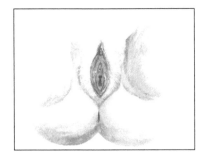

4 Have the resident check the water temperature to make sure that it is not too warm.

5 Apply soap to a wet washcloth.

6 Wash the perineal area using downward strokes from the front to the back on each side of the labia. Make sure to use a clean area of the washcloth with each stroke.

7 Wash downward in the middle over the urethra and vaginal opening. Always wash downward toward the anus with a clean area of the cloth to prevent the spread of infection.

8 Using a second clean washcloth, rinse the soap from the perineal area using the same technique. Wipe front to back using a clean area of the cloth with each stroke.

9 Dry the perineal area with a towel, and inspect for any redness, swelling, odor, drainage, or areas of irritation.

10 After washing the perineal area, turn the resident onto her side and wash and rinse the anal area, moving with upward strokes toward the back. Make sure to use a clean area of the cloth for each stroke.

11 Dry with a clean towel.

12 Reposition the resident for comfort and help her get dressed.

PERINEAL CARE FOR MALES

1 Put on gloves.

2 Drape the resident to expose only the legs and perineal area by folding back the bath blanket. Apply soap to a wet washcloth.

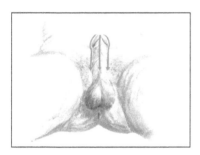

3 Wash the penis from the urethral opening or tip of the penis toward the base of the penis (use a clean area of the washcloth for each downward stroke), and then wash the scrotum. Take care to wash, rinse, and dry between any skin folds. Pull back the foreskin on uncircumcised males and clean under it. Return the foreskin. Check for any redness, swelling, or areas of irritation.

4 Help the resident turn onto his side. Wash, rinse, and dry the anal area, moving upward toward the back.

5 Reposition the resident for comfort and help him get dressed.

COMPLETION STEPS

1. Determine the resident's preferred position for comfort and ask them if they need anything else.

2. Examine the environment for safety and cleanliness.

3. Secure the call light and any other needed items within reach of the resident.

4. Perform hand hygiene.

5. Document the procedure and report any findings to the staff in charge.

Waterless Products

Products are available for bathing a resident without water. You may use individually packaged wet cloths or wipes to clean the body without having to rinse or dry the skin. These products can save time. Waterless products such as dry shampoos are also available for hair care.

Shampooing

Shampooing can be done in the bed, shower, tub, or sink. Washing the resident's hair once a week is usually enough to keep the hair and scalp clean. Some residents prefer to shampoo more often. Many facilities have a hair salon on the premises or may bring in a hair stylist or barber to give haircuts and style residents' hair. Often, you are the one who shampoos a resident's hair, especially those who cannot go to the hair salon. Procedure 5-9 outlines the steps for helping residents with shampooing and conditioning their hair.

Oral Hygiene

Mouth care helps prevent gum disease and tooth loss. Mouth care also improves a resident's appearance, appetite, sense of well-being, and ability to chew food properly. Mouth and gum problems can be contributing factors to many different diseases.

Brushing and Flossing

Help a resident brush at least twice a day and floss at least once a day (Procedure 5-10). Flossing stimulates the gums and removes particles of food from between the teeth that brushing cannot remove. Always encourage residents to do these tasks on their own if they can. During mouth care, inspect the gums for any paleness, discoloration, bleeding, sores, or irritation. Inspect the teeth for decay or looseness.

Dentures

Dentures (false teeth) are worn by people who have lost some or all of their natural teeth. A resident may have full dentures (both upper and lower) or partial plates that replace some teeth (Figure 5-9). Partial plates are usually held in place by an attachment to remaining teeth. Dentures and partial plates are expensive. Handle them carefully to prevent breaking them. Encourage residents to wear their dentures as often as possible to avoid gum

PREPARATION STEPS

1. Check the care plan.
2. Knock, introduce yourself, and address resident by preferred name.
3. Perform hand hygiene.
4. Gather supplies and secure assistance if needed.
5. Explain procedure and ask about resident preferences.
6. Respect privacy and rights at all times.

ITEMS NEEDED

- gloves
- 2 washcloths
- 3 towels
- bath mat
- soap, lotion, shampoo, etc.
- resident's clothing of choice
- bath blanket

1 Assist the resident to the tub room and bring all necessary supplies. Some facilities may use chairs on wheels to transport residents to the tub room. Make sure that the resident is properly dressed and draped to protect their privacy. Use the safety straps if needed and available.

2 Help the resident sit on the chair. Fill the tub halfway with warm water.

3 Remember, always turn off the hot water first. The water temperature should be 98.6°F to 100°F. You can use a thermometer if one is available, or test the water temperature with the inside of your wrist. After you do this, have the resident feel the water to be sure it is comfortable. The resident's physician may order special additives to the bath water, such as bran, oatmeal, starch, sodium bicarbonate, Epsom salts, pine products, sulfa, potassium permanganate, or salt. Always check with the charge nurse about the proper use of any of these substances.

4 Help the resident remove his or her clothing.

5 Check that the bath mat is in place. Help the resident into the tub.

6 Help with bathing as needed. (Put on gloves if you will be assisting with perineal care.) Provide washcloth to cleanse body area; the second washcloth will be used to clean perineal area. Never leave the resident alone in a tub. Always encourage residents to use safety rails. Be sure to check the water temperature during the tub bath to be sure it has not become too cold. Add hot water as needed, not allowing water to run directly on the resident to prevent burns.

7 Place a clean towel on the seat of the chair.

8 Help the resident out of the tub, encouraging the use of safety rails. Cover the resident with a bath blanket.

9 Help the resident with drying, applying personal hygiene products, and dressing.

10 You may give a back rub before dressing, if the resident desires. Remove gloves and perform hand hygiene.

11 Help the resident back to their room. Bring any personal hygiene products back to the room.

COMPLETION STEPS

1. Determine the resident's preferred position for comfort and ask them if they need anything else.
2. Examine the environment for safety and cleanliness.
3. Secure the call light and any other needed items within reach of the resident.
4. Perform hand hygiene.
5. Document the procedure and report any findings to the staff in charge.

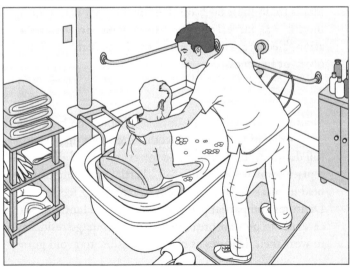

PREPARATION STEPS

1. Check the care plan.
2. Knock, introduce yourself, and address resident by preferred name.
3. Perform hand hygiene.
4. Gather supplies and secure assistance if needed.
5. Explain procedure and ask about resident preferences.
6. Respect privacy and rights at all times.

ITEMS NEEDED

- gloves
- 2 washcloths
- 3 towels (4 if shampooing)
- shower cap (if needed)
- shower chair
- shower mat
- soap, lotion, shampoo, etc.
- bath blanket
- resident's clothing of choice

1. Help the resident to the shower room and bring all necessary supplies.

2. Help the resident sit on the chair.

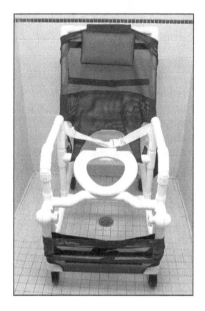

3. Turn on the shower and run with warm water. The water temperature should be 98.6°F to 100°F. You can use a thermometer if one is available, or test the water temperature with the inside of your wrist. After you do this, have the resident feel the water to be sure it is comfortable. Adjust the temperature as needed.

4. Help the resident remove his or her clothing.

5. Help the resident into the shower. Encourage the use of safety rails. Most facilities have shower chairs that lock in place. If the resident needs to shower in a seated position, be sure the shower chair is locked before they sit down.

6. If the resident is not shampooing, use a shower cap to protect hair from getting wet.

7. Help the resident with showering as needed. (Wear gloves if you help with perineal care.) Encourage the resident to participate as much as possible. Give help and verbal cues as needed. Wash from head to toe. Rinse the washcloth as needed. Provide clean washcloth to cleanse perineal area.

8. Place a dry towel on the chair outside the shower.

9. Turn off the shower. Turn off the hot water first to prevent a burn.

10. Help the resident out of the shower and onto the covered chair. Cover the resident with a bath blanket.

11. Help the resident dry off, use personal hygiene products, and get dressed.

12. You may give a back rub before dressing, if the resident desires.

13. Help the resident back to their room. Bring any personal hygiene products back to the room, as well.

COMPLETION STEPS

1. Determine the resident's preferred position for comfort and ask them if they need anything else.
2. Examine the environment for safety and cleanliness.
3. Secure the call light and any other needed items within reach of the resident.
4. Perform hand hygiene.
5. Document the procedure and report any findings to the staff in charge.

PREPARATION STEPS

1. Check the care plan.
2. Knock, introduce yourself, and address resident by preferred name.
3. Perform hand hygiene.
4. Gather supplies and secure assistance if needed.
5. Explain procedure and ask about resident preferences.
6. Respect privacy and rights at all times.

ITEMS NEEDED

- gloves
- 2 washcloths
- 3 towels
- bath blanket
- personal hygiene products
- resident's clothing

If the resident has a wound dressing, ask the nurse to remove it before the bath and apply a clean one afterward.

1. Help the resident to the whirlpool room and bring all necessary supplies.

2. Help the resident sit on a chair.

3. Turn on the water in the whirlpool following the facility's procedure. The water temperature should be 98.6°F to 100°F. You can use a thermometer if one is available, or test the water temperature with the inside of your wrist. After you do this, have the resident feel the water to be sure it is comfortable. Adjust the temperature as needed.

4. Help the resident remove their clothing.

5. Help the resident into the whirlpool bath. Encourage the use of safety rails. Follow the manufacturer and facility guidelines for use of the whirlpool. Before using a mechanical lift, be sure you know how to use it properly. If the physician has ordered an antiseptic solution in the whirlpool bath, the nurse will add the solution or give you specific instructions.

6. Help the resident bathe, and encourage the resident to participate as much as possible. Give help and verbal cues as needed. Wash from head to toe. Rinse the washcloth as needed. Provide clean washcloth for perineal area. Wear gloves if you help with perineal care. Never leave the resident unattended.

7. Place a dry towel on the chair.

8. Help the resident out of the whirlpool bath and onto the covered chair. Encourage the use of safety rails. Cover them with a bath blanket.

9. Help the resident dry off, apply personal hygiene products, and get dressed.

10. You may give a back rub before dressing, if the resident desires. Perform hand hygiene.

11. Help the resident back to their room. Bring any personal hygiene products back to the room, as well.

COMPLETION STEPS

1. Determine the resident's preferred position for comfort and ask them if they need anything else.
2. Examine the environment for safety and cleanliness.
3. Secure the call light and any other needed items within reach of the resident.
4. Perform hand hygiene.
5. Document the procedure and report any findings to the staff in charge.

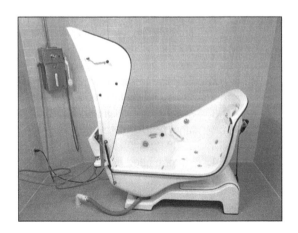

5-9: Shampoo and Conditioning

PREPARATION STEPS

1. Check the care plan.
2. Knock, introduce yourself, and address resident by preferred name.
3. Perform hand hygiene.
4. Gather supplies and secure assistance if needed.
5. Explain procedure and ask about resident preferences.
6. Respect privacy and rights at all times.

ITEMS NEEDED

- comb or brush
- shampoo
- conditioner (if used)
- washcloth
- 1 to 3 towels
- shampoo trough or basin (if needed)
- waterproof bed protector (if needed)

1 Help the resident into a chair.

2 Comb or brush out any tangles before shampooing.

3 Turn on the water to a warm temperature. The water temperature should be 98.6°F to 100°F. You can use a thermometer if one is available, or test the water temperature with the inside of your wrist. After you do this, have the resident feel the water to be sure it is comfortable.

4 Help the resident take off their clothes for showering or tub bathing. Wash the resident's hair first or last, as the resident prefers.

5 If a resident is shampooing at the sink, put the back of the chair against the front of the sink. Pad the rim of the sink with a towel. Position the resident for the method you are using: upright in a shower chair, flat in bed with pillows placed under the shoulders, or tilted in shampoo chair. Protect the resident's clothes with a towel draped over the shoulders. If you are shampooing in bed, you need a shampoo trough, basin, or pail, and a waterproof bed protector.

6 Place a washcloth over the resident's eyes to prevent shampoo or water from getting into the eyes.

7 Wet the hair entirely. Pour a small amount of shampoo into your palm and apply it to the resident's wet hair. Massage the shampoo gently throughout hair and scalp. Some residents use special shampoos or conditioners, which may be prescribed to treat a specific condition. Ask the nurse for instructions and read the labels carefully before using these products.

8 Rinse the hair well with warm water.

9 Apply conditioner, if used.

10 Rinse the hair well with warm water.

11 Help the resident out of the shower or tub into the chair and cover with a bath blanket. Wrap a towel around the hair.

12 Help the resident dry off and get dressed.

13 If the resident is in bed, help them wipe their face with the cloth used to protect their eyes. Remove the trough or basin and remove the waterproof pad. Change the linen as necessary. Position the resident with the head of the bed up.

14 Dry the hair thoroughly and quickly to prevent chilling. Use a hair dryer on a low setting.

15 Style the resident's hair as they prefer. Check the scalp for any flaking, reddened areas, or other problems. Perform hand hygiene.

16 Help the resident back to their room. Bring any personal hygiene products back to the room, as well.

COMPLETION STEPS

1. Determine the resident's preferred position for comfort and ask them if they need anything else.
2. Examine the environment for safety and cleanliness.
3. Secure the call light and any other needed items within reach of the resident.
4. Perform hand hygiene.
5. Document the procedure and report any findings to the staff in charge.

PREPARATION STEPS

1. Check the care plan.
2. Knock, introduce yourself, and address resident by preferred name.
3. Perform hand hygiene.
4. Gather supplies and secure assistance if needed.
5. Explain procedure and ask about resident preferences.
6. Respect privacy and rights at all times.

ITEMS NEEDED

- 1 or 2 towels
- soft-bristle toothbrush
- toothpaste
- paper cup half filled with cool water
- mouthwash
- dental floss
- emesis basin
- gloves and other PPE as needed

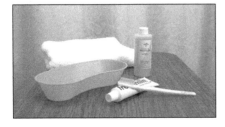

You can help residents with brushing and flossing at the bedside table or the resident's sink, as they prefer. Maintain clean technique with placement of the toothbrush throughout the procedure.

1. Wet the toothbrush, apply a small amount of toothpaste, and set it aside. Mix water and mouthwash in a cup. A solution of half water, half mouthwash is best. (Mouthwash is strong and can harm sensitive gums.) Set this aside.

2. Break off at least 18 inches of floss. Set this aside.

3. Put on gloves. If you know that the resident's gums bleed, talk with the charge nurse about other personal protective equipment you may need, such as protective goggles and a face mask.

4. Put a towel over the resident's chest to protect clothing.

5. Give the resident a small amount of mouthwash solution to swish around to rinse the mouth. Place the emesis basin under the resident's chin so they can spit out the solution after use.

6. Brush the resident's upper teeth and gums first, moving the brush in a downward direction from the gums to the teeth. Then brush the lower teeth and gums, moving upward from the gums to the teeth. Be sure to brush the back of the teeth. Inspect the teeth and gums while brushing.

7. Brush the tongue gently.

8. Help the resident rinse with a small amount of the mouthwash solution.

9. Wrap the ends of the floss around the middle fingers of each of your hands to get a good grip. Gently insert the floss between each tooth and the next. Move the floss to the gum line and down between the teeth. Wrap the floss around your fingertips so you use a clean section of floss as you move from tooth to tooth.

10. Have the resident rinse their mouth thoroughly.

11. Dry off any solution or water around the resident's mouth or chin.

12. Clean and store equipment.

13. Remove gloves and perform hand hygiene.

COMPLETION STEPS

1. Determine the resident's preferred position for comfort and ask them if they need anything else.
2. Examine the environment for safety and cleanliness.
3. Secure the call light and any other needed items within reach of the resident.
4. Perform hand hygiene.
5. Document the procedure and report any findings to the staff in charge.

shrinkage, help them chew food, and to improve their speech and appearance. Dentures should be cleaned at least twice daily (Procedure 5-11). When providing denture care, use toothpaste specifically for dentures, regular toothpaste can damage the dentures. When dentures are removed, always store them in a denture cup in cool water or a denture cleansing solution if the resident prefers.

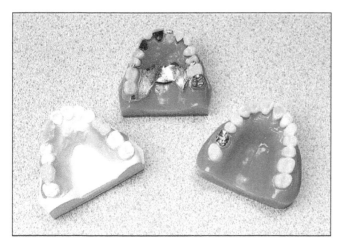

Figure 5-9 Some residents may have partial dentures while others have full dentures.

Mouth Care for Unconscious Residents

You may care for residents who are unconscious. These residents are not aware of their surroundings and cannot respond. Unconscious residents need mouth care every two hours (Procedure 5-12). Because they often breathe through their mouth, the mouth and lips become dry. When performing mouth care for an unconscious resident it is important to position the resident properly to prevent the resident from aspirating. The resident should be positioned so any liquid drains out of their mouth instead of draining to the back of their throat. Aspiration occurs when fluid or foreign material is inhaled into the lungs.

A soft toothbrush can be used to remove plaque if available. Always follow facility policies and procedures for providing mouth care to unconscious residents.

Grooming

Grooming care includes shaving (the face, legs, and/or underarms), trimming facial hair, hair care, and care of fingernails and foot care.

Shaving

Shaving the face is a daily activity for many male residents (Procedure 5-13 and 5-14). Some female residents may want their underarms and legs shaved during a shower or bath (Procedures 5-15 and 5-16). It is important to ask your resident about their shaving preferences. Certain cultures have specific days or time periods when shaving is not permitted.

Residents can use an electric razor or a safety razor (Figure 5-10). Never share the same razor among different residents or recap disposable razors.

Discard disposable razors in a sharps container. Always check with the charge nurse before shaving a resident to learn if there are any special medical considerations. For example, residents who are taking blood-thinning medications must use electric razors because their medication could cause too much bleeding if an accidental cut occurs. Follow facility policy and all safety measures when using an electric razor, including additional measures for when a resident is receiving oxygen therapy.

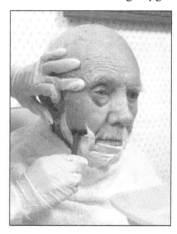

Figure 5-10 Shaving is a daily activity for many male residents.

Facial and Other Hair

Some female residents have a small amount of facial hair. This is common on the chin, the upper lip, and under the lower lip. Never trim or shave this facial hair unless the resident requests it. Always check with the charge nurse before trimming facial hair (Procedure 5-17). Some residents or family members may request hair removal using a cream hair remover (depilatory). These products contain strong chemicals, so follow the manufacturer's directions for storage and use. A physician's order may be required.

Some male residents may have excess hair in the nose or ears that they would like to have trimmed. Use very small safety scissors or a nose hair clipper for this task.

PREPARATION STEPS

1. Check the care plan.
2. Knock, introduce yourself, and address resident by preferred name.
3. Perform hand hygiene.
4. Gather supplies and secure assistance if needed.
5. Explain procedure and ask about resident preferences.
6. Respect privacy and rights at all times.

ITEMS NEEDED

- denture cup (or paper cup half filled with cool water)
- mouthwash
- swab moistened with water and mouthwash
- 1 or 2 pairs of gloves
- 1 or 2 towels
- denture cleaning paste or solution
- denture adhesive (if used)
- paper towels
- emesis basin

If the resident has a partial plate with only a few artificial teeth, handle it using the steps shown below for complete set of dentures. Be careful when you remove the partial plate, which has wires that support the teeth in place. Maintain clean technique with placement of the toothbrush throughout the procedure.

1. Put on gloves. Place a towel over the resident's chest.

2. Ask the resident to remove their dentures and place them in the denture cup. If the resident cannot remove their own dentures, remove them using the following steps.

a. Rinse the resident's mouth with mouthwash solution to moisten it. Ask them to swish the solution around, and put the emesis basin under the chin so the resident can spit out the solution.

b. Remove the upper denture using a paper towel for a better grip. Loosen the denture by gently rocking it back and forth to help break the seal. Put it in the denture cup.

c. Remove lower denture using a paper towel for a better grip. Loosen it by gently rocking it back and forth. Put it in the denture cup.

3. Rinse the resident's mouth with mouthwash solution.

4. If the resident cannot rinse, use a swab moistened with water and mouthwash to clean the entire mouth, including the tongue and gums.

5. Explain that you will clean the dentures and then return them.

6. Take the denture cup with dentures, toothbrush, and toothpaste to the resident's bathroom.

7. Put cleaning paste on the toothbrush. Make sure paste used is one made specifically for dentures.

8. Turn on cool water (hot water can damage dentures), put a small towel or face cloth on the bottom of the sink, and fill the sink halfway. (This helps prevent dentures from breaking if they slip from your hands.)

9. Hold the dentures over the sink and brush all surfaces.

10. Rinse the dentures with cool water.

11. Rinse the denture cup and lid. Return the dentures to the denture cup.

12. If the resident uses denture adhesive, apply it to the dentures before putting them back in the mouth. If the resident does not want the dentures put back at this time, store them safely. Put them in a denture cup half filled with cool water and labeled with the resident's name.

13. Inspect the resident's mouth for dryness, bleeding, sores, a dry coated tongue, or mouth odor. Report any changes to the nurse.

14. Clean and store equipment.

15. Remove gloves and perform hand hygiene.

COMPLETION STEPS

1. Determine the resident's preferred position for comfort and ask them if they need anything else.
2. Examine the environment for safety and cleanliness.
3. Secure the call light and any other needed items within reach of the resident.
4. Perform hand hygiene.
5. Document the procedure and report any findings to the staff in charge.

PREPARATION STEPS

1. Check the care plan.
2. Knock, introduce yourself, and address resident by preferred name.
3. Perform hand hygiene.
4. Gather supplies and secure assistance if needed.
5. Explain procedure and ask about resident preferences.
6. Respect privacy and rights at all times.

ITEMS NEEDED

- 1 or 2 towels
- gloves
- oral swabs or soft toothbrush
- cup with mouthwash
- protective jelly or lip balm
- plastic trash bag

1. Gently turn the resident's head toward you and elevate the head of the bed (if they can tolerate it) to prevent aspiration.

2. Put a towel over the resident's chest to protect clothing.

3. Put on gloves.

4. Gently open the resident's mouth and inspect the mouth, teeth, gums, and tongue for changes or signs of injury: bleeding, sores, loose or broken teeth, dry coated tongue, or mouth odor.

5. Using an oral swab dipped in mouthwash or soft toothbrush, clean the inside of the mouth (gums, tongue, teeth, roof of the mouth, and insides of the cheeks). Tap off excess mouthwash. Excess fluid can drip back into the throat and potentially cause aspiration (inhaling fluid or foreign material into the lungs).

6. Use a towel to dry any solution from around the mouth and chin.

7. Dispose of used swabs by placing into the plastic trash bag.

8. Apply protective jelly or lip balm on the resident's lips to moisten them.

COMPLETION STEPS

1. Determine the resident's preferred position for comfort and ask them if they need anything else.
2. Examine the environment for safety and cleanliness.
3. Secure the call light and any other needed items within reach of the resident.
4. Perform hand hygiene.
5. Document the procedure and report any findings to the staff in charge.

Hair Care

Hair care includes regular shampooing and conditioning plus daily brushing, combing, and styling. Daily brushing or combing, along with good nutrition and adequate fluid intake, promotes healthy hair and scalp (Procedure 5-18). Hairstyle is a personal matter. Many facilities offer hair salon services. Make sure to offer these services to your residents. Sometimes preferences in hair care and style are influenced by a resident's ethnic or cultural background. Listen to residents' preferences and honor their requests. Ask the resident or a family member about their hair care preferences and hairstyles. Encourage residents to brush and comb their own hair when they are able.

Care of Fingernails

Fingernail care includes daily cleaning and regular nail trimming (Figure 5-11). Although the visible part of the nail is not living tissue, the skin around and under it is, and you must protect this area from injury and infection.

Trimmed, smooth nails prevent a resident from accidentally scratching and injuring their skin. If residents cannot clean and trim their own fingernails, you can assist with this process (Procedure 5-19).

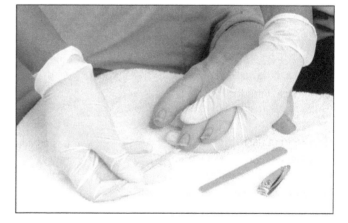

Figure 5-11 Fingernail care involves daily cleaning and regular nail trimming.

5-13: Shaving a Male Resident's Face Using an Electric Razor

PREPARATION STEPS

1. Check the care plan.
2. Knock, introduce yourself, and address resident by preferred name.
3. Perform hand hygiene.
4. Gather supplies and secure assistance if needed.
5. Explain procedure and ask about resident preferences.
6. Respect privacy and rights at all times.

ITEMS NEEDED

- gloves
- razor
- aftershave liquid or lotion (if used)
- basin half filled with warm water
- towel
- washcloth
- mirror
- plastic trash bag

1. Observe the resident's face for any moles, rashes, or cuts. Do not shave those areas, or use extra care if you do.

2. Place a towel over the resident's chest to protect his clothing.

3. Put on gloves.

4. Pull the skin taut and begin shaving the resident's face and neck. Shave using circular motions when using a rotary razor. For foil razors, use a back and forth motion in the direction the beard grows.

5. Rinse the resident's face with the washcloth, dry his face, and apply aftershave liquid or lotion, if he prefers.

6. Remove the towel from the resident's chest. Remove gloves and perform hand hygiene.

7. Give the resident a mirror to view his face to make sure he is satisfied with his appearance.

8. Clean the razor according to the manufacturer's guidelines.

COMPLETION STEPS

1. Determine the resident's preferred position for comfort and ask them if they need anything else.
2. Examine the environment for safety and cleanliness.
3. Secure the call light and any other needed items within reach of the resident.
4. Perform hand hygiene.
5. Document the procedure and report any findings to the staff in charge.

5-14: Shaving a Male Resident's Face

PREPARATION STEPS

1. Check the care plan.
2. Knock, introduce yourself, and address resident by preferred name.
3. Perform hand hygiene.
4. Gather supplies and secure assistance if needed.
5. Explain procedure and ask about resident preferences.
6. Respect privacy and rights at all times.

ITEMS NEEDED

- gloves
- razor
- soap or shaving cream
- basin half filled with warm water
- towel
- washcloth
- plastic trash bag

1. Observe the resident's face for any moles, rashes, or cuts. Do not shave those areas, or use extra care if you do.

2. Place a towel over the resident's chest to protect his clothing.

3. Put on gloves.

4. Using a washcloth, wet the beard with warm water. Apply shaving cream with your hands.

5-14: Shaving a Male Resident's Face (continued)

5 When the beard is covered with shaving cream and softened, begin shaving. Shave in the direction the beard grows. Hold the skin taut and smooth by pulling the skin upward with one hand and shaving with a downward stroke with your other hand. Use short, even strokes. Be particularly careful with the neck, chin, and upper lip. Use upward strokes for the neck, downward and slightly diagonal strokes for the chin, and very short downward strokes above the lip.

6 Rinse the razor in warm water after each stroke.

7 Rinse the resident's face with the washcloth, dry his face, and apply aftershave liquid or lotion, if he prefers.

8 Remove the towel from the resident's chest. Remove gloves and perform hand hygiene.

9 Give the resident a mirror to view his face to make sure he is satisfied with his appearance.

COMPLETION STEPS

1. Determine the resident's preferred position for comfort and ask them if they need anything else.
2. Examine the environment for safety and cleanliness.
3. Secure the call light and any other needed items within reach of the resident.
4. Perform hand hygiene.
5. Document the procedure and report any findings to the staff in charge.

5-15: Shaving a Female Resident's Underarms

PREPARATION STEPS

1. Check the care plan.
2. Knock, introduce yourself, and address resident by preferred name.
3. Perform hand hygiene.
4. Gather supplies and secure assistance if needed.
5. Explain procedure and ask about resident preferences.
6. Respect privacy and rights at all times.

ITEMS NEEDED

- gloves
- razor
- soap or shaving cream
- basin half filled with warm water
- towel
- washcloth

1 Put on gloves. Put the towel under the resident's shoulder on the side on which you are working.

2 Raise the resident's arm to expose the underarm.

3 Wash the area with warm water.

4 Lather some soap and apply it over the area to be shaved or apply shaving cream.

5 Carefully shave the area, using downward strokes.

6 Rinse the underarm area thoroughly and pat dry.

7 Move the towel to under the opposite shoulder and repeat the steps above.

8 Clean or discard equipment according to facility policy.

9 Remove gloves and perform hand hygiene.

COMPLETION STEPS

1. Determine the resident's preferred position for comfort and ask them if they need anything else.
2. Examine the environment for safety and cleanliness.
3. Secure the call light and any other needed items within reach of the resident.
4. Perform hand hygiene.
5. Document the procedure and report any findings to the staff in charge.

5-16: Shaving a Female Resident's Legs

PREPARATION STEPS

1. Check the care plan.
2. Knock, introduce yourself, and address resident by preferred name.
3. Perform hand hygiene.
4. Gather supplies and secure assistance if needed.
5. Explain procedure and ask about resident preferences.
6. Respect privacy and rights at all times.

ITEMS NEEDED

- gloves
- razor
- soap or shaving cream
- basin half filled with warm water
- towel
- washcloth
- plastic trash bag

1. Put on gloves. Place a towel under the resident's leg to be shaved.

2. Wash the part of the leg to be shaved with warm water.

3. Lather some soap or use shaving cream. Spread it over the entire area to be shaved.

4. Carefully shave the leg, using upward strokes from the ankle to the knee. Be especially careful around the bony kneecap. Ask the resident if she wants the thigh area shaved. If so, shave the thigh using upward strokes from the knee to the upper thigh.

5. Be sure to rinse the leg thoroughly and pat dry.

6. Move the towel under the other leg and repeat the steps above.

7. Clean or discard equipment according to facility policy.

8. Remove gloves and perform hand hygiene.

COMPLETION STEPS

1. Determine the resident's preferred position for comfort and ask them if they need anything else.
2. Examine the environment for safety and cleanliness.
3. Secure the call light and any other needed items within reach of the resident.
4. Perform hand hygiene.
5. Document the procedure and report any findings to the staff in charge.

5-17: Trimming Facial Hair

PREPARATION STEPS

1. Check the care plan.
2. Knock, introduce yourself, and address resident by preferred name.
3. Perform hand hygiene.
4. Gather supplies and secure assistance if needed.
5. Explain procedure and ask about resident preferences.
6. Respect privacy and rights at all times.

ITEMS NEEDED

- gloves
- safety scissors
- towel

1. Put on gloves and place a towel over the resident's chest. Using safety scissors, carefully trim the facial hair. Be careful not to nick the skin.

2. Remove the towel from the resident's chest. Remove gloves and perform hand hygiene.

3. Give the resident a mirror to view her face to make sure she is satisfied with her appearance.

COMPLETION STEPS

1. Determine the resident's preferred position for comfort and ask them if they need anything else.
2. Examine the environment for safety and cleanliness.
3. Secure the call light and any other needed items within reach of the resident.
4. Perform hand hygiene.
5. Document the procedure and report any findings to the staff in charge.

PREPARATION STEPS

1. Check the care plan.
2. Knock, introduce yourself, and address resident by preferred name.
3. Perform hand hygiene.
4. Gather supplies and secure assistance if needed.
5. Explain procedure and ask about resident preferences.
6. Respect privacy and rights at all times.

ITEMS NEEDED

- resident's brush and/or comb
- mirror
- personal items for styling such as clips, barrettes, or ponytail holders
- styling products such as gel, mousse, or hairspray

1. Brush hair gently. If the resident's hair is long and tangled, gently remove tangles with a wide-tooth comb before brushing. Start at the ends and work your way up to the scalp.

2. Gently brush and style the hair to the resident's preference. Use any personal items they may request, such as hair clips or styling products.

3. Give the resident a mirror so they can view their hair and confirm that they are satisfied with their appearance.

COMPLETION STEPS

1. Determine the resident's preferred position for comfort and ask them if they need anything else.
2. Examine the environment for safety and cleanliness.
3. Secure the call light and any other needed items within reach of the resident.
4. Perform hand hygiene.
5. Document the procedure and report any findings to the staff in charge.

Foot Care

Foot care is important because older residents are more prone to infection if skin breakdown occurs due to poor circulation in the feet (Figure 5-12). Toenails are thicker than fingernails, especially in older adults. A podiatrist, nurse, or physician usually trims toenails. Follow your facility's policy on trimming toenails.

When you assist with bathing or dressing, inspect residents' feet and between the toes to determine the skin condition. Look for corns, calluses, or other problems. Report any signs of poor circulation (very cold feet, swollen feet, or pale color of the toenail bed), reddened areas, skin breakdown, or cracking of the skin between the toes (Procedure 5-20).

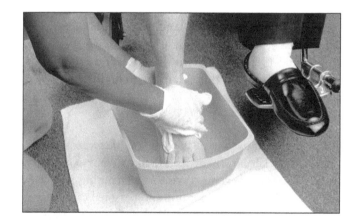

Figure 5-12 Foot care is an important part of a resident's personal care routine to ensure health and comfort.

5-19: Care of Fingernails

PREPARATION STEPS

1. Check the care plan.
2. Knock, introduce yourself, and address resident by preferred name.
3. Perform hand hygiene.
4. Gather supplies and secure assistance if needed.
5. Explain procedure and ask about resident preferences.
6. Respect privacy and rights at all times.

ITEMS NEEDED

- gloves (if needed)
- basin half filled with warm water
- 2 towels
- washcloth
- soap
- lotion
- orange wood stick
- nail clippers
- nail file or emery board

If resident is a diabetic, check with the nurse to see if nail care is to be performed by a licensed staff.

1. Place the basin of warm water on the over-bed table. Have resident check water temperature.

2. Ask the resident to soak their nails in the basin for 3 to 5 minutes.

3. Put on gloves. Leaving one hand in the water, wash and rinse the resident's other hand. Dry the hand and place it on a dry towel.

4. Clean under the nails using the orange wood stick.

5. Repeat steps 3 and 4 for the other hand.

6. Inspect the resident's hands for cracks in the skin, unusual spots or discoloration, and rough areas.

7. Trim the resident's fingernails using the nail clipper. Clip nails straight across. Shape and remove rough edges using an emery board or nail file.

8. Put lotion on the resident's hands and gently massage the hands from fingertips toward the wrists to stimulate circulation. Remove gloves and perform hand hygiene.

9. Tell the nurse about any redness, irritation, broken skin, or loose skin you have observed.

COMPLETION STEPS

1. Determine the resident's preferred position for comfort and ask them if they need anything else.
2. Examine the environment for safety and cleanliness.
3. Secure the call light and any other needed items within reach of the resident.
4. Perform hand hygiene.
5. Document the procedure and report any findings to the staff in charge.

Assisting with Dressing and Undressing

Some residents can dress and undress on their own, while others need your help. Procedure 5-21 outlines the steps for assisting a resident in getting dressed, and Procedure 5-22 outlines the steps for helping with undressing.

Preparing for an Event

Just as you want to look nice when you have visitors or attend a social event, residents also like to look good for visitors and special events. If visitors are coming, you may help the resident with grooming and personal care before they arrive. Remove any clutter in the room, and bring in extra chairs, if needed.

If a resident is leaving the facility for an outing, talk with the family in advance. A family member may want to help the resident prepare that day. If not, find out what time the resident needs to be ready and where they are going. Do they need to wear special clothes? If the weather is rainy or cold, be sure they have the right outerwear, including a warm coat, hat or cap, gloves, boots, scarf, etc.

Preparing for a big event may be confusing for some residents. Remind them what is going to happen on this occasion, especially if the resident has memory loss. This keeps them from being surprised and gives them something to look forward to. If a resident will be away overnight, prepare an overnight bag with essential items they will need. Make a checklist to be sure you do not forget anything.

The extra attention you give a resident in preparing for a visit or an outing helps both the resident and the family feel good. They will appreciate your efforts.

PREPARATION STEPS

1. Check the care plan.
2. Knock, introduce yourself, and address resident by preferred name.
3. Perform hand hygiene.
4. Gather supplies and secure assistance if needed.
5. Explain procedure and ask about resident preferences.
6. Respect privacy and rights at all times.

ITEMS NEEDED

- gloves
- bath basin half filled with warm water
- 2 towels
- soap
- washcloth
- orange wood stick
- lotion
- resident's shoes and socks or stockings

1. Put on gloves and help the resident remove shoes and socks or stockings.

2. To give foot care to a resident sitting in a chair, put a towel on the floor and the basin of water on the towel. Foot care can also be done while a resident is in bed, usually during a bed bath. Put a towel on the bed and the basin on the towel. Ask the resident to flex the leg to soak one foot at a time (3 to 5 minutes each).

3. For seated residents, place both feet in the basin of warm water and soak for 3 to 5 minutes.

4. Clean under the toenails with the orange wood stick. Scrub callused areas with a warm wash cloth.

5. Wash, rinse, dry, and inspect the feet thoroughly. Report any redness, irritation, or cracked, broken, loose, dry, or discolored skin. Report any callused areas, corns, or loose or broken nails.

6. Apply lotion to the tops of the feet, soles of the feet, and heels. Do not apply lotion between the toes. Remove gloves and perform hand hygiene.

7. Help the resident put on clean socks or stockings and shoes.

8. Tell the charge nurse if the resident needs toenail trimming or care for corns, calluses, or other foot problems.

COMPLETION STEPS

1. Determine the resident's preferred position for comfort and ask them if they need anything else.
2. Examine the environment for safety and cleanliness.
3. Secure the call light and any other needed items within reach of the resident.
4. Perform hand hygiene.
5. Document the procedure and report any findings to the staff in charge.

5-21: Assistance with Dressing a Dependent Resident

PREPARATION STEPS

1. Check the care plan.
2. Knock, introduce yourself, and address resident by preferred name.
3. Perform hand hygiene.
4. Gather supplies and secure assistance if needed.
5. Explain procedure and ask about resident preferences.
6. Respect privacy and rights at all times.

ITEMS NEEDED

- clothes, undergarments
- stockings or socks, shoes
- accessories (belt, tie, jewelry)
- plastic-covered pad (if resident is in bed)

As a general rule, if a resident has a weak or paralyzed limb, dress the weak side first. Dress the upper body first, then the lower body.

1 Remove the resident's nightgown or pajamas and offer a choice of clothing. For privacy and to prevent chill, remove the top portion of the resident's gown or pajamas first.

2 Help the resident put on an undershirt or bra, shirt or blouse, or dress. If a resident has a weak or paralyzed arm or has an IV in place, assist with putting that arm in a sleeve first. With an IV, move the solution through the sleeve first and hang it on the pole. Gently guide the resident's arm through the sleeve, being careful not to dislodge the IV needle or tubing. If the resident has an IV pump, call the nurse for assistance.

3 Help the resident put on underwear, socks or stockings, and pants or a skirt.

To put on a garment that opens in the back:

a. Slide the sleeve onto the resident's arm on the weaker side.

b. Slide the sleeve onto the arm of the stronger side.

c. Bring the sides of the garment to the back.

d. Turn the resident toward you, and bring one side of the garment to the back.

e. Turn the resident away from you, and bring the other side of the garment to the back.

f. Fasten the buttons, snaps, ties, or zipper.

g. Place the resident in the supine position (lying on their back).

To put on a garment that opens in the front:

a. Slide the sleeve onto the resident's arm on the weaker side.

b. Bring the resident to a sitting position, and bring the garment around the back. Lower the resident to the supine position.

c. Slide the sleeve onto the resident's arm on the stronger side.

d. Fasten buttons, snaps, ties, or zipper.

To put on a pullover garment:

a. Place the resident in the supine position.

b. Open any zippers or other closures, and place the garment over the resident's head.

c. Slide the sleeve of the garment onto the arm on the resident's weaker side.

d. Raise the resident to a semi-sitting position, bring the garment down over the shoulder, and slide the sleeve of the garment on the arm on the resident's stronger side. If the resident cannot sit upright, turn him/her toward you and pull the garment down on the back. Then turn the resident to the other side, and slide the stronger arm and shoulder into the sleeve. Pull the garment down in the back.

e. Fasten the buttons, snaps, ties, or zipper.

To put on pants or slacks:

a. Slide each pant leg over the resident's foot and up the leg.

b. Ask the resident to raise their hips and buttocks off the bed.

c. Bring the pants up over the hips and buttocks. If the resident cannot raise their hips and buttocks, turn them onto their stronger side. Then pull the pants up over the hips and buttocks on the weaker side. Turn the resident onto the other side and repeat the process.

d. Fasten the buttons, snaps, ties, or zipper.

5-21: Assistance with Dressing a Dependent Resident (continued)

4 Help the resident put on socks or stocking and shoes or non-skid slippers before they stand so they do not slip on the floor. When putting shoes on a resident who is in bed, first place a pad on the bed to protect the bedding.

5 Help the resident stand so you can smooth out their clothing, fasten any remaining closures, and neatly tuck in their shirt or blouse.

6 Help them put on any accessories they want to wear.

7 If a resident wears eyeglasses, dentures, or a hearing aid, help the resident with these items. If a resident uses a prosthesis (artificial body part or limb), you will need to ask the resident or the nurse if this should be put on before or after clothing.

8 Collect soiled garments, and place them in a hamper for the laundry according to the facility's procedure. Perform hand hygiene.

9 If the resident is in bed, after dressing, help him or her out of bed.

COMPLETION STEPS

1. Determine the resident's preferred position for comfort and ask them if they need anything else.
2. Examine the environment for safety and cleanliness.
3. Secure the call light and any other needed items within reach of the resident.
4. Perform hand hygiene.
5. Document the procedure and report any findings to the staff in charge.

5-22: Assistance with Undressing a Dependent Resident

PREPARATION STEPS

1. Check the care plan.
2. Knock, introduce yourself, and address resident by preferred name.
3. Perform hand hygiene.
4. Gather supplies and secure assistance if needed.
5. Explain procedure and ask about resident preferences.
6. Respect privacy and rights at all times.

ITEMS NEEDED

- pajamas, nightgown, or other clothing to be worn after taking off daytime clothes

This procedure is easier if the resident is sitting on the side of the bed. As a general rule, undress and dress the upper body first, then the lower body. If a resident has a weak or paralyzed arm or an IV, remove clothing from the other side first and then from the weak side or the side with the IV. If the resident has an IV, carefully guide the tubing and solution through the sleeve as the resident's arm moves.

1 Help the resident remove garments from the upper body (shirt, dress, blouse, and undergarments).

2 Help the resident put on a pajama top, t-shirt, or a nightgown.

3 Help the resident remove their shoes and socks or stockings. Then help with removing the pants or skirt and undergarments, if those are to be removed.

4 Help the resident put on pajama bottoms or other bottoms such as underpants, boxer shorts, or sweat pants.

5 Help the resident into bed.

6 Perform hand hygiene.

COMPLETION STEPS

1. Determine the resident's preferred position for comfort and ask them if they need anything else.
2. Examine the environment for safety and cleanliness.
3. Secure the call light and any other needed items within reach of the resident.
4. Perform hand hygiene.
5. Document the procedure and report any findings to the staff in charge.

Points to Remember

- Infection control principles and personal care skills are a major part of a nurse assistant's job.

- Microorganisms are tiny organisms that can only be seen with a microscope. They are usually single cells or infectious particles and include bacteria, viruses, fungi, and parasites.

- The chain of infection is how infectious disease is spread. It begins with a microorganism that is capable of causing disease (pathogen) and includes a reservoir, portal of exit, mode of transmission, portal of entry, and a susceptible host.

- Standard precautions are practices designed to prevent the transmission of infectious disease. They represent the minimum infection-prevention measures that apply to all patient (resident) care in any health care setting.

- Proper hand hygiene is one of the most important things you can do to prevent the spread of infection.

- Personal protective equipment is used to prevent the spread of infection. This includes gowns, aprons, gloves, masks, eye shields, and face shields.

- You must follow your facility's guidelines for handling sharps, soiled linen, regular waste, and hazardous waste to protect residents, other staff, and yourself.

- Isolation precautions are used to keep microorganisms from spreading from an infected resident to others. You will need to learn the isolation precautions used in your facility.

- Cleaning is the removal of soil from objects using water, detergent, and scrubbing. Disinfection kills or inhibits the growth of virtually all microorganisms on objects and surfaces using heat, special chemicals, or ultraviolet rays. Sterilization completely eliminates all microorganisms from a surface or object.

- Personal care includes bathing, mouth care, grooming, and dressing. How much help you provide depends on the unique needs and capabilities of each resident. You must take the time to learn residents' personal preferences and tailor your care accordingly.

- Observation is essential in providing care. Nurse assistants observe residents to monitor their physical health and emotional status and to ensure that the care provided meets residents' needs.

- You must learn the common preparation and completion steps and make them part of your daily routine.

Key Terms

airborne precautions — measures taken to prevent the airborne transmission of pathogens

airborne transmission — infection spread by microorganisms contained in particles or droplets suspended in air

antibiotic — drug that inhibits the growth of or kills certain microorganisms

asepsis — the absence of bacteria

aspiration — when fluid or foreign material is inhaled into the lungs

bacteria — single-celled microorganisms; some are beneficial and others may cause infection (singular = bacterium)

biohazardous waste — waste containing blood or other potentially infectious substances; includes needles, blades, and other sharps

chain of infection — process by which infection is spread

cleaning — removing soil from a surface or object

comatose — describes a person who is a coma (unconscious)

contact precautions — measures taken to prevent the spread of infection caused by microorganisms transmitted by direct or indirect contact

contraindicated — when a condition is present that provides a reason for not recommending a medical treatment

diarrhea — feces passed frequently and in liquid form; loose stool

direct transmission — spread of infection from one person to another or when infected blood or body fluids come in direct contact with broken skin or mucous membranes

disinfection — process that kills or inhibits the growth of virtually all microorganisms on objects and surfaces

droplet precautions — measures taken to prevent the spread of infection caused by microorganisms transmitted by droplets produced by coughing, sneezing, talking, or performing procedures

droplet spread — infected oral or nasal secretions transmitted via the eyes, nose, or mouth of another person, most commonly passed through coughing, sneezing, or talking

emesis — the action of vomiting

exposure — being in the vicinity of or in contact with an infectious microorganism

fungus — type of microorganism that can cause infection; examples are yeast and mold (plural = fungi)

healthcare-associated infection (HAI) — infection contracted while in an inpatient, outpatient, or residential health care facility

immunization — administration of a vaccine to prevent a specific infectious disease

indirect transmission — infection spread when a microorganism is transferred from one person to another via a vehicle (inanimate object) or a vector (living host such as a tick or mosquito)

infection — invasion and multiplication of microorganisms such as bacteria and viruses that are not normally present in the body; may or may not produce symptoms

isolation precautions — measures taken to prevent the spread of infection from an infected resident to other people

medical asepsis — reduces the number of microorganisms, also known as clean technique

microorganisms — organisms that cannot be seen with the naked eye; some are capable of causing infection

mode of transmission — the means by which a microorganism is transferred from one carrier to another

multidrug-resistant organism — describes microorganisms that have evolved in a way that makes them resistant to the action of antibiotic

natural flora — microorganisms that are always present, that usually do not cause disease

nonpathogenic — describes microorganisms that do not cause infection

outbreak — sudden increase in cases of a disease within a certain geographic area

parasite — organism that lives in or on another organism

pathogen — microorganism or substance that can produce disease

perineal care — cleaning and care of the area between the anus and external genitals

personal care — care provided for residents that includes bathing, mouth care, hair care, grooming, and dressing

personal protective equipment (PPE) — is equipment worn to minimize exposure to hazards that cause serious workplace injuries and illnesses

podiatrist — physician specializing in the care and treatment of the feet

portal of entry — the opening by which a microorganism enters the host

portal of exit — route taken by microorganisms leaving the body

reservoir — person, animal, or environment in which an infectious agent lives

routine care — daily care activities

safety data sheet (SDS) — sheet containing information about products and chemicals; includes guidelines for safe handling and emergency response

sanitation — promotion of hygiene and prevention of disease by maintaining clean conditions

secretions — substances such a saliva, mucus, perspiration, tears, etc. that come out of the body

standard precautions — evidence-based practices designed to prevent transmission of infectious disease

sterilization — process that completely eliminates all microorganisms from a surface or object

surgical asepsis — known as sterile technique, eliminates all microorganisms

susceptible host — a person who at risk of developing an infection from a microorganism

therapeutic — referring to a treatment

vector — living agent that transmits infection

vehicle — some type of inanimate object that acts as a carrier for microorganism

virus — a type of microorganism that survives only in living things

vomiting — also known as emesis, is when stomach contents exit through the mouth

1. **In the chain of infection, a microorganism leaves an infected person through:**
   a. The reservoir
   b. The portal of exit
   c. The portal of entry
   d. Direct transmission

2. **The best way to break the chain of infection at each link is by:**
   a. Sterilizing all bed linen every morning
   b. Not touching a resident
   c. Wearing a gown and protective eyewear at all times
   d. Performing hand hygiene before and after every contact with a resident

3. **Which type of infection can be transmitted through the air?**
   a. Syphilis
   b. Hepatitis
   c. HIV
   d. Tuberculosis

4. **Standard precautions require that gloves be worn:**
   a. When touching intact skin
   b. When touching non-intact skin, blood or body fluids, secretions, excretions, or contaminated items
   c. When opening the door of a resident room
   d. Standard precautions do not apply to use of gloves

5. **What type of PPE can protect against inhaling droplets in the air?**
   a. Gown
   b. Gloves
   c. Shoe Coverings
   d. Mask

6. **What is a benefit of observing residents carefully while providing care?**
   a. It frees you from having to observe residents at other times
   b. You have the opportunity to talk with residents about your home problems
   c. You may note both physical and psychological changes in residents
   d. You can decide whether or not to give residents their medications, depending on how they feel

7. **What are the three main purposes of bathing?**
   a. To decrease circulation to the skin, to make a resident feel better, and to remove dirt
   b. To remove dirt, perspiration, and microorganisms from the skin, increase circulation to the skin, and to help the resident feel better and more comfortable
   c. To dry out the skin, decrease circulation to the skin, and to remove microorganisms from the skin
   d. To make the resident smell better, to remove perspiration only, and to increase circulation to the skin

8. **Airborne transmission can occur when:**
   a. Microorganisms are carried in aerosols and a susceptible host inhales the particles
   b. Passing microorganisms by touching an inanimate object
   c. Microorganisms are transferred from one person to another through skin-to-skin contact
   d. Microorganisms are ingested by infected food

9. **Using medical aseptic practices, you would:**
   a. Perform oral care without the use of gloves
   b. Wear PPE during perineal care
   c. Use sterile technique to change a soiled brief
   d. Wash gloves so they can be used on multiple residents

10. **How could autonomy be promoted while assisting a resident with dressing?**
    a. Choose the clothes that they will wear
    b. Allow the resident to choose what they would like to wear
    c. Provide a bed bath instead of a shower since it is close to the end of your shift
    d. Enter the resident's room without knocking

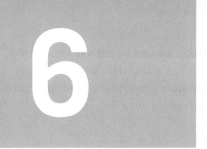

6

Safety and Emergency Care

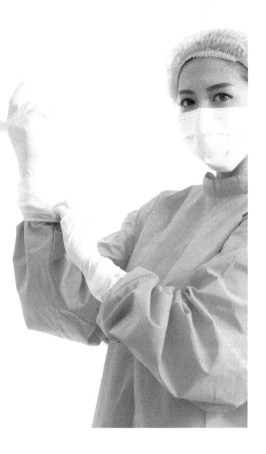

Safety is a critical issue in all health-care settings. Ensuring the safety of residents and protecting yourself as you provide care are your most important roles as a nurse assistant. Each year, billions of dollars in costs are associated with occupational injuries affecting workers in health-care professions. These injuries can be prevented by staying alert and following guidelines for working safely with those in your care. The key to injury prevention is to use common sense and the right equipment for your assigned tasks.

Learning how to prevent workplace injuries improves the quality of your work. Before beginning any task, ask yourself:

- "Am I at risk for exposure to any body fluids?"
- "Is there a better way to do this?"
- "What equipment or help do I need to complete the task safely?"

In this chapter, we discuss personal safety for you and the residents, how to protect yourself from bloodborne pathogens, and how to handle emergency situations and disasters. You will learn about ergonomics, injury-prevention practices, and your role in facility safety programs. You will be introduced to potential hazards and learn how to be prepared for common emergency situations.

OBJECTIVES:

- Define *standard precautions* as it relates to bloodborne pathogens.

- Explain the OSHA Bloodborne Pathogens Standard and how it applies to the actions of health care staff.

- Define *ergonomics,* and demonstrate proper body mechanics for daily care tasks.

- List at least 10 common sense strategies for preventing injury to yourself and residents.

- Describe your role in disaster preparedness and your responsibilities during an actual emergency.

- State general guidelines that should be followed in an emergency situation.

- Identify the signs of choking and demonstrate how to perform the Heimlich maneuver.

- Explain the correct emergency care measures for a resident experiencing a heart attack, cardiac arrest, seizure, burns, hemorrhaging, and shock.

Protecting Yourself from Bloodborne Infections

Microorganisms in blood that are capable of causing disease are called **bloodborne pathogens**. Those of major concern in health-care settings include two types of the **hepatitis** virus (hepatitis B and hepatitis C) and the human immunodeficiency virus (HIV), which causes AIDS.

Hepatitis B and C

Hepatitis is a disease characterized by inflammation of the liver. The hepatitis B virus (HBV) is present in high concentrations in the blood of an infected person. This means there is a greater chance of infection from HBV exposure than there is with exposure to HIV. Hepatitis B is one of the most common infectious diseases worldwide, but there is a vaccine to prevent it. Medications are currently available to treat HBV, but there is no cure.

Some people infected with HBV experience no symptoms and do not realize that they carry the virus in their blood. Symptoms include fever, weakness and fatigue, abdominal and/or joint pain, loss of appetite, nausea and/ or vomiting, dark urine, and jaundice (yellowing of the skin and whites of the eyes). HBV is transmitted via contact with infected blood, through sexual contact with an infected person, and can be passed from mother to infant during birth.

Hepatitis C (HCV) can also be a "silent" disease, with symptoms that emerge only after years or decades of infection. Symptoms are similar to HBV and may also include bruising and bleeding easily and swelling of the abdomen and/or legs. HCV is transmitted in the same ways as HBV. Chronic HCV is now curable with medications taken for two to six months.

The most serious problem with HBV and HCV infections is that some people with these infections never get well. Their liver damage may be so serious that they eventually need a liver transplant.

HIV/AIDS

The **human immunodeficiency virus (HIV)** attacks the immune system and, if untreated, can lead to **acquired immunodeficiency syndrome (AIDS)**, a potentially fatal condition. HIV is transmitted through blood and other body fluids via sexual contact, contact with infected blood, by sharing needles, or from mother to child during pregnancy or breastfeeding. There is no cure for HIV/AIDS, but medications can slow its progression.

Symptoms vary and may include fever, headache, sore throat, muscle and joint pain, rash, and swollen lymph glands. HIV infection can be detected with an antibody-screening test but often, signs and symptoms do not occur for 10 or more years. During this time, an infected person can spread the infection to others.

OSHA Bloodborne Pathogens Standard

In Chapter 5, you learned about standard precautions that must be used to prevent the transmission of infection. The Occupational Safety and Health Administration (OSHA) was created by Congress to ensure safe and healthful working conditions for workers by setting and enforcing standards and by providing training, outreach, education, and assistance.

Bloodborne Pathogens

OSHA Bloodborne Pathogens Standard requires all health-care agencies, including long term care facilities, to follow the CDC standard precautions for bloodborne pathogens. The OSHA standard protects workers from all known and unknown diseases transmitted by blood. In addition, there are several other requirements, which are described in the following sections.

Preventing Needlesticks

Microorganisms in blood can enter another person's body through an accidental needlestick.

In this case, the needle is an intermediate object that transfers the resident's blood to you through your skin. OSHA requires that safety needles and syringes with attached safety devices be used (Figure 6-1). After using the needle, the shield can be pressed against a hard surface to cover the needle.

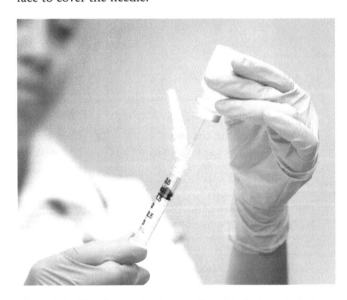

Figure 6-1 Needles and syringes with safety features help to prevent needlesticks.

If a needlestick occurs, you must follow the facility policy for evaluation and follow-up. Diabetic residents may sometimes be allowed to self-inject their insulin, so being aware of your facility's policy is important in helping residents and ensuring proper disposal of needles and other supplies.

Exposure Control Plan

OSHA requires that all facilities have a written exposure control plan to eliminate or minimize employees' exposure to blood and body fluids. Every department is covered by this plan, and every employee should be aware of the plan and be able to review it at any time.

Engineering and Work-Practice Controls Engineering controls use various devices to reduce hazards. For example, a needle-disposal container (sharps container) should be located near places where needles, blades, and other sharp items are used. By doing so, sharps can be disposed of directly without the need to transport them to another location.

Personal Protective Equipment

OSHA mandates the use of personal protective equipment (discussed in detail in Chapter 5), which provides barriers that prevent contact between infectious microorganisms and a susceptible host. Gloves, masks, eye protection, face shields, and gowns or aprons protect you from contact with blood and other body fluids (Figure 6-2).

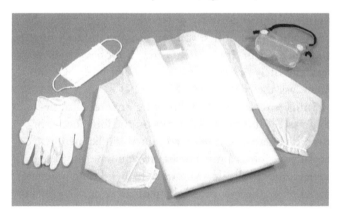

Figure 6-2 Examples of personal protective equipment.

Housekeeping

The facility environment must be kept clean and sanitary. OSHA requires a written cleaning schedule for each facility. This includes the methods for decontaminating surfaces or equipment soiled with blood or body fluids. If you have questions about how the OSHA Bloodborne Pathogens Standard is implemented in your facility, ask the infection control practitioner.

Hepatitis B Vaccination and Follow-Up

OSHA requires that all facilities provide the hepatitis B vaccine free of charge to all employees who may have occupational exposure to blood or other infectious materials. OSHA also requires that facilities offer a free blood test one to two months after employees have received the last shot in the HBV vaccine series. This test determines if the vaccine will be effective. The facility cannot require that employees receive the vaccine or blood test. If exposure occurs, the facility must provide immediate post-exposure evaluation and follow-up, either on site or at another health-care facility. (The LTC facility covers the cost of any outside services.)

Information and Training

The OSHA Bloodborne Pathogens Standard requires that facilities provide information and training to all employees during working hours. This training must include information about bloodborne pathogens, tasks that involve occupational exposure, and ways to reduce the risk of exposure.

Nurse Assistant Tasks Involving Exposure to Blood

Because you provide most resident care, you may notice blood in a resident's stool, urine, or vomit or in drainage from a wound. Always wear gloves when handling any resident's body secretions and excretions.

The risk of being splashed in the eyes, nose, or mouth with any fluid containing blood can be minimized by following standard precaution procedures. If you are at risk of being splashed with any body fluids — even just a little — always wear the appropriate eye, nose, and mouth barrier protection.

You may sometimes clean up spills on the floor or in a resident's bathroom, which may include blood or other body fluids. Follow the facility's procedure for cleaning up spills, using the correct detergent and disinfectant. Wear a gown or plastic apron if your skin or clothing may be soiled. Always wear gloves when cleaning any type of spill. The infection control practitioner or head housekeeper can teach you the best way to clean up spills.

Sharps Safety Equipment

Nurse assistants do not usually perform tasks using needles or other sharps, but some may be tasked with changing sharps disposal containers. Injury and exposure to infection can occur if needles are improperly disposed of, are sticking out the top of the container, or have punctured the side of the container. To prevent injury, examine the sharps disposal container carefully before you touch it.

Punctures from needles and other sharps and cuts from used scalpels put health-care workers at risk for many infections. All facilities have procedures for handling and disposing of used sharps. Sharps containers should be located as close as possible to where they are used. Usually these containers are on medication carts and in medication rooms. Some facilities have sharps containers on the walls of residents' rooms. Know the location of all the sharps containers in your facility.

Wastes Requiring Special Handling

The OSHA Bloodborne Pathogens Standard defines **regulated waste** and includes rules for waste handling, storage, and shipping. Regulated waste is discarded in specially marked red bags or bags with a biohazard label (Figure 6-3). Many types of waste require special handling, including:

- Pathological wastes
- Lab cultures
- Liquid waste
- Human blood and products of blood
- Items saturated with blood or body fluids
- Items contaminated with blood, such as used sharps

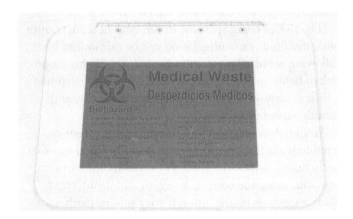

Figure 6-3 The biohazard label is used to identify waste that requires special handling.

Injury Prevention

Studies have shown that on-the-job injuries can result from repetitive body movements, incorrect posture, lifting residents or items that are too heavy, using the wrong equipment, and using equipment incorrectly. When caring for a resident, injuries can be prevented by using a five-step approach:

1. Determine the resident's capabilities.
2. Determine the equipment you need.
3. Determine and communicate to other staff the steps needed for safe handling.
4. Follow the care plan.
5. Evaluate the success of tasks performed.

Ergonomics

Ergonomics is the scientific study of how people can function safely and efficiently at work. Its principles are the basis for the policies, equipment, and staff training needed to provide quality care. You are not responsible for implementing these steps alone. The interdisciplinary team helps to determine the right steps for you and the resident.

You may encounter situations in which you must lift or help someone, but the physical demands are beyond your capability. If you rely on proven ergonomic principles, consider your capabilities and those of the resident, and use the appropriate equipment, you will make the task easier and safer for both of you. You must make sure that you know how to use all equipment before you begin the task.

Repetitive motions such as bending, lifting, turning, and reaching put you at risk of injury. A resident's unpredictable actions also increase the risk. If you don't use the right equipment correctly or you misuse your body when performing your duties, you can seriously injure yourself and the resident. If you are unsure about how to move a resident safely or how to use a particular piece of equipment, ask the charge nurse for help.

Injuries result from not knowing how to do something safely and from bad habits on the job. Sooner or later, if you are not careful, an injury will happen. As you begin your job as a nurse assistant, you have the perfect opportunity to develop safe work habits. Using practices based on ergonomic principles reduces your risk of being injured now and throughout your career.

Being Aware Prevents Injuries

Safety-related decision making begins with your participation as part of the interdisciplinary team in assessing a resident's capabilities. Categorizing residents' abilities provides information that guides you in knowing the best way to move, transfer, or reposition them. It also helps in determining how to help with their daily care. As part of your training and orientation, you will learn your facility's system for communicating this information. This communication must not violate the resident's right to privacy but should give staff the information they need to work safely with the resident.

Using the right equipment for each resident is an important part of preventing injuries. Many kinds of equipment can help you move residents from bed to chair, chair to toilet, and chair to bed (Figure 6-4). Other equipment is used to help position and reposition residents in their beds and chairs. The key is to know what is available and to follow the manufacturer's directions for its use. Table 6-1 provides examples of equipment that is commonly used to help move, transfer, or reposition residents and help with activities of daily living.

Never put yourself or the resident at risk. Being safety-conscious requires being observant, paying attention to details, and continually evaluating the situation. You must be willing to ask questions and to change your way of doing things, if necessary. Ask the charge nurse about any procedure or equipment you do not completely understand. Ask the charge nurse for help in evaluating situations until you gain more experience. Remember, each resident and situation is different, so you must adapt your actions to meet the resident's unique needs.

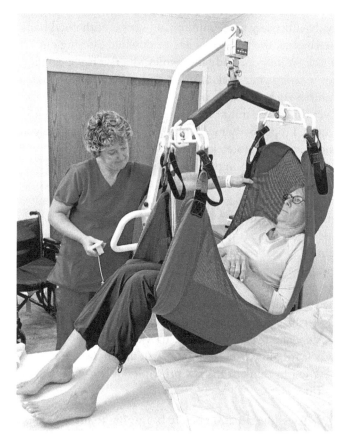

Figure 6-4 Mechanical lifts help move a resident from one place to another, such as from bed to chair.

Table 6-1   Equipment Used to Help Move Residents

Type of Equipment	Uses
Mechanical lifts, including: ■ total body lifts ■ stand-assist lifts ■ ambulation lifts ■ bath/shower lifts	Move residents from one location to another, such as from the bed to a chair, from the chair to the toilet, or off the floor
■ Slide boards ■ Transfer mats ■ Slippery sheets (friction-reducing devices) ■ Draw sheets ■ Trapeze bars	Lateral transfers between two horizontal surfaces, such as when you move from the bed to a stretcher
■ Gait belt ■ Transfer belt with handles ■ Pivot discs ■ Range-of-motion machines	■ Positioning ■ Ambulation ■ Repositioning ■ Transfer from bed to chair ■ Manipulation of a body part
■ Shower/toilet combination chairs ■ Extension-hand tools ■ Pelvic-lift devices	Help with activities of daily living (ADLs) (bathing, dressing, transferring, toileting, and eating)

Rules for Safety

Following are common sense rules that promote safety for you and your residents. These rules are grouped by how they affect residents, you, and the environment. Some rules involve all three. Consider each resident's individual safety needs. The needs of residents with visual impairments are different from those with hearing impairments. The key is to know your residents and their special needs, the equipment you can use, and other staff who can help. With this knowledge you can adjust the rules to fit each situation.

Residents

- Before walking with a resident, check their path for potential fall hazards, such as water on the floor.
- Ensure that proper footwear is worn during transfers and when walking with a resident.
- Encourage residents to use handrails and grip rails.
- Use a **gait belt** (also called a transfer belt) when walking or transferring a resident, unless otherwise noted on

their care plan. This device is used to help steady a resident during transfers or walking. Always check with the charge nurse before using a gait belt on a resident who has open or surgical wound, trauma, or medical devices on the abdomen or chest.

To apply a gait belt:

1. Assist the resident to a sitting position, if possible.

2. Apply gait belt snugly around the resident's waist, over their clothing. You should be able to fit your fingers between the belt and the resident. Tuck the end of the gait belt strap inside the belt so it is not hanging down.

3. After completing the task, with the resident in a seated position, remove the gait belt carefully. Avoid pulling which can cause shearing or tearing of the skin.

- When bathing residents, test the water temperature carefully to be sure it is not too hot or too cold.

- Always turn off the hot-water faucet before the cold one, to prevent hot water from dripping on a resident's skin or on you.

- Encourage residents to use their assistive and prosthetic devices (such as glasses or a walker) when they get up at night to use the bathroom.

- Always respond to call lights immediately. Be sure the call light button is close by each resident and that residents know how to use it.

- Familiarize residents with all furniture and equipment in their surroundings.

- Always keep each resident's bed in its lowest position.

- Frequently inspect residents' assistive devices, such as walkers and canes. Be sure that the rubber tips are in place and that the device fits the resident correctly.

- When moving a resident to or from movable equipment such as wheelchairs, shower chairs, beds, etc., always lock the wheels first.

- Only use side rails according to facility policy.

Nurse Assistants

- Wear nonskid shoes.

- Always use good body mechanics (discussed in the following section). For example, avoid jerky movements, such as abrupt turns. When you turn, move your feet so that your body can follow smoothly. Avoid twisting motions. Never reach high overhead for something. Instead, use a stool.

- Use equipment to lift and move residents instead of relying solely on your physical strength. Always ask for help when you need it.

- Never run down a hallway. Use caution when turning a corner because someone may be there.

- Never use electrical equipment near water.

- Report any nonworking equipment.

- Keep yourself healthy.

Environment

- Clean up spills immediately.

- Keep residents' rooms and hallways free of clutter.

- Make sure hallways are well lit.

- Use night lights in residents' rooms.

- Always store chemicals such as cleaning solutions and medications in their proper place.

Body Mechanics

Body mechanics is the way in which the body balances and moves while engaged in daily activities. Proper body mechanics increase your efficiency and safety by using the body effectively while minimizing stress. With good body mechanics, the body does less work while carrying out a task. With poor body mechanics, the risk is increased for injuring your back or other body areas. Even though injuries such as strains and sprains may not seem serious, over time these minor injuries can lead to a more serious injury. Proper body mechanics ensure that every time you move, you are protecting yourself from injury.

It is important to pay attention to protecting your back all day long. Before you lift a person or an object, take a moment to assess the situation. If you are about to lift a resident, first find out if they can help you. Use the appropriate equipment when needed. If you have any doubt about your ability to lift someone with or without equipment, get help before you attempt it. You will learn many different techniques for helping a resident move in bed and between bed and chair. You can injure your back if you are careless about body mechanics. Be aware of your posture and make sure you are moving and lifting the right way (Procedure 6-1). Your body will thank you for it.

You can think of the key principles of body mechanics as three steps:

1. Assess the situation before beginning to lift, move, or position a resident.

2. Prepare yourself by considering your body mechanics.

3. Determine how to do the lift, move, or position.

6-1: Moving and Lifting a Resident Using Proper Body Mechanics

PREPARATION STEPS

1. Check the care plan.
2. Knock, introduce yourself, and address resident by preferred name.
3. Perform hand hygiene.
4. Gather supplies and secure assistance if needed.
5. Explain procedure and ask about resident preferences.
6. Respect privacy and rights at all times.

ITEMS NEEDED

- Extra sheet or towel
- Gait belt or transfer belt
- Sliding board

This process involves three phases, and each phase includes a sequence of steps.

PHASE 1: ASSESS THE SITUATION.

1 Adjust the height of the bed. Move it up to the height of your elbow when giving care (as when giving a complete bed bath) and down when moving someone out of the bed. Changing the height reduces the amount of bending you have to do.

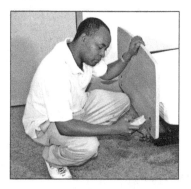

2 To avoid reaching injuries, bring any items you need close to you.

3 If you are moving a resident in bed, consider putting your knee up on the bed. This allows you to get closer to residents without reaching.

4 You may want to use a friction-reducing device. Place a barrier such as a sheet or towel between your knee and the bed sheets.

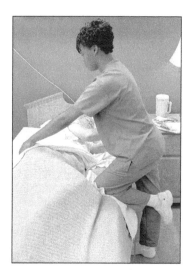

PHASE 2: PREPARE YOURSELF.

1 Place your feet about shoulder-width apart, one foot slightly in front of the other, for a stronger base of support and better stability.

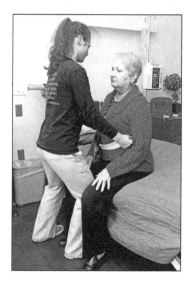

2 Tighten your abdominal muscles. This supports your spine.

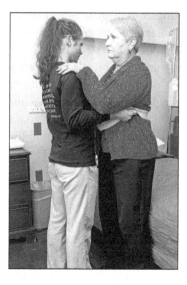

3 Keep your back neutral.

6-1: Moving and Lifting a Resident Using Proper Body Mechanics (continued)

PHASE 3: DETERMINE HOW TO MOVE, AND EXECUTE THE LIFT.

1 Get as close as possible to the resident. The "hug" position is very supportive. Use a gait or transfer belt with handles for a secure grip.

2 Keep your palms up when lifting. Lift from underneath, using your biceps (muscles of the upper arm).

3 Inhale deeply before you begin the lift, and exhale while you lift. This helps pump blood and oxygen to your muscles.

4 Rock to gain momentum for a lift or move. Rocking is moving your body very slightly, either back and forth or side to side. This rocking motion increases your strength.

5 Bend your knees and lift the resident using your leg, arm, and abdominal muscles, not your back.

6 Always be careful not to move a resident too quickly, which can cause injury. When possible, use a sliding board as a bridge between the bed and chair and a friction-reducing device.

COMPLETION STEPS

1. Determine the resident's preferred position for comfort and ask them if they need anything else.
2. Examine the environment for safety and cleanliness.
3. Secure the call light and any other needed items within reach of the resident.
4. Perform hand hygiene.
5. Document the procedure and report any findings to the staff in charge.

Preventing Resident Falls

CMS defines a fall as unintentionally coming to rest on the ground, floor, or other, lower level, but not as a result of an overwhelming external force (e.g., resident pushes another resident). Falls can cause serious injuries at any age. When an elderly person falls, it can be extremely dangerous (Figure 6-5). Falls can result in cuts and bruises and serious injuries such as bone fractures and head injuries. According to the CDC, more than one out of four older people falls each year. Even if an injury does not occur or is relatively minor, a resident who has fallen may become fearful and less independent. They may stop walking by themselves or getting out of bed to use the bathroom. This loss of mobility can lead to number of other problems. Maintaining the resident's independent mobility as long as possible is important for their health and quality of life.

Falls occur for a number of reasons. As we age, our bodies change. Changes in the musculoskeletal and nervous systems, which affect posture and balance, make falls more likely. Many residents in long term care are frail and have health conditions that affect their posture, balance, and mobility. Other factors that increase the chance of falling include poor vision, sensory problems, and the use of certain medications. Falls are more likely in residents with increased toileting needs and when the resident's surroundings are cluttered and crowded. A fall can also occur if you are not moving correctly or using the correct equipment when moving, transferring, or walking with a resident.

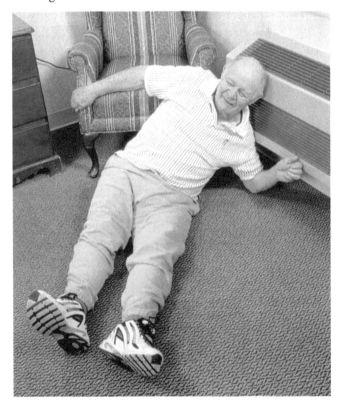

Figure 6-5 Falls can cause serious injuries in older adults.

Guidelines for Preventing Falls

Many long term care facilities have fall prevention programs. To prevent or minimize falls, consider all the factors involved. Work with the interdisciplinary team — talk with other staff and share your ideas about how to make the environment safer. For example, you may notice that after receiving their evening medication, a resident has trouble maintaining their balance. This is something you should report.

You can discuss the resident's routines with the team. You might share the information that a resident drinks a lot of fluids late in the day, goes to bed early, and often gets up during the night to use the bathroom. If the night staff is aware of this resident's habits, they can assist with toileting more often and thereby prevent a fall. You can also make sure that no obstacles such as furniture or equipment block the pathway to the bathroom. Ensuring that the bed is locked and in the lowest position is also your responsibility.

Here are some tips for preventing resident falls:

- Encourage residents with glasses to wear them.
- Encourage residents to wear well-fitting nonskid footwear.
- Answer call lights in a timely manner.
- Assist to the toilet as needed.
- Keep all pathways clear and well-lit.
- Eliminate clutter in the resident's room and bathroom.
- Keep residents' personal items within their reach.
- Use mechanical devices for transfers.
- Report changes in a resident's behavior.
- Report any broken or malfunctioning equipment and any lighting problems.

Devices and Equipment Used to Prevent Falls

An interdisciplinary approach is needed to help prevent resident falls. You will participate in meetings to discuss residents with a history of falls or who have fallen recently. You may be asked about how a resident sits in a wheelchair or chair. Does he slide forward or slouch in the chair, lean over to one side, or lean forward?

Your knowledge of the residents will help the team determine whether a piece of equipment or a device can be used to help prevent a fall. For example, seating devices can support a resident's posture. Motion-detection devices can be used to turn on lights or alarms when a resident approaches stairs or opens a door. Support handles can

be installed in the resident's bathroom. A raised toilet seat makes it easier to get on and off the toilet. All these devices can help prevent a resident from falling.

You have learned that residents must not be restrained. Keep residents' rights in mind, and never restrain a resident because you think that will prevent a fall. Residents must be able to move freely. Seat belts on wheelchairs may be used to remind the resident to call the nurse when they want to get up from the chair. These straps usually fasten together with Velcro and may be used only if the resident can easily open the belt.

Side rails (or bed rails) may be used when they are part of the resident's care plan. Side rails can be useful in helping residents turn and reposition in bed. They can provide a handhold for getting into or out of bed. They give some residents a feeling of comfort and security.

Remember that side rails should never be raised automatically for any resident. In fact, some residents may become injured or even die if they become caught in the rails or between the mattress and rails. Residents can be seriously injured if they try to climb over the rails and fall. Residents who are frail or elderly or those who are confused, in pain, or have uncontrolled body movements or other conditions, are at greater risk of injury when side rails are used. Always follow your facility's policy for the use of side rails. Your facility may require a health care provider order for their use.

Environmental Safety

The environment in a long term care facility may present some safety hazards. The good news is that by being aware and taking proper action, you can avoid and control these hazards and prevent injuries.

Wet Floor and Other Hazards

Everyone is responsible for cleaning up spills. Regardless of whether you create a spill or see one that is already there, you must clean it up immediately. If you see a spill while responding to a medical emergency, you can call out to alert someone else that the spill must be cleaned up before anyone slips and is injured. You must be alert to anything on the floor that could cause a person to slip or trip, such as urine, water, broken floor tiles, soap, paper clips, bed cranks, food, and other items.

Floor cleanup is simple. First, make sure that everyone is alerted to the danger by placing a "Wet Floor" sign in the area. Then use the appropriate supplies and equipment to wipe up the spill (paper towels, sponge, mop, etc.) making sure to follow facility requirements when cleaning up body fluids.

When working with water, as when helping a resident with bathing, showering, or washing hair, be extra careful. Falls are much more likely to occur when the resident is on a wet surface or water is being used. Keep your work area as clean and dry as possible.

Electrical Safety

Electrical safety is also everyone's concern. When working with or around electricity, follow these guidelines:

- Never use electrical devices near water.
- Always dry your hands before using electrical equipment.
- Never use extension cords or outlet expanders (devices with multiple outlets that plug into a single outlet). Laws prohibit their use in facilities.
- If you're not currently using an electrical device, turn it off.
- Report any electrical shock from a device to your supervisor. The device should not be used again until it is repaired.
- Never try to repair an electrical device yourself.

Pay attention to electrical items brought in by residents and their family members. Items such as electric razors, televisions, radios, stereos/CD players, fans, and lamps should be examined by maintenance staff to avoid potential electrical problems. Some facilities have a policy requiring an inspection before an electrical device can be used. Supervise any resident's use of equipment.

Always make sure that electrical devices are in working order. Frayed cords, missing safety guards, exposed wires, and cracks are signs of a problem. Sparks, excessive heat, or a hissing or buzzing sound are also signs that the device is not working properly. Do not use or allow a resident to use any device with these problems, and report any such conditions to your supervisor immediately.

Chemical Safety

By law, all employers and employees must know about any chemical hazards in the workplace and how to protect themselves from these hazards. Employers must communicate this information through employee training programs.

The most common chemicals in long term care facilities are disinfectants and cleaning products. If you follow the manufacturer's directions for their use, you and your residents will be safe. Your training will include understanding container labels. You must get in the habit of reading and following the label directions. Labels contain most of the information you need to protect you and your residents. If you find a container without a label, do not use it or smell it to guess what it is. Take it to the charge nurse immediately.

If any hazardous chemicals are used in your facility, you will receive specialized training on their proper use. The OSHA Hazard Communication Standard requires this training, which includes safety information you need to know.

All facilities must also make available a *safety data sheet* (SDS) for every chemical used on the premises (Figure 6-6). Each sheet lists the product's chemical contents, fire and health hazards, use precautions, clean-up procedures, disposal requirements, necessary personal protective equipment, and first-aid procedures (see Procedure 6-2). These sheets are kept in an accessible location, such as the nurses' station. If you are exposed to a chemical and have a reaction, go to the emergency room of the nearest hospital and take the SDS with you.

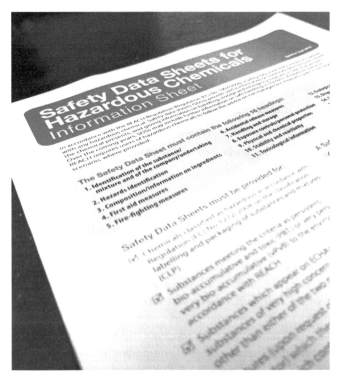

Figure 6-6 Facilities must have safety data sheets on hand for all chemicals used on the premises.

GENERAL EMERGENCY FIRST AID:

1 Follow the guidelines in the safety data sheet for the chemical.

2 See your supervisor immediately, who will contact the local poison control center or the American Association of Poison Control Centers Poison Helpline (1-800-222-1222), if needed, to find out what actions to take.

3 If you or a resident inhale a chemical, get into fresh air as soon as possible.

4 If you or a resident get a chemical on your skin, rinse it off with lots of running water.

5 If you or a resident swallow a chemical, do not induce vomiting. Rinse out your mouth or theirs.

6 If applicable, follow the poison center or helpline instructions.

FOR CHEMICAL SPILLS OR SPLASHES IN YOUR EYES:

1 Immediately flush your eyes with cool running water for at least five minutes. Remove contact lenses.

2 Continue flushing for at least 15 minutes, holding the eyelids open to ensure that the entire eye is rinsed.

Employees' Right to Know

As an employee, you have a legal right to see certain kinds of personnel and safety records. In addition to your employment and medical histories and job description, you have the right to see documents affecting safety in the facility. You can request to see your department's chemical inventory list, safety data sheets, and the OSHA publication "Access to Employee Exposure and Medical Records Standard." You may want to read these if you have questions about which chemicals you may be exposed to on the job or what to do in an emergency.

Safety Around Oxygen

Oxygen (O2) is an important gas in your facility. Oxygen itself is not flammable, but it can make other things ignite and burn. Its use increases the risk of fire and explosion. Because of these risks, you must follow certain precautions in areas where oxygen is being used.

Oxygen can come from several different sources. It may come from a valve in the wall, from tanks of compressed gas, or from a machine called an oxygen concentrator. Regardless of the source, these precautions always apply:

- Keep all flames and potential sources of sparks away from oxygen. There must be no smoking when oxygen is in use.
- Place a "No Smoking — Oxygen in Use" sign on any door to a room where oxygen is being used (Figure 6-7).

- Never put any kind of lubricant on hoses or fittings used with oxygen, because this could start a fire. If the pieces don't go together smoothly, tell the charge nurse. Never try to force a fit. The tank may be labeled incorrectly.

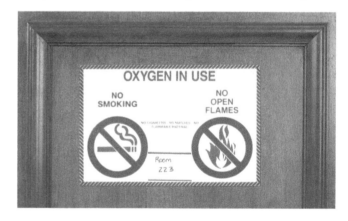

Figure 6-7 Oxygen in Use signs must be posted in plain view.

Disaster Preparedness

Disasters include natural events such as tornadoes, hurricanes, tropical storms, floods, and earthquakes. Explosions, fires, and acts of violence that disrupt the normal functioning of a facility are also considered disasters. All facilities have written disaster plans in case of an emergency. These plans usually say that employees must first move residents to safety and then care for them. Regardless of problems caused by the disaster, you must still meet the needs of your residents.

Disaster plans do not assign tasks to people by name because different staff members are on duty at various times. Emergency tasks are assigned by job title (job description). You must be familiar with your facility's disaster plan and know the role of nurse assistants in the event of a disaster.

Weather-Related Disaster

Possible weather events depend on the region in which you are located. Emergencies can occur suddenly, as with a violent storm, or with advance warning, such as with a hurricane. The charge nurse will tell you when to evacuate residents following either the shelter in place (internal evacuation) or external evacuation plan.

Every facility has an evacuation plan that contains a "priority of movement." This is the order in which residents should be moved (Figure 6-8). As a nurse assistant, you need to be aware of the policy and confident of your role in the evacuation. During an evacuation, a senior nurse or administrative staff member will be giving instructions. It is important for the safety of everyone that you stay alert and follow directions.

To evacuate bedridden residents, you use emergency transfer methods that are quick, efficient, and safe. These methods are different from your usual transfer techniques (see Procedure 6-3).

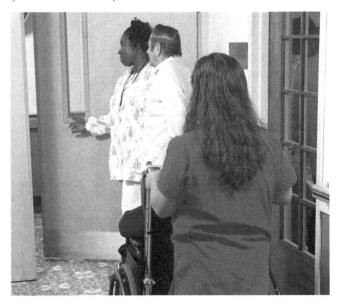

Figure 6-8 Residents must be evacuated in priority order in the event of a disaster or other emergency.

PROCEDURE

6-3: Emergency Transfer Techniques

ITEMS NEEDED

- Blankets

ONE NURSE-BLANKET CARRY

This carry should be used for a resident who is smaller than you when you must transport the person without assistance.

1. Fold the blanket diagonally with the point downward and the long ends on either side of the resident.

2. Help the resident into a sitting position on the bed.

3. Wrap the blanket around the resident's back and under the arms (like a shawl), and then tie the ends of the blanket in a knot. Cross the resident's arms.

4. Insert your right arm between the knotted blanket (below knot) and the resident's chest.

5. Turn your back to the resident, bend your knees, and adjust the blanket comfortably over your right shoulder.

6. Straighten your knees to lift the resident from the bed with a minimum amount of strain or effort. Carry the resident on your back. Support the resident's legs with your left arm.

7. Carry the resident to safety.

6-3: Emergency Transfer Techniques (continued)

BLANKET DRAG

1 Unfold the blanket on the floor.

2 Help the resident onto the blanket diagonally.

3 If the resident is wearing shoes, remove them. This eliminates the possibility of the heels catching on stairs or floor obstructions.

4 Lift the corner of the blanket nearest the resident's head, keeping the resident's head off the floor.

5 Using one or both hands, pull the resident, head first, to a place of safety.

PACK STRAP METHOD

1 Help the resident to a sitting position.

2 Grasp the resident's right wrist with your left hand and left wrist with your right hand.

3 Place your head under the resident's arms (without releasing their wrists) and turn, placing your back against the resident's chest so that your shoulders are lower than their armpits.

4 Pull the resident's arms over your shoulders and across your chest for leverage. Keep the resident's wrists firmly grasped.

5 Lean forward slightly, straighten your knees, and transport the resident to safety.

HIP METHOD

1 Turn the resident on their side, facing you.

2 Sit on the bed, and place your back against the resident's abdomen.

3 Grasp the resident's knees with one arm, and slide your other arm down and across their back.

4 Stand up slowly while drawing the resident up onto your hips.

5 Carry the resident to safety.

CRADLE DROP (TO BLANKET)

1 Unfold the blanket on the floor, facing the side of the bed.

2 The resident should be in the supine position.

3 Lift under the resident's knees with one arm and under the shoulders with the other. Guide the resident toward you.

4 Bend one knee and press it against the bed, keeping your foot firmly on the floor.

5 Lower the resident to the floor by bending your back leg to the floor. Keep your other knee against the bed. Your raised knee will support the resident's knees and legs, and your arm will support their shoulders and head. The cradle formed by your arm and knee will protect their shoulders and head.

6 Pull the resident toward you and ease them onto the blanket.

KNEEL DROP

1 Unfold the blanket on the floor. The resident should be in the supine position.

2 Face the side of the bed and lower yourself to a kneeling position.

3 Grasp the resident's knees with one arm, and their head and shoulders with the other.

4 Pull the resident straight out from bed until their body contacts your chest. Allow the resident to slide downward to the cushion formed by your knees.

5 Ease the resident onto the blanket and move to safety.

COMPLETION STEPS

1. Determine the resident's preferred position for comfort and ask them if they need anything else.
2. Examine the environment for safety and cleanliness.
3. Secure the call light and any other needed items within reach of the resident.
4. Perform hand hygiene.
5. Document the procedure and report any findings to the staff in charge.

Fire

Fire safety and preparedness are a major responsibility for all employees. Your role in emergency preparedness is important. Stay on the alert for potential problems and participate in all prevention activities to help keep everyone safe.

In your new employee orientation, you will learn your facility's fire plan. Fire procedures are posted in each department and at each nurses' station near the phone. In areas that do not have 911 response systems, local emergency phone numbers should be posted for the fire department, police or sheriff, ambulance, and Poison Control Center.

Fire drills should be held at least every three months on each shift. You must participate in these drills to ensure that you and all staff are as prepared as possible.

To prevent fires, follow these guidelines:

- Report any unsafe condition so that corrective measures can be taken right away.
- Enforce no-smoking regulations.
- In smoking areas, safety ashtrays should be used, and cigarettes must always be out when discarded.
- Never store anything within 18 inches of a water sprinkler head. Do not park linen hampers or food carts where they will block or hide a wall-mounted fire alarm pull station.
- Keep corridors and exits free of equipment that cannot be wheeled out of the way.
- Exit doors and fire doors should never be locked or blocked.
- Doors to maintenance areas, elevators, equipment rooms, and boiler rooms should always be kept closed.

First to Notice a Fire

If you enter a room where there is a fire or you are the first person to see a fire, do this:

1. Stop and quickly assess the situation.
2. Yell for help and sound an alarm if one is present.
3. Immediately remove all residents from the area. Do this quickly because smoke inhalation causes most deaths in fires, not the fire itself. If possible, turn off residents' oxygen.
4. Do not open the windows.
5. When everyone is out, close the door to the room. Most doors in health care facilities are fire doors. They help contain a fire for one to two hours.

6. Evacuate the residents from rooms on both sides of the room that is on fire.
7. Never open a closed door during a fire unless you have no other choice. If you must open a door, place your hand on it first to check if it is warm, and look for smoke coming from underneath. If the door is warm or you see smoke, do not open the door. Opening the door allows oxygen into the room, strengthening the fire and risking an explosion and serious injury.
8. Move residents at immediate risk to the end of the wing farthest from the fire or remove them from the wing or unit entirely if instructed to do so.
9. Use a fire extinguisher only if the fire is very small and contained, such as in a wastebasket. Do not try to fight a larger fire because it can get out of control quickly.

Fire Alarm on Another Wing or Unit

1. Follow your facility's emergency plan and the charge nurse's instructions.
2. Clear residents out of hallways into their rooms and close the doors. Remember that these are fire doors.
3. If several residents are in a gathering area, close the door to that room instead of moving them through fire doors to return them to their rooms. Act calmly and reassure the residents.
4. Make sure the halls are free from obstructions.

Evacuation

Evacuate residents per facility policy. The reason for having a priority order is that if evacuation began with bedridden residents who take more time to be moved, the process would take longer and more residents could potentially be trapped in the burning area. Moving ambulatory residents first means that more residents will be saved if the fire spreads quickly. Priority order for evacuation:

1. Those nearest the fire first
2. Ambulatory residents
3. Ambulatory residents who need assistance
4. Residents who use wheelchairs
5. Residents who are bedridden
6. Residents' charts and medication carts

Many facilities incorporate the RACE and PASS acronyms into the fire plan. The RACE acronym provides directions for responding to a fire.

R - Rescue/Remove all residents in immediate danger.

A - Alarm/Alert - activate the alarm and alert others of the fire.

C - Confine/Contain the fire if possible by closing doors.

E - Extinguish/Evacuate - if the fire is small, attempt to extinguish the fire. If the fire is too large to extinguish, leave the area and close the doors. The staff in charge or the fire department will give directions to evacuate if necessary.

The PASS acronym provides directions for using a fire extinguisher.

P - pull the pin the fire extinguisher.

A - aim the nozzle at the base of the fire.

S - squeeze the handle.

S - sweep from side to side.

Incident Reporting

Sometimes, no matter how careful everyone is in their efforts to prevent injuries, an accident does happen. As human beings, we're not perfect. Even if you follow the rules, a problem can occur. If an accident or injury does occur, you may need to complete an incident report. An incident is defined as something that goes wrong that should not happen again. Regardless of whether the incident involves equipment, staff, or a procedure failure, tell your supervisor immediately. The sooner a problem is reported, the sooner it can be corrected.

The Nurse Assistant Role in Emergency Care

As a nurse assistant, you must be prepared for emergencies and know how to respond. Being prepared helps prevent or at least control the chaos that often surrounds emergencies. When your facility holds emergency drills, treat the practice situation as you would a real emergency. When you are completely prepared and know what to do, the steps to take will be natural to you during an actual crisis. Know your facility's policies and procedures and where emergency equipment is located on the floor or unit where you work.

A resident's condition may suddenly worsen, or a resident may be injured unexpectedly or develop a life-threatening condition. These situations are medical emergencies. The first aid given to a resident in a medical emergency — before a physician or emergency medical professionals arrive — can prevent serious problems and even save their life. The goal of this initial treatment is to save the resident's life, prevent disability, and prevent an injury or sudden illness from getting worse. First aid is administered by a nurse assistant only until health care personnel with more training arrive and provide additional care.

What to Do

When an emergency situation arises with a resident, you must remain calm, stay with the person, call for help, and begin first aid. When help arrives, you are expected to assist as needed. When you first realize that an emergency is happening, ask yourself these questions:

- What exactly is the emergency?
- Do I know what to do?
- What should I do first?

The following are general guidelines for action in an emergency situation:

- If possible, use standard precautions and put on gloves.
- Remain calm, and let the resident know that you are there to help them.
- Do not move the resident unless you must remove them from a dangerous situation. Moving a resident if you are not properly trained could cause further injury.
- Know the codes your facility uses to identify emergencies. When a code is called, all staff must know what is happening so that valuable time is not lost.
- Keep an injured or suddenly ill resident warm by covering them with a blanket. If it is very hot, lightly cover them with a sheet.
- After the charge nurse arrives, you may be asked to call 911 or your local emergency number.
- When you speak with an emergency operator, provide this information: name, address, and telephone number of the facility, the nature of the emergency, and what type of first aid has been given.

Heart Attack

The heart is a muscular, hollow organ with four chambers (Figure 6-9). The heart pumps blood containing oxygen and nutrients to the entire body. The heart muscle itself needs a blood supply, and the coronary arteries supply it with oxygenated blood. When this blood supply is interrupted due to a blockage, a heart attack occurs. The clinical term for a heart attack is **myocardial infarction (MI)**. Blockage can occur due to **plaque** or protein, along with **cholesterol** in the lining of the arteries, breaking off and forming a clot. This clot then blocks the flow of blood.

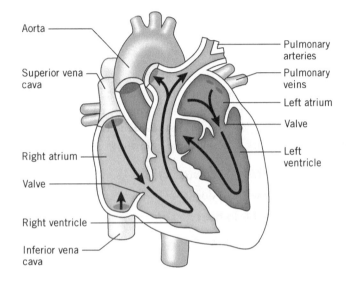

Figure 6-9 Major structures of the heart.

If a resident tells you that he or she is having chest pain, this is very serious. You must report it immediately. Chest pain is always considered a sign of a heart attack until the responding medical team determines the exact cause. The charge nurse may ask you to monitor the resident's pulse and blood pressure during the episode. You should immediately report any change in the resident's vital signs.

Many people having a heart attack do not experience chest pain, and women often experience symptoms that are different from those of men. Other signs and symptoms include:

- Dizziness (lightheadedness)
- Nausea or abdominal pain
- Anxiety
- Shortness of breath
- Pain in the head, neck, or upper body
- A sense of tightness or fullness in the chest
- Pain in one or both arms
- Weakness

- Pale skin color in a light-skinned person or an ashen skin tone in a dark-skinned person
- Cold, clammy sweat
- Palpitations (rapid or irregular heartbeat)

Residents may downplay their symptoms because they do not want to believe that something serious is wrong. If a resident shows any of these signs and symptoms, report them to the charge nurse immediately. Early treatment improves the chance of survival and can minimize damage to the heart muscle. Once you have notified the charge nurse, take the resident's vital signs, and help them to a comfortable position. Loosen tight clothes. Stay with them. Often the resident is frightened, so stay calm and reassure them that help is on the way.

Cardiac Arrest

Cardiac arrest is the sudden loss of heart function (no heartbeat). Cardiac arrest may result from various causes, including a heart attack. The signs include:

- No pulse
- Lack of normal breathing
- Pale, grayish skin color and blue lips
- Loss of consciousness

The treatment for cardiac arrest is **cardiopulmonary resuscitation (CPR)**. Many facilities have an automated external defibrillator (AED) that is used during cardiac arrest. An AED analyzes the heart rhythm and if necessary delivers an electrical shock to the heart. Each facility has its own protocol for treating a resident who is experiencing cardiac arrest. Know the procedure where you work.

Not all residents want to receive CPR. Some residents have signed a living will or advance medical directive stating that they do not wish to be resuscitated if their heart stops. If you find a resident who is not breathing and has no pulse, call for help immediately. Every second counts. The charge nurse knows which residents should receive CPR and those who should not. While all staff should be aware of do-not-resuscitate directives, the charge nurse can confirm the resident's status.

Depending on your facility's policy, you may need to learn how to assist with CPR. To administer CPR, you need special training and certification. If your facility does not offer CPR training, you can take a CPR course from the local American Red Cross, American Heart Association, or community hospital.

Choking

Many people die each year by choking. Choking usually happens when food or another object gets stuck in the throat. Residents are at risk of choking when:

- Their bites of food are too large or are poorly chewed.
- They talk or laugh too much while eating.
- Their dentures do not fit well.
- They have a chronic illness or stroke, which causes weakness and difficulty swallowing.

If the throat is completely blocked, this is called an airway obstruction. You must act quickly. You have only four to eight minutes to save the resident's life. A choking victim who is still conscious will usually grab or gesture at their throat (Figure 6-10). In some cases, the resident may already be unconscious when you find them.

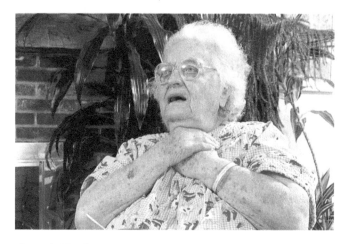

Figure 6-10 People who are choking tend to clutch at their throat.

PROCEDURE

6-4: First Aid for Choking

FOR A PERSON WHO IS SITTING OR STANDING:

1 Stand behind the resident.

2 Wrap your arms around the resident's waist, and lean the resident slightly forward.

3 Make a fist with one hand and place it on the resident's stomach below the rib cage and a little above the navel. Keep your thumb on their stomach, and place your other hand over your fist.

4 Sharply thrust your fist inward and upward. This causes a burst of air from the lungs that should dislodge the food or object.

5 Repeat the thrusts until the blockage is dislodged.

FOR A PERSON WHO HAS BECOME UNCONSCIOUS AFTER CHOKING:

1 If the resident is not already on the floor, gently lower them to the floor and call for help.

2 Once the resident is on the floor, position them on their back.

3 Kneel at the resident's side.

4 CPR should be initiated based on the facility's policy and patient directives.

5 Medical staff may ask you to monitor and assist with CPR, depending upon facility policy and your training

Signs of a complete airway obstruction include:

- Bluish skin, lips, and nails.
- Difficult, noisy breathing or not breathing at all.
- Inability to speak or cough with force.

With a partial airway obstruction, the resident can speak, breathe, and cough but may have difficulty breathing and may not be getting enough oxygen.

If the resident cannot eject the object from their throat by forceful coughing, assistance is likely needed from an emergency medical team. The charge nurse may ask you to call 911. It is important that you are familiar with the emergency equipment used in your facility because you may also be asked to get items such as oxygen and suction equipment.

When a resident is choking, you should:

1. Ask "Are you choking?" The resident will not be able to answer if his or her airway is completely blocked.
2. Call for help.
3. Never leave the resident. This is a life-threatening situation.
4. Administer first aid for choking (Procedure 6-4). When performed properly, the **Heimlich maneuver** (Figure 6-11) will dislodge the object from the resident's throat.

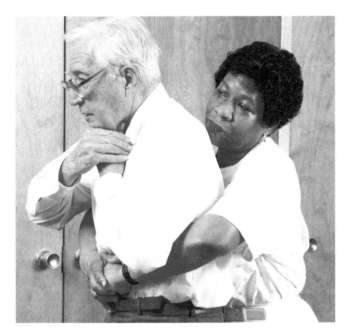

Figure 6-11 The Heimlich maneuver is used as part of first aid for choking victims.

Fainting is a temporary loss of consciousness caused by decreased blood flow to the brain. Residents who feel like they are going to faint, usually feel lightheaded, dizzy or nauseous. If a resident is feeling like they are going to faint, assist them to a lying or sitting position. If they are sitting you can have them put their head between their knees. If they are in a lying position, raise their legs about 12 inches off of the floor and loosen any constrictive clothing. If a resident faints, lower them to the floor and position them on their back and raise their feet unless injuries are noted to their head, spine or abdomen. Once a resident recovers encourage them to get up slowly. Notify your charge nurse immediately so the resident can be assessed.

Seizure

A **seizure** can be caused by many different conditions, including a brain tumor, infection in the brain or spinal cord, head injury, medications, poisoning, or a seizure disorder such as epilepsy. Often, residents with a seizure disorder are on medication. A seizure is abnormal electrical activity in the brain that produces sensory and behavioral changes and changes in consciousness.

Seizures may be classified as simple or complex. With a simple seizure, there is usually no loss of consciousness. A complex seizure usually involves a change in the level of consciousness. Seizures are also classified as generalized and partial seizures. The type of seizure depends on how much of the brain and body is affected. With generalized seizures, the entire brain is affected, and the resident may experience massive muscle spasms, fall to the floor, involuntarily urinate or defecate, and/or lose consciousness. **Epilepsy**, sometimes called a seizure disorder, is when seizures are not caused by a temporary medical condition.

To help a resident having a generalized seizure, you must remain calm and call for help immediately. Do not leave the resident alone, and reassure the resident that you are there to protect them. First aid measures are described in Procedure 6-5.

In a partial seizure, the abnormal activity happens in only part of the brain. In this case, symptoms are specific to the part of the brain affected, and only one side or part of the body is involved. A resident having a partial seizure may have a dazed, blank look and experience jerking movements of one part or side of the body. Sensory changes may also occur such as a prickling sensation or numbness. First aid may not be needed for this type of seizure, but you should remain with the resident and observe, report, and record what you see during the seizure.

6-5: First Aid for Generalized Seizure

1 To prevent a fall, help the resident to the floor.

2 Place something soft such as a folded towel, folded clothing, or a pillow (if one is available) under the resident's head.

3 Remove any nearby objects that could cause injury.

4 Turn the resident on his/her side to prevent aspiration and allow for drainage of saliva and vomit.

5 Do not put anything in the resident's mouth.

6 Do not try to hold the resident down or to stop the convulsions. The resident is not aware and cannot control the seizure activity.

7 Remove any tight jewelry the resident is wearing, especially around the neck.

8 Loosen any tight clothes (such as a belt or tie) to help the resident breathe better.

9 Do not give CPR unless the resident does not have a pulse or respirations after the seizure.

10 Do not give the resident anything by mouth until the seizure has stopped and they are fully awake and oriented.

11 Remain with the resident until the seizure is over. Reassure and comfort them as best you can. They may be confused, disoriented, frightened, or embarrassed.

12 Record the time the seizure began, the parts of the body involved, the strength of the activity, whether the resident lost bowel and bladder control, the resident's mental status, and how long the seizure lasted.

COMPLETION STEPS

1. Determine the resident's preferred position for comfort and ask them if they need anything else.
2. Examine the environment for safety and cleanliness.
3. Secure the call light and any other needed items within reach of the resident.
4. Perform hand hygiene.
5. Document the procedure and report any findings to the staff in charge.

Minutes or hours before a seizure, a resident may experience an aura. Often the aura involves one or more senses. For example, the resident may tell you that they smell a certain smell, have an odd taste in their mouth, see an odd light or spots before their eyes, or hear a particular sound. If the resident recognizes an aura from a past seizure, you can take measures to protect them from injury during the coming seizure.

Stroke

A stoke or cerebral vascular accident occurs when a blood vessel that carries blood to the brain becomes blocked or ruptures. According to the American Stroke Association, strokes are the fifth leading cause of death and a leading cause of disability in the United States. They report that 80 percent of strokes are preventable. As a nurse assistant, it is important to know the warning signs of a stroke. Early treatment increases survival rates and decreases disabilities.

The American Stroke Association uses the letters F. A. S. T. as warning signs to spot a stroke.

F - facial drooping
A - arm weakness
S - slurred speech
T - time to call 911

Other warning signs:

- Difficulty walking
- Sudden, severe headache
- Vision problems

- Confusion
- Numbness

You will learn more about strokes in chapter 11.

Burns

Burns may be caused by many different things such as a hot object, fire, hot water, too much sun, electricity, or chemicals. The first aid for all burns other than electrical burns is the same (Procedure 6-6). Electrical burns require different treatment (Procedure 6-7).

Hemorrhage

Hemorrhage is uncontrolled bleeding that results in excessive blood loss. The human body normally contains 5 to 6 quarts of blood. Losing a small amount of blood usually causes no harm. But if 1 to 2 quarts or more is lost, the situation is life threatening. This much blood loss may lead to shock and death.

Bleeding can be internal or external. While you cannot see internal bleeding, it may be indicated if the resident vomits blood, coughs up blood, or has blood in the urine or stool. They may complain of pain, lose consciousness, and go into shock. See Procedure 6-8 for first aid for internal hemorrhage. External hemorrhage results from a wound that is bleeding profusely. First aid for external hemorrhage is shown in Procedure 6-9.

Shock

Shock is a medical emergency in which the body's organs and tissues are not receiving enough blood and therefore are deprived of oxygen. This allows a dangerous build-up of waste products in the blood. There are many causes of shock, including an allergic reaction, an injury or wound, a heart problem or heart attack, a severe infection, and internal or external bleeding.

A resident who goes into shock may have these signs and symptoms:

- Pale, ashen, or bluish skin color
- Skin cool to the touch
- Vomiting
- Excessive thirst
- Weak, rapid pulse
- Decreased blood pressure
- Increased respirations
- Unconsciousness

Shock is an emergency that requires immediate medical attention. You need to call for help. The charge nurse may ask you to call 911. First aid steps for shock are described in Procedure 6-10.

Managing Your Emotions in an Emergency

When an emergency happens, it is natural to be nervous. You may feel yourself reacting with increased pulse and respiration. You may feel lightheaded and scared, especially at the sight of a wound that is bleeding. You may begin to sweat or have a sudden burst of energy. Whatever you feel, know that this is normal. The most important thing is to remain calm. Take a few deep breaths and steady yourself, if needed, as you prepare to give first aid.

Never let residents know that you are nervous or afraid. Remember your training. It is your job to comfort and reassure them while following the correct protocol for the situation. When you remain calm and in control, you are helping the resident feel confident that you are doing everything possible to assist them through a frightening episode.

6-6: First Aid for Burns

FOR BURNS NOT FROM AN ELECTRICAL SOURCE:

1 Remove the resident from the fire or the source of heat and call for help.

2 Depending on the size and degree of the burn, the charge nurse may ask you to run cool water over the burn.

3 If possible, remove any jewelry or clothing in the burned area that has not adhered to the burn.

4 Apply a clean, cotton cloth over the burn. Do not use a towel or blanket because loose fibers can stick to the burn.

5 Do not put soap, ointment, butter, oil, or margarine on the burn.

6 Keep the resident warm. The charge nurse will determine if the resident needs emergency help.

COMPLETION STEPS

1. Determine the resident's preferred position for comfort and ask them if they need anything else.
2. Examine the environment for safety and cleanliness.
3. Secure the call light and any other needed items within reach of the resident.
4. Perform hand hygiene.
5. Document the procedure and report any findings to the staff in charge.

6-7: First Aid for Electrical Burns

1 Make sure the resident is no longer in contact with the power source (electricity can travel to you if the power is still on). If the resident is in contact with the electricity, the power source must be turned off before you touch him or her.

2 Call for help, and lay the resident down. Raise the lower portion of the resident's body to reduce shock, if possible.

3 Check for breathing and circulation. Perform CPR if the resident has no pulse and respiration (depending upon facility policy and your training).

4 Once the charge nurse has determined that the resident is stable, you may be asked to run cool water over the burn.

5 If possible, remove any jewelry or clothing in the burned area that has not adhered to the burn.

6 Cover the burn with a clean, cotton cloth. Do not use a towel or blanket because loose fibers can stick to the burn.

7 Do not put soap, ointment, butter, oil, or margarine on the burn.

8 Keep the resident warm. The charge nurse will determine if the resident needs emergency help.

COMPLETION STEPS

1. Determine the resident's preferred position for comfort and ask them if they need anything else.
2. Examine the environment for safety and cleanliness.
3. Secure the call light and any other needed items within reach of the resident.
4. Perform hand hygiene.
5. Document the procedure and report any findings to the staff in charge.

6-8: First Aid for Internal Hemorrhage

1 Keep the resident warm, and call for help.

2 Do not try to move the resident unless the resident is vomiting.

3 If the resident is vomiting, place them on their side to prevent aspiration and maintain an open airway.

4 Elevate the resident's legs about 12 inches off the bed or floor if they are on their back and there is no injury to the neck, back, or legs.

5 Do not give the resident anything to eat or drink.

6 The charge nurse will determine what other steps to take.

COMPLETION STEPS

1. Determine the resident's preferred position for comfort and ask them if they need anything else.
2. Examine the environment for safety and cleanliness.
3. Secure the call light and any other needed items within reach of the resident.
4. Perform hand hygiene.
5. Document the procedure and report any findings to the staff in charge.

6-9: First Aid for External Bleeding

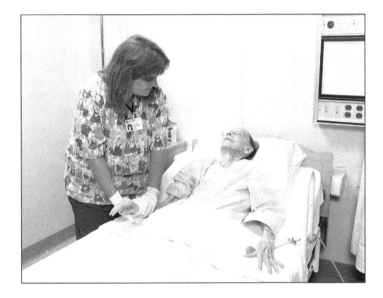

1 Call for help, but do not leave the resident alone.

2 If possible, use standard precautions.

3 Place a clean cloth over the bleeding wound.

4 Put pressure on the wound with the palm of your hand until the bleeding stops.

5 If you can, elevate the wound above the level of the resident's heart to slow the bleeding

6 Do not apply a tourniquet to stop the bleeding. Applying a tourniquet may cause unnecessary tissue death or even loss of a limb. The charge nurse will determine what additional steps to take.

COMPLETION STEPS

1. Determine the resident's preferred position for comfort and ask them if they need anything else.
2. Examine the environment for safety and cleanliness.
3. Secure the call light and any other needed items within reach of the resident.
4. Perform hand hygiene.
5. Document the procedure and report any findings to the staff in charge.

1 Call for help. The charge nurse may ask you to call 911.

2 Keep the resident warm and do not try to move the resident unless they are vomiting.

3 If the resident is vomiting, place them on their side to prevent aspiration and maintain an open airway.

4 If they are on their back and there is no injury to the neck, back, or legs, then elevate their legs slightly off the bed or floor.

5 If the resident is bleeding externally, place a clean cloth over the wound, put pressure on it, and elevate the wound above the level of the resident's heart, if possible.

6 Do not give the resident anything to eat or drink unless instructed to do so. The charge nurse will determine if emergency help is required.

COMPLETION STEPS

1. Determine the resident's preferred position for comfort and ask them if they need anything else.

2. Examine the environment for safety and cleanliness.

3. Secure the call light and any other needed items within reach of the resident.

4. Perform hand hygiene.

5. Document the procedure and report any findings to the staff in charge.

Points to Remember

- Protecting residents, staff, and yourself from bloodborne pathogens is an important part of your job. You must exercise care in the handling of sharps and follow facility procedures for all care activities to prevent the spread of infection.

- Injury prevention involves using proper body mechanics when lifting and moving objects and residents and in all daily care tasks.

- You can prevent resident falls through careful monitoring and the use of assistive devices when needed.

- Being aware of chemical, electrical, and other environmental hazards is part of your role in preventing injury to yourself and others.

- Disaster preparedness includes knowing the facility's disaster plan and what your responsibilities are in keeping residents safe.

- The nurse assistant has a specific role in an emergency. You must understand emergency procedures and first aid guidelines and know how to assist if a resident experiences situations such as choking, falling, bleeding, burns, seizure, stroke, or heart attack.

acquired immunodeficiency syndrome (AIDS) — severe disorder of the immune system caused by the human immunodeficiency virus (HIV)

antibody — protein produced by the body to fight infection or illness

aura — a sensation that often precedes a seizure

bloodborne pathogens — pathogen present in blood that can be transmitted via blood or body fluids

body mechanics — principles of proper body movement for efficiency and injury prevention

cardiac arrest — complete cessation of heart activity (no heartbeat)

cardiopulmonary resuscitation (CPR) — emergency procedure to restore cardiopulmonary function

cholesterol — fatty substance produced by the body and ingested in food

epilepsy — sometimes called a seizure disorder, a disorder in which the seizures are not caused by a temporary medical condition

ergonomics — study of the interaction of workers and their environment; its principles drive the design of equipment and work environments

external evacuation — moving residents out of the facility to another site for safety

fainting — a temporary loss of consciousness caused by decreased blood flow to the brain

fall — unintentionally coming to rest on the ground, floor, or other. lower level, but not as a result of an overwhelming external force

gait belt — also known as a transfer belt, used to help steady a resident during transfers or walking

Heimlich maneuver — emergency procedure to dislodge food or an object obstructing the airway

hemorrhage — excessive or uncontrolled bleeding

hepatitis — viral infection of the liver

human immunodeficiency virus (HIV) — virus that causes AIDS

internal evacuation — moving residents to another location within the facility for safety

myocardial infarction — damage to an area of the heart due to lack of blood supply and oxygen; commonly called a heart attack

plaque — fatty deposit on blood vessel walls

regulated waste — contaminated waste that must be disposed of according to facility policies and government regulations

seizure — abnormal electrical activity in the brain that causes sudden, involuntary muscle movements

shock — medical emergency in which body tissues and organs are not receiving adequate blood and oxygen

stroke — also known as a cerebral vascular incident, occurs when a blood vessel that carries blood to the brain becomes blocked or ruptures

▷ Check Your Knowledge

1. **Which of these actions will help to prevent resident falls?**

   a. Eliminate clutter in the resident's room
   b. Be sure all residents eat their meals
   c. Limit the number of times you move the resident
   d. Move the resident's personal things, like eyeglasses, out of the way

2. **The purpose of ergonomics is:**

   a. To help workers buy better health insurance
   b. To help workers cope with stress
   c. To design better care plans for residents
   d. To prevent injuries in the work place

3. **What is the first step you take to prevent being injured when caring for a resident?**

   a. Determine the resident's capabilities
   b. Weigh the resident
   c. Ask someone to help
   d. Stand straight and bend at the knee

4. **What device is used to help steady a resident during transfers or walking?**

   a. A footboard
   b. A transfer board
   c. A gait belt
   d. A pivot disc

5. **Safety Data Sheets (SDS) list a substance's chemical contents, fire and health hazard and:**

   a. Precautions
   b. Clean-up procedures
   c. Disposal requirements
   d. All of these

6. **If a resident is hemorrhaging from a leg wound, what should you do to control bleeding?**

   a. Put firm, steady pressure on the wound with your gloved hand
   b. Put an ice pack on it
   c. Leave the resident alone and go get help
   d. Start CPR immediately

7. **The Heimlich maneuver is used with a resident who is:**

   a. Vomiting
   b. Feeling nauseated
   c. Having a seizure
   d. Choking

8. **One of the residents has burned his hand on a hot light bulb. You should:**

   a. Put butter on the burn
   b. Take the resident outside in the cool air
   c. Run cool water over the burn
   d. Put rubbing alcohol on it

9. **If an evacuation is ordered due to a fire, residents should be evacuated in this order:**

   a. Ambulatory residents
   b. Those nearest the fire first
   c. Bedridden residents
   d. Residents who use wheelchairs

10. **In addition to chest pain, some other signs and symptoms of a heart attack include:**

    a. Shortness of breath
    b. Cold, clammy skin
    c. Both of these
    d. Neither of these

7

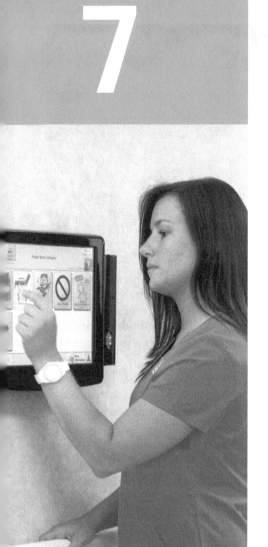

Documentation and Core Nursing Skills

From your first minute on the job, you are flooded with information. You are listening, observing, and reading and also talking, being observed, and recording information. Providing the highest quality care depends on clear, thorough, and accurate information. Residents and other health care team members depend on the information you communicate.

Centers for Medicare and Medicaid Services (CMS) guidelines require that facilities collect standard data for every resident using an instrument called the Minimum Data Set (MDS). The interdisciplinary team uses the MDS to develop the resident's care plan. It is also used by state and regulatory officials to evaluate the facility and to obtain Medicare or Medicaid reimbursement.

It is important to accurately record your observations about residents' physical and psychological status, as well as about their social and recreational activities. Much of the information collected about residents comes from the physical examination, including the resident's vital signs, height, and weight. Data collection begins when the resident is admitted to the facility. It is an ongoing process in which you will play a critical role. The information you collect becomes part of the resident's medical record.

In this chapter, you will learn why accurate **documentation** is critically important and how information should be recorded. You will also learn your role in the admission, transfer, and discharge processes and how to make each a positive experience for the residents you care for.

OBJECTIVES:

- Name the sources of information about residents.

- Explain the difference between objective and subjective information.

- Explain your role in the care planning process.

- Explain when and how to report and document information about the resident.

- Explain your role in the history and physical examination and the admission process.

- Demonstrate methods for taking vital signs: temperature, pulse rate, respiration rate, and blood pressure.

- Demonstrate how to measure height and weight using an upright scale.

- Explain why protecting residents' privacy is so important and describe measures you can take to ensure their privacy.

- Demonstrate how to make an unoccupied and an occupied bed.

- Demonstrate the use of a call system.

- Describe your role in transferring and discharging a resident.

Gathering Information

Gathering information is an important job responsibility required by regulations. The health care team relies on the information you record as you care for residents. Some documentation may be used months or years later. You and other staff members can verify facts with certainty at a later time because you recorded them accurately.

You have learned that giving the best care possible means that you must get to know the resident. As you provide care, you will receive information from residents and others. This information will be used to create the resident's care plan, which provides an interdisciplinary approach for each resident's care. If you are unsure of anything when talking with members of the team, the resident, or family members, just ask. Don't make assumptions. Asking questions and clarifying information are important forms of communication for the whole team. There are many sources of information about residents. The following sections describe the most common sources.

Residents

Residents are the main source of information about themselves. They can give you valuable information about their needs and care preferences. Some residents might be confused or tell you something that they wish were true. When you have questions, you must verify facts with the charge nurse. It is especially important to listen to and report or document residents' feelings and preferences. This enables other members of the health care team to better understand the residents and give more personalized care.

The Medical Record

A resident's health record is also known as the medical record or the chart. The medical record is the primary communication tool used by the interdisciplinary team. It is also a legal record of a resident's stay in the facility. The chart can be in the form of an **electronic medical record (EMR)**. In this case, information is documented using a computer system and specific software. Or the chart can be maintained as a paper record (Figure 7-1).

As the basic tool for planning, recording, and evaluating a resident and their care, the chart helps organize the information gathered about a resident. All information in a resident's chart is confidential and belongs to the facility. Because it is a record of each resident's condition and care, it must be complete and accurate.

[handwritten note: not in record, legally didn't happen]

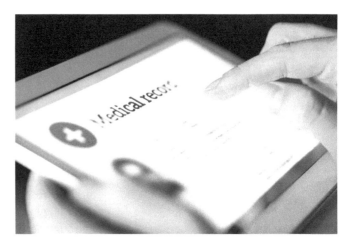

Figure 7-1 The resident's medical record (chart) includes information such as the medical history, care plan, and documentation of ongoing care.

There is a common saying: "If it isn't in the record, it didn't happen." Weeks, months, or years later, no one will clearly remember facts that are not properly documented.

It will be as if a situation never happened. The purpose of the resident's chart is to provide accurate, permanent information about the resident that can be used by the facility, the staff, and the resident.

A typical chart has many different sections or components, including the resident's medical history (past conditions and events), current records, and care plans. All team members record information in the chart. Most charts include the following types of information:

- Identifying information (resident's name, medical record number, birth date, etc.), often on a form called the **face sheet** *[handwritten: NEVER ERASE]*
- Admission papers outlining the reason for admission
- Permission forms signed by the resident or his/her representative, such as a consent for treatment form, and legal documents such as a do-not-resuscitate order
- Physician's orders that may include orders and notes from a clinical nurse practitioner, physician assistant, and other consulting physicians
- Progress notes from various health care team members, such as nurses, the dietician, respiratory therapist, and physical therapist
- Test results such as lab test and hearing test reports and X-rays and other diagnostic imaging results
- Graphs or **flow sheets** used for recording nursing activities, such as vital signs, weights, bowel movements, activities of daily living (ADLs), and intake and output (I & O) of food and fluids

[handwritten note: – line through it, initial + date]

Nurse assistants often document information by using an electronic device called a **kiosk**. or writing it out on a hard copy form. Electronic documentation may consist of information about the resident's functional status and flow sheets may be used to document objective information. This information consists of facts based on what you can see, hear, smell, or touch. Each flow sheet is used for only one type of information, such as the vital signs record, the intake and output record, and the weight chart. Flow sheets make it easier to see changes in residents over time. You can evaluate your observations by comparing them with previous findings. As you record facts about residents, you and other members of the care team can monitor their progress and notice changes that could become problems if not addressed in a timely manner.

Other departments also document information in the medical record. These parts of the chart describe how the team is working together to help a resident reach their goals.

In some facilities, paper records are kept together in a holder like a notebook. When EMRs are used, the information can be accessed and updated using a computer system. In your orientation, you will learn your facility's requirements for documentation.

Other Means of Communication

Other communication devices may be used to provide additional information about residents. Different facilities use different systems. You will learn about these in your orientation.

Words and symbols on residents' door cards may be used. A *door card* is the name sign on or beside the door to a resident's room. In some facilities, colored dots on door cards identify blind or deaf residents who would need special help in an emergency. Other signs with words or symbols that are posted by the resident's bed may provide additional information. Be sure you understand all this information.

Staff, Family, and Friends

Other staff members will tell you about residents. Facility staff in other departments who have worked with a resident often have valuable information. Other nurse assistants also have information you can use in providing individualized care. Family members and visitors can also tell you a good deal about residents. Be sure to verify any information obtained from family or friends because they may not always know the full situation.

Policies and Procedures and Privacy Laws

Facility **policies and procedures (P&Ps)** are rules for how work is to be performed in the facility. P&Ps spell out how and why things are done; they provide guidance that helps you care for residents in specific situations. Always follow facility policies and procedures to ensure that your actions are correct. The Health Insurance Portability and Accountability Act (HIPAA) of 1996 is a federal law that set standards to protect patients' health information. This law covers privacy issues related to the resident's care, including who has access to personal health information (PHI); also known as protected health information. During your orientation, your facility will provide you with more information about HIPAA and the guidelines that you must follow.

Assessing the Resident

> vital signs

Your observation of a resident is an excellent source of information. Objective information is factual information. You obtain objective information by looking, listening, smelling, and touching. Good observation skills involve focusing on detail. You will know more about the situation if you use all your senses. Objective information includes vital signs or lab results.

Subjective information is your guess or opinion about what you observe. Subjective information also includes what residents tell you about how they feel, such as when they complain about pain or dizziness. Subjective information can be very helpful as long as you identify it as resident's feeling or your own feeling or opinion. Accurate observations and reports incorporate both subjective and objective information. The key is to use language that clearly differentiates facts from feelings.

Health care includes many assessments of a resident and their condition. The first step in assessment is to gather data. This includes objective information. As a nurse assistant, you are a key part of this process, especially gathering data, because you spend so much time with residents. All other departments depend on your careful and accurate observations. You will hear the nurse talk about this assessment process, which is often called "completing the MDS."

The most important assessment tool used for all residents in a Medicaid or Medicare facility is the **Resident Assessment Instrument (RAI)**. This assessment was developed to improve resident quality of care. The RAI has three components (Figure 7-2):

- The Minimum Data Set (MDS)

- Care Area Assessment (CAAs)
- RAI Utilization Guidelines

The MDS is a standardized assessment that is the foundation of the RAI process and provides for a more thorough assessment and development of the care plan. As a nurse assistant, you have an important role in providing accurate documentation that will be used when completing the MDS. You will be required to document how each resident performs specific activities of daily living (ADL's) and how much assistance you are providing. ADLs include toileting, transferring, eating, walking, bed mobility, and dressing. Since a resident's abilities may change throughout the day, it is important to document immediately after care is provided. For example, a resident may be more independent or require less assistance with ADL's in the morning, but by bedtime they are tired and require more assistance from staff. It is a best practice to document as soon as possible after care is provided.

The completed MDS will provide a list of potential problems for the resident. The nurse will use the CAA process for every problem that is identified. The CAAs are used to develop the residents' individual care plan. The RAI utilization guidelines are instructions on when and how to use the RAI.

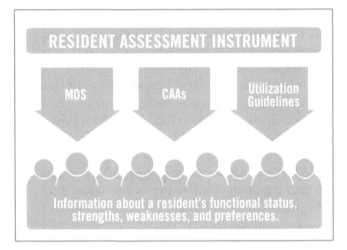

Figure 7-2 The MDS and CAAs are part of the Resident Assessment Instrument (RAI).

Resident Care Plan

A **care plan** is a document that lists a resident's needs and goals as well as the actions and approaches the interdisciplinary team will use to help the resident to meet their goals. Many health professionals in the facility have input into the plan, and all staff use the plan to ensure consistent care.

The care plan is based on assessments of the resident done upon admission and ongoing assessments throughout their stay. However, the plan is never considered "finished" because it must be updated as the resident changes. Change means either improvement or decline in any area. It also changes because of information that you and other staff gather about the resident's needs, preferences, strengths, weaknesses, and goals.

The care plan lists each resident's medical, nursing, and psychosocial needs, often listed as problems. For each problem, an objective or goal is written. Your observations and experience with a resident are especially important for developing the care plan and keeping it up to date. By observing the resident, you can report whether the care plan is working.

How to Report Information

You report different information in a number of different ways. Usually, you report to the charge nurse, but sometimes you need to report to other staff members. Since all staff must maintain the confidentiality of information about a resident, you can safely report to other members of the interdisciplinary team. However, when reporting verbally, use a private location so others will not overhear you.

Most of your reports are made directly to another staff member, and you must be careful to not reveal confidential information when talking with family members and visitors. If you are ever unsure about sharing information, then check with the charge nurse before you speak with anyone else.

Types of Reporting

You will provide three main types of reports: routine reports, immediate reports, and "by a certain time" reports:

- **Routine reporting** — At the end of your shift, you report to the charge nurse about the residents you cared for and the care you provided. Report information that is not time-sensitive and can wait until the end of the shift.
- **Immediate reporting** — Some observations must be reported immediately. You must immediately report any situation that would be considered dangerous for the resident (Figure 7-3), staff, or visitors.
- **"By a certain time" reporting** — This type involves information that is needed by a set time. Examples are set times for vital signs to be recorded or weights to be documented, per physician's orders.

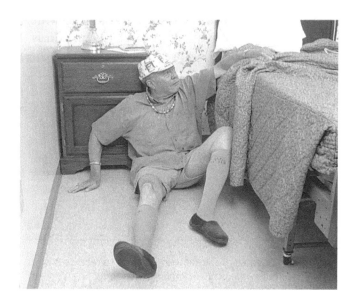

Figure 7-3 Some information must be reported immediately, such as a resident's fall.

Your Role in Documentation

The facility maintains many kinds of written information and reports. In addition to residents' charts, you will also document information using worksheets and forms such as incident reports. Most written records communicate information to other staff. But documentation may be used for other purposes, such as by an insurance company or in a court case. Review of a resident's medical records can occur months after the documentation was completed so having precise accurate records eliminates the need to rely on memory for specific details. Nurse assistants follow the same guidelines for documentation as all other health professionals.

Even documentation that seems routine is important. When you are documenting, you may discover something that also needs to be reported. You report this information to the nurse in addition to documenting it in the resident's record. Documentation involves watching for trends and changes to assist the staff in identifying potential problems early on.

Each facility has their own processes for how a nurse assistant can document. You must be sure that you understand your facility's policies and procedures for your role in creating and maintaining documentation.

In some facilities, nurse assistants write progress notes. These are notes about a resident and the care you give. This information is listed by date and may include:

- General statements of care given
- The resident's appointments and activities
- Any complaints from the resident
- General statements about the resident's psychological well-being
- Reports of visitors, including physician visits

Some facilities use checklists that require only your initials and simple documentation. You may record intake and output numbers directly in the chart or on worksheets that the unit clerk or charge nurse later records in the chart. Your facility may use a combination of different charting methods; some items may be documented on paper, while others are recorded electronically.

Electronic Documentation

As the world of health care advances, changes will occur in the methods and systems you use. Each year, more facilities make the shift to electronic documentation systems. You will need to understand the specifics of your facility's system. Timely and precise reporting of residents' condition is one of your priorities. When using an electronic system, accuracy becomes even more important. When documenting electronically, entries are time and date stamped automatically. Refer to your facility's policy for documenting late entries or if an entry was recorded in the wrong medical record. It can be difficult to correct a mistake within an electronic system and may require the assistance of your charge nurse. If you are uncertain what to do or how to use the system, check with your supervisor for guidance.

Guidelines for Documentation

Common sense rules apply to chart documentation. Chart entries must be clear and easy to read. Follow the documentation guidelines shown in Box 7-1 to ensure accuracy and prevent misunderstandings. Remember that the chart is a legal record. If entries in the chart cannot be read or seem incorrect or as if they have been altered, it makes it difficult to be certain of the facts.

Documentation should be completed at the point-of-care, or as soon as possible after care was provided. Documenting immediately after caring for the resident gives a more accurate account of when the care was provided and what care was given. Documentation should occur more than once a shift. For example, if you assist a resident to the bathroom three times during your shift, there should be three entries to reflect the care provided.

Box 7-1

GENERAL GUIDELINES FOR WRITTEN DOCUMENTATION

- The resident's name should appear on every page of the chart. It is written on each new page before any other information is entered.
- Write all entries in permanent blue or black ink. Do not use pencil or felt-tip markers (can smear when wet).
- Write each entry clearly so it is easy to read. Print or write neatly.
- Record the date and time of each entry as required.
- Document only your own actions and observations.
- Use standard medical terminology and abbreviations.
- Charting is continuous. Do not leave spaces or skip lines between entries.
- Sign each entry and include your title after your name. In some cases, you may initial the entry when your signature is somewhere else on the form.
- Do not make changes to chart entries unless you have made an error. If you make an error, correct it immediately and properly.

Correcting an Error in Written Documentation

The resident's chart and most forms that you use are legal records. People who look at records for legal purposes examine alterations closely. Attorneys, state surveyors and other inspectors, and insurance company officials may carefully inspect residents' records. To prevent problems and misunderstandings, all health professionals use a standard method for correcting mistakes in hard-copy documentation.

If you make a mistake, you must correct it so that accurate information is recorded. For example, if you misspell a word, you must correct it to prevent a possible misunderstanding. Follow facility policy when making corrections. These steps to explain how to make corrections in written documentation:

1. Draw a single line through the incorrect word or entry. Do not cover an error with an X or scribble over it, because readers must be able to tell what was originally written.
2. Print "Void, or Mistaken Entry" above or beside the incorrect word or entry
3. Add your initials and the date above it.
4. Clearly write the correct word before continuing (Figure 7-4).
5. For mistakes in flow charts, circle the mistake, write in the correction, and add the date and your initials in the margin or on the back of the sheet.

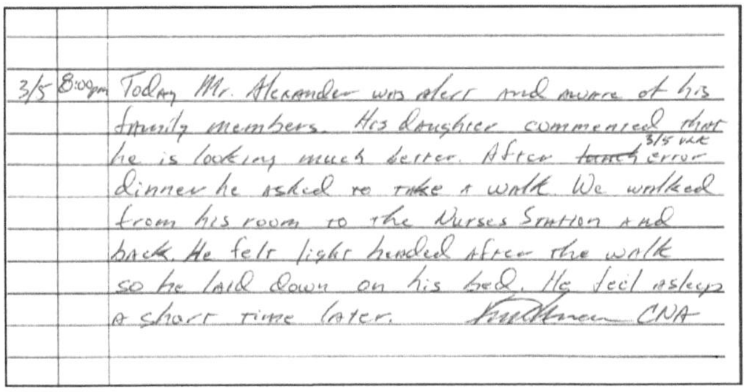
3/5 8:00pm Today Mr. Alexander was alert and aware of his family members. His daughter commented that he is looking much better. After ~~lunch~~ 3/5 MK error dinner he asked to take a walk. We walked from his room to the Nurses Station and back. He felt light headed after the walk so he laid down on his bed. He fell asleep a short time later. CNA

Figure 7-4 Example of a correction in a written record. Always follow the proper procedure for correcting errors in paper and electronic records.

Common Medical Terms and Abbreviations

Medical terminology is a language of its own. You will need to master many of these terms and abbreviations because they are used throughout the medical record. As you gain more experience, the language will become familiar to you. Keep in mind that the "medical speak" that is appropriate in the medical record is most likely not understandable to people who are not in the health professions. Residents, family members, visitors, new staff members, and employees in other departments may find the terminology to be very confusing.

Most facilities use many of the same standard terms and abbreviations. Some facilities use their own variations of certain terms. Never be embarrassed to ask what something means. It is much worse not to ask and guess wrong. Commonly used medical terms are included in the Glossary (Appendix A), and common abbreviations are shown in Appendix B.

Remember that it is more important to document information clearly than to use complicated medical terms. Sometimes health professionals think that they must use an "official" medical term when they could have used a simpler term that communicated the information more clearly to the rest of the staff.

History and Physical Examination

To clearly understand a resident's total physical, psychological, and social needs, a history must be taken and a physical examination performed. Together, this process is known as the **history and physical (H&P)**. The exam is always performed by a physician or designated health care provider when a resident is admitted to a facility. An examination is also done when a resident becomes ill. Your role is to assist the resident and the physician (or nurse) before and during the examination. You may be responsible for gathering information, providing equipment and supplies, and handling laboratory specimens. During the exam, health care team members use communication, documentation, and reporting skills while collecting subjective and objective information.

Along with the physical examination, the resident's vital signs are taken, and height and weight are measured — these provide basic information about the resident's health status. Later in this chapter you will learn these skills. At the beginning of the resident's first physical examination, a history is usually taken.

Purpose of the History

The purpose of obtaining an accurate history is to learn as much about the resident as possible. An accurate history is the basic foundation for collecting data and understanding the resident's needs or problems. Residents who can provide information have an opportunity to share information about their past and present health issues and how they feel at the time of the exam. The staff gains insight into the person's habits, lifestyle, and beliefs. With permission of the resident, ask the physician if you can listen in while the history is taken. This is a good way for you to get to know the resident if he or she is comfortable with your participation.

Sometimes the resident's health problems mean that the person cannot provide information to the team. Instead, information in the resident's record and from family members and friends is used. In such cases, the physician will explain to the person providing information why accurate data is needed to ensure that the resident receives the best possible care.

Many residents now have a personal health record (PHR). This record may be in written or electronic form. An electronic PHR may be stored with a web-based service or on a memory card or flash drive. Before taking a resident's history, a health care professional should always ask them or their health care representative if a PHR exists. If a PHR does exist, the health care professional should first review the PHR and then ask questions to clarify or update that information.

Collecting the History Data

The history includes certain categories of information. It usually includes the following components:

- Identification information (name, date of birth, previous address, etc.)
- Chief complaint (also called chief concern) — if the resident has an immediate medical issue
- History of present illness (background on current health issues)
- Past medical and surgical history
- Allergies
- Current medications (prescription and over-the-counter)
- Social history (occupation, marital status, and lifestyle information such as diet, exercise, drug/alcohol/tobacco use, and sexual activity)
- Family history (age and cause of death of close relatives; family history of disease)
- Subjective review of systems (questions about the various body systems)

Nurse Assistant's Role in the Physical Examination

Once the history is complete, the physician proceeds with the physical examination. This begins with an objective review of body systems. This systematic approach provides both subjective and objective information about the residents' health.

Your role in the physical examination is to ensure the resident's safety, comfort, and privacy. You are also responsible for:

- Applying the principles of standard precautions
- Preparing the equipment the physician will use
- Covering the examination table with clean disposable paper
- Measuring the resident's height and weight and accurately recording this information
- Taking the resident's vital signs and accurately recording this information
- Assisting the resident with undressing, putting on the gown, and dressing after the exam
- Helping the resident onto the examination table and providing pillows and a warm blanket, if needed
- Assisting the physician with positioning the resident safely during the exam
- Draping the resident during the exam
- Collecting, labeling, and depositing specimens in the area designated for pick-up and transport to the lab (Figure 7-5)

- Providing the physician with equipment needed during the examination
- Reassuring and comforting the resident, if necessary
- Assisting the resident as needed after the examination

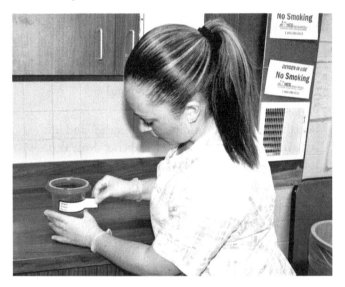

Figure 7-5 Nurse assistant labeling a specimen immediately after collection.

Techniques Used in Physical Examination

The physician uses various techniques to assess the resident's physical health during the physical examination. Inspection (observing the resident's body) provides valuable visual information about the resident's health status. Palpation (a method of touching) helps the physician determine the condition of internal structures and organs by feel. This technique also enables the physician to locate any areas of tenderness or pain. Percussion (tapping on a body area) helps to determine if an area or organ is solid, air-filled, or fluid-filled. Auscultation (listening to body sounds using a stethoscope) can reveal abnormalities in function. The sense of smell is also used during the physical exam. Abnormal odors can help determine whether a resident has an infection, liver problems, or other conditions.

After the physical examination, you have a very important role — to listen to and acknowledge any fears or concerns the resident has and to explain what the next steps will be. The resident may be very anxious about the findings and any tests that are ordered. If you know the time frame, tell the resident when to expect more information. You can play an important role in assisting the physician and making the exam process as comfortable as possible for the resident.

Taking and Recording Vital Signs

As the nurse assistant helping with the physical examination or admitting the resident to the facility, you are responsible for taking and recording the resident's vital signs. Vital signs is the term used to describe a person's temperature, pulse rate, respiration rate, and blood pressure. The inclusion of the word "vital" shows their importance — they are crucial measurements of life functions.

Vital signs are always taken (measured) as part of the initial admission physical examination and during the resident's stay as ordered by the physician. Vital signs are always taken if a resident has any physical, mental, social, or other change that might signal an illness. Facilities usually have a protocol for how often vital signs are taken. Vital signs are recorded in the resident's record or on a special form so that the health care team can evaluate the significance of any changes or abnormalities.

Take vital signs correctly and record them accurately. Vital signs are usually recorded with abbreviations: T for temperature, P for pulse, R for respiration, and BP for blood pressure. For example: T 98.6, P 86, R 20, and BP 120/80.

Nurses and physicians rely heavily on accurate records to decide whether and how to treat a resident's condition. Medications are often ordered based on records of vital signs. If a resident's vital signs change, cannot be taken, or seem abnormal to you, tell the charge nurse immediately. If you are ever unsure about the vital signs you take, get immediate help from your supervisor.

Temperature

Body temperature is a measurement of body heat, and normal temperature may vary by person, age, activity, or time of day. A person's temperature normally changes a bit over the course of a day. The lowest reading is usually in the morning before the person wakes. The highest is in the late afternoon and evening. Normal body temperature has always been considered to be 98.6°F, but some studies have shown that body temperature can vary from 97°F to 99°F. Since a normal temperature may vary by person, it is important to establish a baseline temperature for each resident.

A higher-than-normal temperature is commonly called a fever. Fever may indicate an infection or an allergic reaction to a medication, food, or other substance. An older resident's temperature does not fluctuate as much as a younger person's, even in these situations. A resident with a fever often has other signs and symptoms of infection or illness.

There are six ways to measure body temperature with a thermometer:

- Oral (in the mouth)
- Rectal (in the rectum)
- Axillary (under the arm)
- Tympanic (in the ear with a probe)
- Temporal scan (on the forehead with a probe)
- Non-Contact Infrared (NCIT) (usually directed toward the forehead)

Normal temperature ranges vary by body site. The thermometer is also kept in place for different lengths of time in different locations. Table 7-1 shows the normal ranges using various methods, and Table 7-2 summarizes information on the different types of thermometers.

When reporting and recording temperatures, it is important to note what method was used to measure the temperature since normal ranges may vary.

Table 7-1 Normal Temperature Ranges

Method of Measuring Temperature	Normal Temperature Range	Average
Oral (in the mouth)	97.6°F to 99.6°F	98.6°F
Axillary (under the armpit)	96.6°F to 98.6°F	97.6°F
Rectal (in the rectum)	98.6°F to 100.6°F	99.6°F
Tympanic (in the ear)	96.6°F to 98.6°F	97.6°F
Temporal (on the forehead)	98.6°F to 100.6°F	99.6°F

Table 7-2 Types of Thermometers

Type of Thermometer	Description	Guidelines
Oral glass thermometer	■ Blue top and long, narrow or small, rounded tip	■ Non-mercury glass thermometers are used. ■ Non-lubricated disposable cover is used.
Axillary glass thermometer	■ Has a long bulb	■ Non-mercury glass thermometers are used. ■ Non-lubricated disposable cover is used.
Rectal glass thermometer	■ Red top and a rounded tip to prevent injury to rectal tissue	■ Non-mercury glass thermometers are used. ■ Lubricated disposable cover is used.
Electronic digital thermometers (most commonly used type)	■ Various types may be used to take oral, axillary, and rectal temperatures. ■ Temperature is displayed on the front of the device. ■ Some have a battery and an auto-shut-off mechanism that turns off after 60 seconds; others are recharged on a charging base.	■ Disposable probe covers are used. ■ Use a blue tip for oral/axillary temps and a red tip for rectal temp. ■ Insert thermometer, wait for beep; after the beep, temperature is displayed.
Tympanic (ear) probe	■ Electronic device that measures heat from blood vessels in the eardrum	■ Probe is placed in the ear. Wait for beep; after the beep, temperature is displayed.
Temporal scan	■ Electronic device	■ Probe is placed in the middle of the forehead. User presses Scan button and slides the probe across the forehead toward the hairline. After 30 seconds, the scan shuts off and the temperature is displayed.
Disposable thermometer	■ Has a chemical dot that changes color when heated	■ Chemical change can be seen in 45 to 60 seconds.
Temperature-sensitive tape	■ Tape strip for use on the forehead or abdomen	■ Tape changes color in about 15 seconds in response to body heat.
Non-contact infrared thermometer (NCIT)	■ Electronic device that is pointed toward the forehead and measures skin or surface temperature	■ Device is pointed toward the forehead. Trigger is pressed and temperature is displayed.

Precautions When Using a Glass Thermometer

Electronic digital thermometers are the type most commonly used. Because glass thermometers are easily broken, most facilities do not use glass thermometers. If glass thermometers are used, they do not contain mercury.

Oral Temperature

An oral temperature is the method used most often (Procedure 7-1). An oral temperature should not be taken when a resident:

- Is receiving oxygen with a mask or has trouble breathing
- Is confused or combative
- Has a mouth disorder or gum disease or has had recent oral surgery
- Is paralyzed on one side of the mouth (as after a stroke) and cannot hold the thermometer in place
- Is in a coma

PROCEDURE

7-1: Taking an Oral Temperature with an Electronic Thermometer

PREPARATION STEPS

1. Check the care plan.
2. Knock, introduce yourself, and address resident by preferred name.
3. Perform hand hygiene.
4. Gather supplies and secure assistance if needed.
5. Explain procedure and ask about resident preferences.
6. Respect privacy and rights at all times.

ITEMS NEEDED

- Electronic thermometer and probe cover
- Chart or form for recording temperature
- Pen
- Gloves (if there is a possibility of contact with body fluids)

1. First, check with the resident to make sure that they have not consumed anything hot or cold or smoked within the last 10 minutes. If they have, wait 5 to 10 minutes before proceeding.

2. Put on gloves if there is a possibility of contact with body fluids.

3. Ensure that the thermometer is reset, and then put on the plastic probe cover.

4. Insert the thermometer probe under the resident's tongue, and ask them to close their lips around it. (The resident may want to hold onto the end of the thermometer to keep it in place.) Do not allow the resident to walk while the thermometer is in their mouth.

5. Wait for the signal (beep) that the temperature reading is complete. As you wait, you can take the person's pulse and respiratory rates.

6. Remove the thermometer and the plastic cover. If there is an excessive amount of mucus on the thermometer when you remove it, use gloves or another barrier to remove the cover.

7. Read the temperature and record the result.

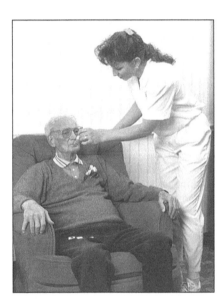

COMPLETION STEPS

1. Determine the resident's preferred position for comfort and ask them if they need anything else.
2. Examine the environment for safety and cleanliness.
3. Secure the call light and any other needed items within reach of the resident.
4. Perform hand hygiene.
5. Document the procedure and report any findings to the staff in charge.

- Has a nasal tube for feeding
- Has a history of seizures

Rectal Temperature

The rectal temperature (Procedure 7-2) is considered to be the most accurate temperature because it registers the body's core temperature. A rectal temperature is taken when ordered by the physician or when a resident is confused or very restless and may bite a thermometer if placed in the mouth. The rectal method is also used when a resident can breathe only through their mouth.

Taking rectal temperature is not advised or must be done using extreme caution when a resident has diarrhea or hemorrhoids or has had recent rectal surgery. In these situations, check with the nurse to make sure that the temperature should be taken rectally. Be sure to use a rectal thermometer. It usually has a red stem and a short, rounded bulb. Use a disposable thermometer cover for the electronic probes.

PROCEDURE

7-2: Taking a Rectal Temperature with an Electronic Thermometer

PREPARATION STEPS

1. Check the care plan.
2. Knock, introduce yourself, and address resident by preferred name.
3. Perform hand hygiene.
4. Gather supplies and secure assistance if needed.
5. Explain procedure and ask about resident preferences.
6. Respect privacy and rights at all times.

ITEMS NEEDED

- Electronic thermometer and probe cover
- Tissue or gauze pad
- Chart or form for recording temperature
- Pen
- Gloves
- Lubricant
- Sheet or blanket

1. Be sure to wear gloves. Always cover the resident with a sheet or blanket when taking a rectal temperature.

2. Make sure the electronic thermometer has been reset.

3. Position the resident on either side. Help the resident bend up the upper leg as far as possible.

4. Put a plastic cover over the thermometer and lubricate it. Separate the person's buttocks with one hand. Use your other hand to insert the thermometer ½ to 1 inch into the rectum.

5. Hold the thermometer in place until the temperature reading is complete. You must stay with the resident during this time to prevent them from rolling off their side and being injured by the thermometer. Talk with them to take their mind off the procedure.

6. Remove the thermometer, and wipe any excess lubricant from the rectum with a tissue or a gauze pad.

7. Remove the cover, read the temperature, and record the result.

COMPLETION STEPS

1. Determine the resident's preferred position for comfort and ask them if they need anything else.
2. Examine the environment for safety and cleanliness.
3. Secure the call light and any other needed items within reach of the resident.
4. Perform hand hygiene.
5. Document the procedure and report any findings to the staff in charge.

Non-Contact Infrared Temperature (NCIT)

This method has become more commonly used to reduce cross-contamination and the spread of infection. Using a NCIT is quick and easy but must be used according to manufacture guidelines (Procedure 7-3). This type of thermometer should not be used in direct sunlight or near a radiant heat source.

Axillary Temperature

The axillary temperature (the armpit) is the least reliable method. Use it only when the other methods cannot be used, such as when a NCIT in not available or with a confused resident who will not allow you to take a temperature by other methods. To take an axillary temperature, use an oral thermometer in the armpit (Procedure 7-4).

Temperature can be measured in two different scales, Fahrenheit (F°) or Celsius (C°). The U.S. typically uses the Fahrenheit scale but most electronic thermometers have an option to measure in both scales. When taking a temperature, make sure that the thermometer is set to the appropriate setting. Refer to Appendix E for information on converting between Fahrenheit and Celsius.

Pulse Rate

The pulse rate is the number of times the heart beats in a minute. The **pulse** is the rhythmic throbbing of an artery that coincides with the contractions of the heart. You can feel the pulse in several body areas. Figure 7-6 shows common pulse sites.

Usually, you take the pulse at the wrist. This is called the **radial pulse**. It is quick and easy to take and usually gives an accurate reading. The normal pulse rate in an adult at rest is 60 to 100 beats per minute. The pulse normally has a regular rhythm, beating at regular intervals with pauses in between.

PROCEDURE

7-3: Taking a Non-Contact Infrared Temperature

PREPARATION STEPS

1. Check the care plan.
2. Knock, introduce yourself, and address resident by preferred name.
3. Perform hand hygiene.
4. Gather supplies and secure assistance if needed.
5. Explain procedure and ask about resident preferences.
6. Respect privacy and rights at all times.

ITEMS NEEDED

- Non-Contact Infrared Thermometer
- Chart or form for recording temperature
- Pen

The NCIT should be used in a draft-free area, out of direct sunlight, and away from any radiant heat sources

1. The forehead should be clean, dry, and free from obstruction, such as hair or a headband.

2. If the resident has been in a cold or hot environment or had something on their forehead that could change the surface temperature, allow time for their temperature to stabilize.

3. Ask the resident to remain still while measuring their temperature.

4. Read the thermometer and record the results.

5. Clean the device according to manufacture guidelines.

COMPLETION STEPS

1. Determine the resident's preferred position for comfort and ask them if they need anything else.
2. Examine the environment for safety and cleanliness.
3. Secure the call light and any other needed items within reach of the resident.
4. Perform hand hygiene.
5. Document the procedure and report any findings to the staff in charge.

The pulse rate may be faster than normal due to exercise or other physical exertion, anxiety, anger, a heart condition, or certain medications. It may be slower than normal due to a heart condition, a pacemaker, certain medications, or when a person is in a very calm, resting state (as when meditating). A pulse rate that is faster than normal is known as tachycardia and a pulse rate that is lower than normal is called bradycardia.

When taking a pulse, the resident should be sitting or lying calmly. You need to pay attention to any irregularities in the rhythm (the pattern of beats). Note how strong the pulse is. If you can easily feel the pulse with your

7-4: Taking an Axillary Temperature with an Electronic Thermometer

PREPARATION STEPS

1. Check the care plan.
2. Knock, introduce yourself, and address resident by preferred name.
3. Perform hand hygiene.
4. Gather supplies and secure assistance if needed.
5. Explain procedure and ask about resident preferences.
6. Respect privacy and rights at all times.

ITEMS NEEDED

- Electronic thermometer and probe cover
- Chart or form for recording temperature
- Pen
- Washcloth and towel

1. Make sure that the thermometer is reset.

2. Place probe cover on thermometer.

3. Loosen the resident's clothing to be able to reach the underarm area. Wash and dry the axilla (armpit).

4. Place the thermometer in the resident's axilla. Have them place the arm along their side.

5. Wait until you are prompted that the temperature reading is complete. You must stay with the resident during this time to prevent injury. You may want to chat to take their mind off the procedure.

6. Remove the thermometer from the axilla.

7. Read the temperature and record the result.

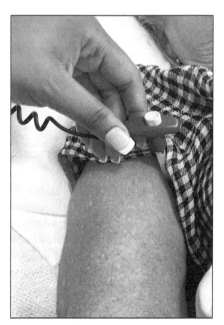

COMPLETION STEPS

1. Determine the resident's preferred position for comfort and ask them if they need anything else.
2. Examine the environment for safety and cleanliness.
3. Secure the call light and any other needed items within reach of the resident.
4. Perform hand hygiene.
5. Document the procedure and report any findings to the staff in charge.

fingertips, it is strong. If the pulse feels very faint under your fingers, it is weak. Report any irregularities to the charge nurse. The best way to learn pulse strength is to practice on a lot of people.

You will use your index and middle fingers to take a pulse (Procedure 7-5). Do not use your thumb because your thumb has a pulse that could be confused with the resident's pulse. An apical heart rate can be obtained by listening to the heart with a stethoscope.

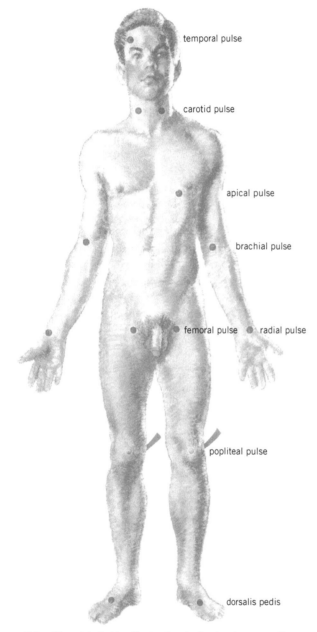

Figure 7-6 The dots in the illustration indicate places on the body where you can feel a pulse.

Respiratory Rate

Respiration is the process of inhaling air into the lungs and exhaling air out of the lungs.

The **respiratory rate** is the number of breaths per minute. Count the respiratory rate by watching a resident breathe in and out (Procedure 7-6). One respiration is equal to one inspiration (breathing in) and one expiration (breathing out). A person's normal respiratory rate changes with physical activity, emotional responses, and with sleep. The normal respiratory rate for an adult at rest is 12 to 20 breaths per minute. When counting a respiratory rate, you must also observe how residents are breathing. Are they taking deep slow breaths or shallow rapid breaths? Are the breaths in a regular pattern, or is there variation between deep, slow breaths and shallow, rapid breaths?

Examples of abnormal respiratory patterns:

- **Bradypnea** is a slower than normal respiratory rate.
- **Tachypnea** is a faster than normal respiratory rate.
- **Dyspnea** means difficult or labored breathing.
- **Apnea** is slow or stopped breathing

Record your findings and report any irregularities to the charge nurse. If a resident is talking or knows you are counting their respirations, they may alter their breathing and make it more difficult for you to obtain an accurate reading. To obtain a full set of vital signs, try this approach: keep your fingers on their wrist after taking their pulse rate and count their respirations.

Blood Pressure

Blood pressure (BP) is the pressure of blood pushing against the walls of the arteries. Changes in blood pressure may signal a change in a resident's health status or disease process. Consistently high blood pressure, known as **hypertension**, can lead to a stroke, heart attack, or other problems. A blood pressure that is too low, known as **hypotension**, can lead to fatigue, or weakness. It may also indicate the need to evaluate or change the resident's medications. A resident may have orthostatic hypotension, also known as postural hypotension, and this can cause their blood pressure to drop when they stand and lead to fainting. If you have a resident with orthostatic hypotension, encourage them to stand or make position changes slowly.

Blood pressure is affected by the force of the heart's contraction, the rigidity of the arterial blood vessels, and the amount of circulating blood. Two numbers are recorded for a blood pressure, such as 170/80. The

PREPARATION STEPS

1. Check the care plan.
2. Knock, introduce yourself, and address resident by preferred name.
3. Perform hand hygiene.
4. Gather supplies and secure assistance if needed.
5. Explain procedure and ask about resident preferences.
6. Respect privacy and rights at all times.

ITEMS NEEDED

- Watch with a second hand
- Chart or form for recording pulse rate
- Pen

1. Place your second and third fingers gently over the radial artery (on the thumb side of the resident's wrist) and note the rhythm of the pulse.

2. Look at your watch, and when the second hand is on the 12, start counting the pulse for 1 minute. Count each beat you feel. Check for abnormalities in the rhythm.

3. Record the result.

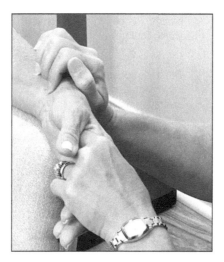

COMPLETION STEPS

1. Determine the resident's preferred position for comfort and ask them if they need anything else.
2. Examine the environment for safety and cleanliness.
3. Secure the call light and any other needed items within reach of the resident.
4. Perform hand hygiene.
5. Document the procedure and report any findings to the staff in charge.

top (first) number is the systolic pressure, which is the pressure in the artery when the heart is pumping. The bottom (second) number is the diastolic pressure, which is the pressure when the heart is at rest between beats.

Many factors can affect a person's blood pressure, including family history, stress, medications, weight and diet, physical position, exercise, smoking, and the arm in which blood pressure is taken. Some factors can be controlled, and others cannot. A resident's BP might be higher on admission because of anxiety. A resident's BP and other vital signs are usually taken often during the first week to determine a normal baseline for this person.

Blood pressure is expressed as millimeters of mercury (mm Hg). The normal blood pressure range for adults is below 120/80mm Hg and above 90/60 mm Hg. In someone over age 50, a systolic blood pressure above 140mm Hg is a much more important cardiovascular disease risk than a high diastolic reading. The systolic BP in older adults tends to be higher than in younger individuals because the arteries become narrower and more rigid with age. Table 7-3 shows the classification of blood pressure for adults.

Table 7-3 Blood Pressure Classification According to the American Heart Association

BP Classification	Systolic BP MMHG	Diastolic BP MMHG
Normal	Lower than 120	And Lower than 80
Elevated	120-129	And less than 80
Stage 1 Hypertension	130-139	Or 80 – 89
Stage 2 Hypertension	140 or higher	Or 90 or higher
Hypertensive Crisis	Higher than 180	And/or higher than 120

PREPARATION STEPS

1. Check the care plan.
2. Knock, introduce yourself, and address resident by preferred name.
3. Perform hand hygiene.
4. Gather supplies and secure assistance if needed.
5. Explain procedure and ask about resident preferences.
6. Respect privacy and rights at all times.

ITEMS NEEDED

- Watch with a second hand
- Chart or form for recording respiratory rate
- Pen

1 Count the respiratory rate immediately after counting the pulse rate.

2 Keep your fingers on the resident's radial pulse but without pressure. You do this so the resident will breathe normally. People tend to hold their breath or breathe deeper if they know you are counting.

3 Watch the chest go up with inspiration and down with expiration. Count the respiratory rate for 1 minute.

4 Record the result.

COMPLETION STEPS

1. Determine the resident's preferred position for comfort and ask them if they need anything else.
2. Examine the environment for safety and cleanliness.
3. Secure the call light and any other needed items within reach of the resident.
4. Perform hand hygiene.
5. Document the procedure and report any findings to the staff in charge.

Blood pressure should be measured when a resident is sitting or lying down. You can manually take the blood pressure in either arm or use an electronic blood pressure monitor (Procedures 7-7 and 7-8). Blood pressure should not be taken in an arm with an intravenous (IV) tube present or in an arm that is injured or has recently undergone surgery. To take a blood pressure, you will need a stethoscope and a sphygmomanometer (blood pressure cuff) (Figure 7-7) or an electronic blood pressure monitor.

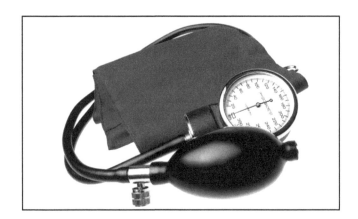

Figure 7-7 Blood pressure cuff

7-7: Taking a Manual Blood Pressure

PREPARATION STEPS

1. Check the care plan.
2. Knock, introduce yourself, and address resident by preferred name.
3. Perform hand hygiene.
4. Gather supplies and secure assistance if needed.
5. Explain procedure and ask about resident preferences.
6. Respect privacy and rights at all times.

ITEMS NEEDED

- Sphygmomanometer with cuff of correct size for resident
- Stethoscope
- Chart or form for recording blood pressure
- Pen

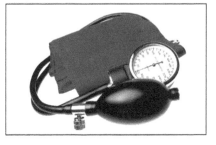

1 Have the resident place one arm on the bed, bedside table, or arm of a chair, with the palm facing up and elbow at the same level as the heart. (If the arm is higher than the heart, the blood pressure can register too low. If the arm is lower than the heart, the blood pressure can register too high.)

2 Expose the resident's arm by rolling the sleeve up to the shoulder, taking care that the sleeve is not too tight on the arm, which could increase the blood pressure.

3 Wrap the blood pressure cuff evenly around the upper arm 1 inch above the elbow. Be sure to use the correct size cuff. The wrong size cuff can result in an incorrect reading. The cuff should fit over the center of the resident's upper arm. It should not extend to the elbow or under the resident's armpit.

4 Make sure that the resident's extended arm is not lying on the tubing and that the tubing is not kinked. The tube attached to the bulb should be on the side closest to the resident's body. The tube to the sphygmomanometer gauge should be on the other side of the arm, away from the body.

5 Close the valve (small metal knob on the bulb) in the air pump by turning it clockwise.

6 Place the stethoscope earpieces in your ears.

7 Locate the pulsation in the brachial artery by placing your second and third fingers over the area. When you find the pulse, place the diaphragm of the stethoscope firmly over the area and hold it in place with your left hand. (Do this with your right hand if you are left-handed.)

8 With your right hand (left, if left-handed), pump air into the cuff by squeezing the bulb until the gauge measures 180–200. If you hear the pulse as soon as you stop pumping, begin again and pump the cuff pressure so the gauge reads higher than 200.

9 Slowly open the valve on the bulb and watch the cuff pressure decrease on the gauge.

10 Listen for the first thumping sound and note the pressure reading; this number is the systolic pressure.

11 Continue to listen for a distinct change in sound (a muffled sound) or the last sound and note the pressure reading; this number is the diastolic pressure.

12 Record the results.

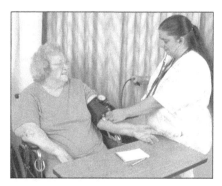

COMPLETION STEPS

1. Determine the resident's preferred position for comfort and ask them if they need anything else.
2. Examine the environment for safety and cleanliness.
3. Secure the call light and any other needed items within reach of the resident.
4. Perform hand hygiene.
5. Document the procedure and report any findings to the staff in charge.

7-8: Taking an Electronic Blood Pressure

PREPARATION STEPS

1. Check the care plan.
2. Knock, introduce yourself, and address resident by preferred name.
3. Perform hand hygiene.
4. Gather supplies and secure assistance if needed.
5. Explain procedure and ask about resident preferences.
6. Respect privacy and rights at all times.

ITEMS NEEDED

- Blood pressure monitor
- Chart of form for recording
- Pen

1. Have the resident place one arm on the bed, bedside table, or arm of a chair, with the palm facing up and elbow at the same level as the heart. (If the arm is higher than the heart, the blood pressure can register too high. If the arm is lower than the heart, the blood pressure can register too low.)

2. Expose the resident's arm by rolling the sleeve up to the shoulder, taking care that the sleeve is not too tight on the arm, which could increase the blood pressure.

3. Wrap the blood pressure cuff evenly around the upper arm one inch above the elbow. Be sure to use the correct size cuff. The wrong size cuff can result in an incorrect reading. The cuff should fit over the center of the resident's upper arm. It should not extend to the elbow or under the resident's armpit.

4. Make sure that the resident's extended arm is not lying on the tubing and that the tubing is not kinked.

5. Press the start button on the blood pressure monitor.

6. Wait for the signal that the blood pressure reading has finished.

7. Remove the blood pressure cuff.

8. Record the blood pressure as displayed on the screen.

9. Clean and store the blood pressure monitor according to facility policy.

COMPLETION STEPS

1. Determine the resident's preferred position for comfort and ask them if they need anything else.
2. Examine the environment for safety and cleanliness.
3. Secure the call light and any other needed items within reach of the resident.
4. Perform hand hygiene.
5. Document the procedure and report any findings to the staff in charge.

Height and Weight

A resident's height is measured as part of the admission physical examination. A resident's weight is measured on admission and regularly thereafter according to the care plan. Some medical conditions may require a resident to be weighed daily. Height and weight measurements made at the time of admission are used as baseline data. Later measurements are compared to these. If this baseline data is wrong, this can affect the person's data collection and plan of care.

It is common for residents to be routinely weighed every month unless otherwise ordered by the physician. These measurements help the nursing staff, dietitian, and others on the health care team know if a resident's weight is normal for their height, sex, and age.

Monitoring Weight

Regular weight checks are done to see if residents are gaining or losing weight. Drug dosages may be calculated based on a person's weight, and weight may be monitored to determine the success of diet, drug, or dialysis therapy.

Weight is one of the most important indicators of nutritional status. Evaluation of a resident's weight status involves comparing their current weight with their usual weight. Weight loss may be desirable for some residents, such as those who have been retaining fluid or who are obese. For others, weight loss is not desirable, as it can be a sign of nutritional deficiencies or disease.

A resident's weight can be interpreted in several ways. Weight is often calculated as either a percentage of ideal weight or a percentage of usual weight. Both are important. The percentage of ideal weight gives a benchmark comparison for evaluating the resident's weight. The dietitian or dietary manager calculates ideal weight.

Accuracy in weighing the resident and recording the data is important because weight is an indication of health. Because accuracy is so critical, a weight change of two to five pounds or more should be rechecked and confirmed before you record and report it.

Underweight residents are less resistant to infection, more sensitive to cold, and may be weaker overall. Tell the nurse immediately about a resident's weight loss. A weight change is considered severe in the following situations:

- Loss of five pounds or more in one month
- Loss of 7.5% of body weight or more in three months (for a 120-pound person, this equates to a nine-pound loss)
- Loss of 10% of body weight or more in six months (for a 120-pound person, this equates to a 12-pound loss)

Weight can be measured in several ways, depending on a resident's mobility. If the person can stand, use a standard bathroom scale or upright scale (Figure 7-8). Scales for wheelchairs are also available. For residents confined to bed, lift scales are used (Figure 7-9).

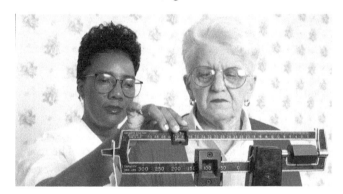

Figure 7-8 An upright scale is used to weight residents who can stand up and maintain their balance.

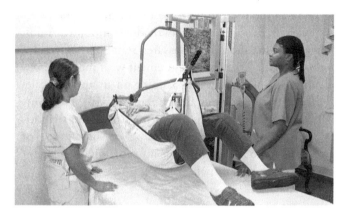

Figure 7-9 Residents who are confined to bed can be weighed using a scale that employs a mechanical lift.

You will learn to use all types of scales in your facility. Follow these guidelines:

- The scale must be checked periodically for accuracy. Follow the manufacturer's procedure for checking the scale's balance. There may be a lever or knob you can adjust.
- Always weigh a resident on the same scale because there may be slight differences between scales.
- Try to weigh a resident at the same time of day and wearing the same amount of clothing.
- If a resident's weight has increased or decreased by more than two to five pounds compared with the previous month, weigh them again and report the weight change to the nurse.

The dietitian may calculate and use the resident's **body mass index (BMI)** to evaluate their nutritional status. A standard formula is used to determine whether a resident is at a desirable weight, underweight, overweight, or obese based on their sex, height, and current weight.

Weight can be measured in pounds or kilograms. When recording a resident's weight make sure to record the weight using the correct system of measurement. Refer to Appendix E for information on converting between pounds and kilograms.

Measuring Height

Weight cannot be properly evaluated without a height measurement. Height is difficult to measure for residents who cannot stand erect or who have a disease such as arthritis or osteoporosis. An alert, oriented resident can be asked to report their height, but height must still be measured because it may decrease with age. The resident's previous height gives you an idea whether your measurement is accurate.

The method used to measure a resident's height, as with weight, depends on the individual's mobility. Ambulatory residents should be measured standing, preferably without shoes. Take the measurement with the resident standing against the wall or standing on an upright scale with a vertical measuring device (Figure 7-10). Procedure 7-9 describes the steps for measuring height and weight using an upright scale. Height can be measured in feet or inches. Refer to Appendix E for information on converting between feet and inches.

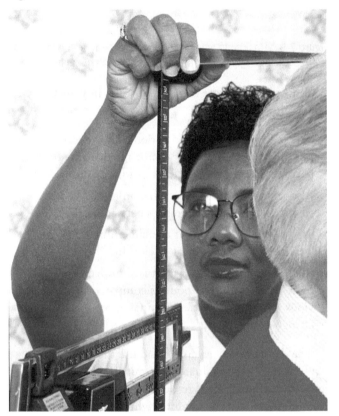

Figure 7-10   For residents who can stand on an upright scale, height is measured using the attached height measurement bar.

If a resident is confined to bed, check with the nurse to make sure you can measure their height as they lie face up, flat on the mattress. Residents with breathing difficulties may not be able to lie flat in bed. Using a tape measure, measure from the crown of the head to the bottom of the heel. Record the measurement in feet and inches. The dietitian will use a formula to calculate an estimate of the resident's standing height.

Residents with contractures or other disabilities that make it difficult to measure height may need to be measured by special means such as a knee-height caliper or by arm span. Alternative ways to measure height may be used by the dietitian or the charge nurse. They will tell you what they need you to do.

Residents with amputated lower limbs (on one or both sides, at any leg level) need careful measurements of their height on admission. If any surgical amputation is performed after admission, height must be measured following surgery. A full or partial loss of limb or height affects the resident's BMI and caloric requirements.

Admission of Residents

Residents are usually admitted to a long term care facility when their physical or mental condition makes it too difficult to remain in their home. Usually the family decides that 24-hour care is needed. This decision is often very stressful for both the resident and the family.

A resident may come directly from their own home or the home of a family member. Sometimes a resident comes from a hospital or another facility. Each new resident will have unique needs and concerns. You must keep in mind the loss the person feels and the difficulty involved in adjusting to their surroundings (Figure 7-11).

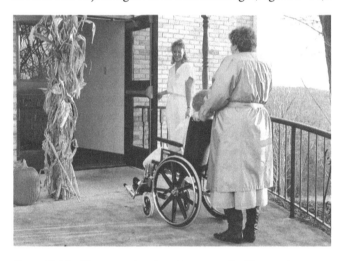

Figure 7-11   The move to a long term care facility may be stressful for both the resident and family.

Being admitted to a long term care facility is a very emotional experience that often causes anxiety. The resident may feel fearful about the unknown. Some new residents experience relocation stress syndrome. A resident's health can deteriorate within a few weeks after entering a facility because of poor adjustment to the new setting. What you and other staff members do can make a dramatic difference. You can make this experience much less difficult for the resident. Remember that residents are often upset about moving. A friendly, home-like, caring, and welcoming atmosphere may help them feel more comfortable (Figure 7-12).

7-9: Measuring Height and Weight Using an Upright Scale

PREPARATION STEPS

1. Check the care plan.
2. Knock, introduce yourself, and address resident by preferred name.
3. Perform hand hygiene.
4. Gather supplies and secure assistance if needed.
5. Explain procedure and ask about resident preferences.
6. Respect privacy and rights at all times.

Special scales are used to weigh a resident in a wheelchair or in bed. Follow your facility's policy and the manufacturer's instructions for using these scales. The following instructions are for the use of a mechanical upright scale.

1. Determine if the resident can walk to the scale or whether you need to bring a portable scale to their room.

2. Before the resident steps on the scale, adjust the height measurement bar so it is positioned higher than the resident's head.

3. Ask the resident what their height is and how long ago it was measured. Reductions in height occur due to aging-related changes in bones, muscles, and joints. It can also be associated with certain disease states.

4. Clear the scale and make sure it is balanced. It should register zero when the weights are moved all the way to the left.

5. Place a paper towel on the scale platform, and ask the resident to remove their shoes.

6. Help the resident step up and stand on the scale. Make sure they are not holding anything.

7. Have the resident stand up straight, with their arms by their sides and eyes facing forward. Slowly lower the height measurement bar to the top of their head. Record their height in feet and inches.

8. Measure the resident's weight by moving the weights to the right until the balance needle is centered. If the weight is five pounds or more higher or lower than the previous measurement, weigh the resident a second time to check for accuracy. If this is still the case, report it to the charge nurse. If the resident is wearing a cast or brace while being weighed, note this and report it to the charge nurse.

9. Help the resident step off the scale.

10. Record the resident's height and weight and report the findings to the charge nurse.

COMPLETION STEPS

1. Determine the resident's preferred position for comfort and ask them if they need anything else.
2. Examine the environment for safety and cleanliness.
3. Secure the call light and any other needed items within reach of the resident.
4. Perform hand hygiene.
5. Document the procedure and report any findings to the staff in charge.

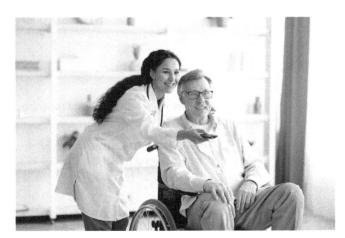

Figure 7-12 It is part of your job to help new residents get oriented to their room and to the facility.

Interdisciplinary Approach to Admission

The admission process includes forms that must be filled out and procedures that must be followed. Admission is a complex effort. The whole interdisciplinary team is involved. All team members work together to make the admission a successful experience.

The following personnel may be involved in the admission of a resident:

- **Admission Director or Coordinator.** This person's main responsibility is to help residents through the admission process. He or she may be a social worker, nurse, or person trained in admission policies and procedures. These staff members often work with discharge planners at hospitals.

- **Social Worker.** This person may also serve as the admissions coordinator. The social worker helps fill out the admission paperwork and takes a social history of the resident. He or she may also help the family with financial issues, such as advising on how to apply for Medicaid funding.

- **Housekeeping Department staff.** They help clean and set up the new room. They may also be involved in helping residents move in.

- **Dietary Department staff.** They interview residents or family members to find out the resident's food preferences.

- **Maintenance Department staff.** They may help move residents into the facility and install equipment such as phones for residents who want one.

- **Front Office staff.** These employees assist with financial concerns and payment schedules. They may provide information about how to apply for Medicaid funding.

- **Nurses.** The charge nurse makes sure that all equipment and medications are ready for a resident upon admission. They assess each resident carefully and document all findings. The charge nurse starts the assessment process. Nurses answer the resident's and family members' questions and helps them feel as comfortable as possible. The nurse also obtains or confirms orders with the resident's physician.

How Do You Prepare for the New Resident?

Because you will spend the most time with the resident, you have an important role in helping the resident feel welcome upon arrival. A room that is properly prepared helps the resident and family feel welcome. It shows that you are ready, organized, and capable of providing excellent care. Before the resident arrives, you may do the following:

- Check that the bed is made, a pillow is on the bed, and a blanket is available in the room.

- Check that a chair and working reading light are present and that the light is working.

- Make sure that the call light/button is in place and working properly.

- Make sure that the bed's electric or manual cranks are working.

- Confirm that personal care supplies such as washcloth, towel, soap, and soap dish are in place. If you already know the person cannot get to the bathroom, have a clean bed pan (and a urinal for a male resident) in the bedside table.

- Make sure that a water glass and water pitcher are ready to fill upon the resident's arrival in the room, unless contraindicated.

- Make sure that the resident's name is posted on or next to the door.

Greeting a New Resident

Greeting a resident warmly when they arrive helps make the admission process more pleasant. Introduce yourself in a way that inspires confidence and creates a sense of well-being.

To help a resident feel comfortable, you should:

- Maintain your professionalism but show warmth in your interactions. You are part of the facility's first impression on residents and family members.
- Greet the new resident by name, for example, Miss or Mrs. Smith. Some residents may prefer to be called by their first names, but never use their first name unless you have been invited to do so. Always ask how they prefer to be addressed.
- Introduce yourself by name. Explain that you are a nurse assistant and will be helping the resident get settled. Assure them you are there to help if they have questions.
- Greet any family members or friends who come with the resident.
- If the room is shared, introduce the new resident to their roommate. This helps both residents feel more comfortable.
- In your initial conversations, make an effort to get to know the new resident.

Orienting a New Resident

After a resident has unpacked and you finish filling out forms such as a personal item inventory and the resident's basic assessment, show them around the facility. You can get them oriented to their surroundings and explain equipment and resources. Your tour should include features of their room such as bathroom facilities, nurse call button, telephone, television, and how the bed functions. You should show new residents and their family other important locations within the facility, including the dining area, activity or recreation area, visitors' or residents' lounge, nurses' station, and the location of the telephone if one is not in the room. If a resident cannot leave the room or bed, show them everything in the room. Describe other areas in the facility that they can visit at a later time.

It often takes a while, sometimes as long as six months, for new residents to feel comfortable in their new home. Remember that it can be very frightening to move from a familiar home to a new place filled with many strangers. Plan to spend extra time with and pay special attention to a resident during this time.

Creating a Home in a Long Term Care Facility

As previously discussed, entering a long term care facility can be an emotional time. In many cases, residents have had to leave their home and part with many cherished belongings. It is your job to help create a sense of home for residents in the facility.

To meet this challenge, you must first learn how the resident wants the room to be arranged. For example, a resident may want to display pictures of grandchildren or to use a favorite bedspread or quilt on the bed. They may want personal items to be within reach or stored in a special place. Understanding the resident's wants and needs is your highest priority. You must do everything possible to help each resident feel like the facility is their home.

You can promote a home-like feeling by encouraging residents to bring in their own things. If there is adequate space, a resident may bring a few small furniture items.

Framed artwork and photos, wall hangings, other decorative items, and plants can personalize the room. Familiar things help create a positive environment and a sense of security for a new resident. You can offer positive comments about pictures and other personal touches in the room.

Caring for Residents' Personal Belongings

In long term care facilities, residents have the right to bring with them and use personal items as space permits. Residents often bring both necessary items such as clothes, shoes, and hearing aids, and personal items that have special meaning.

If a resident's possessions are damaged, lost, or stolen, this can cause great distress for a resident and the family. The resident may feel vulnerable and think that staff members don't care for them and can't be trusted. Residents and family must be able to count on staff to respect and protect personal belongings.

An inventory (listing) of the resident's belongings is completed as part of the admission process (Figure 7-13). Personal items brought into a resident's room after admission must also be recorded on this form, and items that have been removed must be noted.

Keeping track of personal belongings is the responsibility of the entire care team. For example, if a resident's eyeglasses are missing, inform housekeeping, laundry, and dietary staff. The glasses may be in the laundry in a shirt pocket or accidentally left on a dining tray.

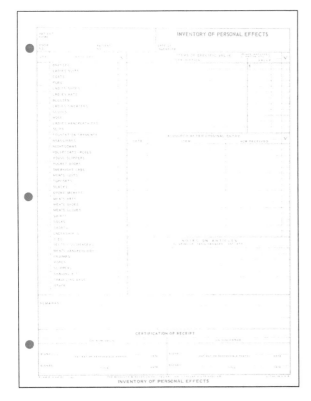

Figure 7-13 When a resident is admitted, an inventory form is completed to document the resident's personal items. This form is updated when new belongings are purchased or received.

Follow these guidelines for handling residents' personal belongings:

- Treat a resident's belongings with care and respect. Have the attitude that a resident's possessions are important and valuable.

- Help safeguard the resident's personal possessions. Valuable items such as cash, jewelry, and heirlooms should not be kept in the facility. The family should take them home. However, if such items are in the room, check with the charge nurse and follow the facility's protocol. Make sure that these items are on the inventory list.

- Talk with every resident to learn how they want the room cared for. Together, you can work out a schedule that meets their needs and complies with facility policy.

- Be careful when cleaning or tidying the room to avoid damaging special belongings. Open the closet and drawers only with the resident's permission.

- Some residents choose not to bring personal items to the facility. In this case, treat the furniture in their room as if it were their own, and encourage them to do the same.

- Family members and friends may bring food gifts for the resident. Follow your facility policy and tell them what type of container the food must be in. Offer to help with storing food, if necessary.

- If a resident's belonging is lost or damaged, report it to the charge nurse immediately. Stay alert and remain aware of the environment to reduce the chance of loss or damage.

Care of a Resident's Clothes

Clothing is an important aspect that contributes to the resident's self-esteem. Follow these guidelines in caring for residents' clothing:

- Make sure that all clothing is labeled with the resident's name; a tag or label should be sewn or affixed on the inside of the garment (Figure 7-14).

- Watch for new clothing brought in by family members and friends, and make sure that every new item is labeled.

- Be especially careful on occasions such as holidays and birthdays. Imagine how a resident and family would feel if a beautiful blouse received as a gift was misplaced or damaged in the laundry.

- Try to keep the resident's clothing from becoming soiled or stained. If a resident tends to spill food, use a large napkin or a fabric or disposable protector to prevent stains during meals and snacks.

- If a spill or other accident does happen, wash the soiled item in a sink as soon as possible to prevent a permanent stain. You may also ask the laundry department to treat the stained clothing, depending on your facility's protocol.

- Place soiled laundry in the appropriate bag or container, following your facility's protocol.

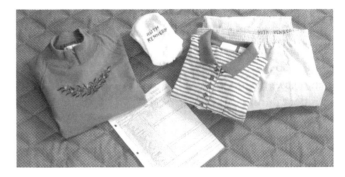

Figure 7-14 The resident's clothing must be labeled with the resident's name.

Care of Other Belongings

Belongings such as hearing aids, eyeglasses, and dentures are necessary for the well-being of residents. Follow these guidelines:

- These items should be labeled or marked with the resident's name. (Kits are available for marking dentures.)

- Keep these items in appropriate cases or containers when not in use. Encourage residents to do the same.

- Hearing aids should be removed at night and placed in a container with the battery door open to conserve battery life. Hearing aids should be cleaned according to manufacture guidelines.

- Eyeglasses should be cleaned at least every morning and when removing at night.

- Dentures should be cleansed and stored in a denture cup and placed in the resident's bedside table when not in use.

- Record the serial number of a hearing aid in the resident's record for future reference.

- Routinely check pockets when collecting clothes for the laundry. It is your job to prevent valuables such as a watch, hearing aid, or wallet from going through the laundry.

- Watch that dentures, eyeglasses, or hearing aids are not left on bedding or food trays.

Respecting Residents' Privacy

Even though many people go in and out of residents' rooms, you and all staff must respect their privacy. The facility is their home. Residents have private lives — they are not just part of your routine. As you get to know residents, be careful not to let this familiarity become routine. Always be mindful.

To show respect for residents' privacy, always follow these guidelines:

- Knock on the door (Figure 7-15), and ask permission to enter. If the resident cannot respond, enter the room and introduce yourself.

- Ask how residents want their rooms arranged and maintained.

- Never move items in the room without a resident's permission.

- Encourage residents to help care for and arrange their room.

- Maintain residents' privacy through respectful and clear communication in everything you do.

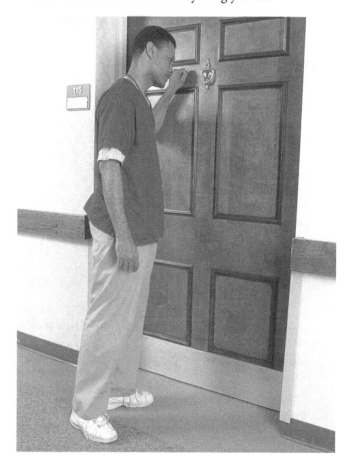

Figure 7-15 Always knock on the resident's door and wait for permission to enter.

Daily Routines

You will become part of a resident's daily routine by assisting with their care and helping to maintain their environment. Always remember to ask the resident's permission before touching or cleaning any item in their room.

Bed Making

As a nurse assistant, you are responsible for caring for all items in a resident's room, especially the bed. Making a neat, wrinkle-free bed is important for the resident's comfort and dignity. It also helps prevent skin irritation and breakdown. Most residents can get out of bed while you make it. This is called making an unoccupied bed (Procedure 7-10). But some residents cannot get out of bed, and then you need to make an occupied bed (Procedure 7-11).

7-10: Making an Unoccupied Bed

PREPARATION STEPS

1. Check the care plan.
2. Knock, introduce yourself, and address resident by preferred name.
3. Perform hand hygiene.
4. Gather supplies and secure assistance if needed.
5. Explain procedure and ask about resident preferences.
6. Respect privacy and rights at all times.

ITEMS NEEDED

- Two flat sheets or one fitted and one flat sheet
- Draw sheet (if used)
- Pillow cases
- Blanket
- Bedspread

1. Look for any belongings in the bed. Residents may fall asleep with personal belongings under the pillow or in the bed.

2. Lower the head of the bed and raise the bed to a comfortable position for you to work, usually about hip level.

3. Remove the bedspread and any blankets. Fold them and place on the chair.

4. Remove soiled linen, including the pillow case. Loosen sheets from under the mattress and carefully roll them into a ball, keeping the soiled side inside and away from your body. (This keeps the cleaner side closer to you and prevents the spread of organisms from dirty linens.) Place the soiled sheets in the laundry bag.

5. Check the mattress for any soiling or wetness. Wash and dry it with paper towels if necessary. Change the mattress pad if it is soiled or scheduled for change.

TO REPLACE A FITTED SHEET:

1. Starting at the top corner of the mattress, fit the corner of the sheet over the edge of the mattress, then go to the bottom of the bed on the same side and fit the sheet over that edge. Do not shake the linen while unfolding it. (Shaking the linen raises dust and organisms.)

2. Go to the opposite corner at the top of the bed and fit the sheet over that edge, and then move to the bottom of the bed and wrap the sheet over the last exposed mattress corner. The sheet should fit the mattress snugly.

TO USE A FLAT SHEET AS THE BOTTOM SHEET:

1. Unfold the flat sheet lengthwise down the center of the bed. Do not shake the linen while unfolding it. (Shaking linen raises dust and organisms.)

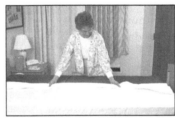

2. Place the hem seams toward the mattress. This keeps rough edges away from the resident.

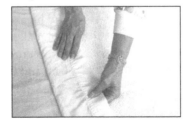

3. Slide the sheet so that the hem is even with the foot of the mattress. Keep the fold in the exact center of the bed. (You want the extra length of sheet at the top to tuck it under the mattress).

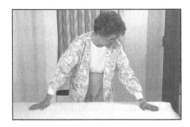

4. Open the sheet from the fold so that the sheet covers the entire mattress and hangs evenly on both sides. Tuck the top hem in tightly under the mattress at the head of the bed by lifting the mattress and sliding the sheet under the mattress.

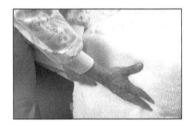

5. Make a mitered corner (also called a hospital corner). Face the side of the bed. Pick up the top of the sheet hanging down the side of the bed, and lay it on top of the bed so it looks like a triangle. Tuck the remaining sheet under the mattress. Drop the section of sheet from on top of the bed over the side of the bed, and tuck it in. Repeat for the other three corners.

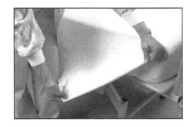

6 Tuck the remaining sheet under the mattress neatly.

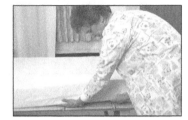

IF A DRAW SHEET IS USED:

A draw sheet is often used for residents needing help with moving and positioning, or sometimes to keep bottom sheets clean and dry.

1 Unfold the sheet and place it in the center of the bed so that it covers the middle part of the bed.

2 Tuck in the draw sheet on the side where you are working. You may also place any needed disposable incontinence pads over the draw sheet.

TO REPLACE THE TOP SHEET AND BEDSPREAD:

1 Place the top sheet on the bed. The wide hem should be even with the head of the mattress, with the seam on the outside. When you fold the hem over, the smooth side will be next to the resident's skin, preventing irritation from any rough edges. The excess sheet will be over the foot of the bed.

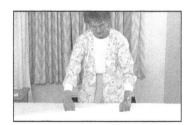

2 Open the sheet from the fold so that the sheet covers the entire mattress and hangs evenly on both sides.

3 Place the bedspread on top of the sheet so that it hangs evenly on both sides. Make sure that the sheet does not stick out below the bedspread on the sides.

4 Tuck in the sheet and bedspread at the foot of the bed, making mitered corners on both sides.

5 Smooth the sheet and bedspread from the bottom to the top of the bed, and fold down the top hem of the sheet over the bedspread.

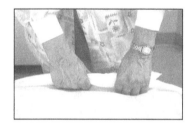

TO REPLACE THE PILLOW CASE:

1 Hold the center of the closed end of the pillow case with your hand and turn it inside out over your hand.

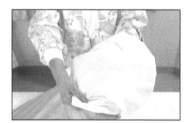

2 Grab the pillow with your hand inside the pillowcase and slide the case over the pillow. Make sure that the corners of the pillow fit into the corners of the case.

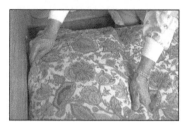

3 Place the pillow(s) at the head of the bed, and fold the spread over them.

TO FINISH:

1 Place the folded blanket at the foot of the bed or in the closet, if the resident prefers.

2 Lower the bed to its normal position.

COMPLETION STEPS

1. Determine the resident's preferred position for comfort and ask them if they need anything else.
2. Examine the environment for safety and cleanliness.
3. Secure the call light and any other needed items within reach of the resident.
4. Perform hand hygiene.
5. Document the procedure and report any findings to the staff in charge.

7-11: Making an Occupied Bed

PREPARATION STEPS

1. Check the care plan.
2. Knock, introduce yourself, and address resident by preferred name.
3. Perform hand hygiene.
4. Gather supplies and secure assistance if needed.
5. Explain procedure and ask about resident preferences.
6. Respect privacy and rights at all times.

ITEMS NEEDED

- Two flat sheets or one fitted and one flat sheet
- Draw sheet (if used)
- Pillow cases
- Blanket
- Bedspread

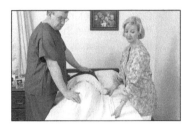

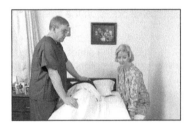

1. If moving the resident will require help from another nurse assistant, make sure that person is ready to assist before you begin.

2. Lower the head of the bed, and remove the pillow from under the resident's head. (Do this only if the resident is comfortable lying completely flat on the bed.)

3. Remove the bedspread and any blankets. Fold them and place them on the chair.

4. Loosen the top and bottom sheets from under the mattress.

5. Help the resident roll over on their side toward you. Make sure the resident stays covered throughout the procedure. Raise the side rail and ask them to hold onto it for support. If there is any risk that the resident could be injured when using the side rail, do not use it.

6. Move around to the other side of the bed.

7. Check for any personal belongings in the bed.

8. Roll lengthwise (top to bottom) the soiled bottom sheet from the side of the mattress to the center of the bed close to the resident's body. (If the linen is damp or wet, wear gloves and place a barrier such as plastic-covered padding over the sheet.)

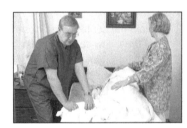

9. Change the mattress pad if it is soiled or scheduled for changing.

TO REPLACE A FITTED SHEET:

1. Starting at the top corner of the mattress, fit the corner of the sheet over the edge of the mattress, then go to the bottom of the bed on the same side and fit the sheet over that edge. Be sure half the mattress is covered and the sheet is tucked close to the resident.

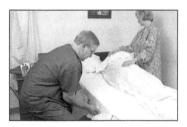

2. If you are using a draw sheet, place it in the center of the bed so it covers the middle part of the bed and is tucked close to the resident. Tuck in the draw sheet on the side you are working. You may also place any needed disposable incontinence pads over the draw sheet.

TO USE A FLAT SHEET AS THE BOTTOM SHEET:

1. Unfold the flat sheet lengthwise down the center of the bed. Do not shake the linen while unfolding it. (Shaking linen raises dust and organisms.)

2. Place the hem seams toward the mattress. This keeps rough edges away from the resident.

3. Slide the sheet so that the hem is even with the foot of the mattress. Keep the fold in the exact center of the bed. (You want the extra length of sheet at the top to tuck it under the mattress).

4. Open the sheet and fan-fold it lengthwise so that one half of the sheet is next to the rolled dirty sheet.

5. Tuck the top hem in tightly under the mattress at the head of the bed by lifting the mattress edge and sliding the sheet under it.

6 Make a mitered corner (also called a hospital corner). Face the side of the bed. Pick up the top of the sheet hanging down the side of the bed, and lay it on top of the bed so it looks like a triangle. Tuck the remaining sheet under the mattress. Drop the section of sheet from on top of the bed over the side of the bed, and tuck it in. Repeat for other three corners.

7 Tuck the remaining sheet under the mattress neatly.

8 If you are using a draw sheet, place it in the center of the bed so it covers the middle part of the bed. Fan-fold the excess and tuck it in with the sheet. Tuck in the draw sheet.

CONTINUE WITH THE NEXT STEPS:

1 Flatten the rolled or fan-folded sheets and help the resident roll over the linen toward you, using the correct procedure for turning them. Don't forget first to remind the resident that the roll of linen is behind them.

2 Move to the opposite side of the bed, lower the side rail, remove the dirty linen, and place it in the laundry bag. Never leave the resident unattended to take away dirty laundry.

3 Pull the clean linen toward you until it is completely unfolded, and tuck the sheets in tightly the same way as you did on the other side.

4 Tuck in the draw sheet, if used.

5 Help the resident roll back to the center of the bed.

TO REPLACE THE TOP SHEET AND BEDSPREAD:

1 Place the top sheet on the bed over the sheet covering the resident. Open the sheet from the fold so that the sheet hangs evenly on each side of the bed. The wide hem should be at the top with the seam on the outside. When you fold the hem over, the smooth side will be next to the resident's skin, preventing any rough edges from touching them. The excess sheet should hang over the foot of the bed.

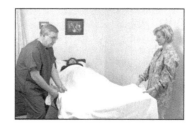

2 Ask the resident to hold onto the clean sheet, then carefully remove the dirty top sheet by placing your hand under the clean top sheet and rolling the dirty sheet down toward the foot of the bed. Remove it and place it with the other dirty linen.

3 Place the bedspread on top of the sheet in the same way you did the top sheet. Make sure that the sheet does not stick out below the bedspread on the sides.

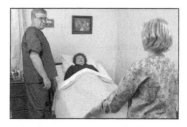

4 Tuck in the sheet and bedspread at the foot of the bed, making mitered corners on both sides.

5 Smooth the sheet and bedspread from the bottom to the top of the bed, and fold down the top hem of the sheet over the bedspread.

6 Make sure that the top linens are not so tight that they are pressing on the resident's feet. To be sure, make a toe pleat. This is done by pulling the top linen up to form a pleat.

TO REPLACE THE PILLOW CASE:

1 Hold the center of the closed end of the pillow case with your hand and turn it inside out over your hand.

2 Grab the pillow with your hand inside the pillowcase and slide the case over the pillow. Make sure that the corners of the pillow fit into the corners of the case.

3 Place the pillow under the resident's head.

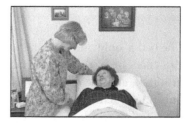

COMPLETION STEPS

1. Determine the resident's preferred position for comfort and ask them if they need anything else.
2. Examine the environment for safety and cleanliness.
3. Secure the call light and any other needed items within reach of the resident.
4. Perform hand hygiene.
5. Document the procedure and report any findings to the staff in charge.

Follow these guidelines when making any bed:

- Always ask the resident's permission first.
- Wear gloves if the linen is soiled.
- Raise the bed to a good working height.
- Make one side of the bed at a time to reduce the steps you have to take.
- Place a draw sheet or lift sheet on the bed for residents who need assistance with bed mobility.
- When making an occupied bed, always roll a resident toward you, which is safer than rolling the resident away from you.
- Make sure there are no wrinkles.
- Follow the facility's policy about when to change linens. Often the routine is a complete change of linens once or twice a week or when soiled.
- Keep soiled linens away from your uniform.
- Never put linens on the floor. Follow the facility's policy for putting soiled linen in proper laundry bags.

If you have a resident coming back from the hospital or a new admission that is being transferred by a stretcher, you may be asked to make an open or surgical bed. To make this type of bed, you would fan fold the top sheets out of the way to the foot or side of the bed. The bed is usually placed in a high position to transfer the resident to the bed from the stretcher.

Finishing Touches

The bed is only one part of a resident's environment. You also take care of the bedside table, over-bed table, other furniture, and the resident's belongings. Think about finishing touches you can contribute to make a resident's room feel warm, friendly, and more comfortable. Simple actions can make a difference:

- Keep the noise level down as you work.
- Eliminate clutter such as disposable cups, tissues, and old newspapers and magazines. Ask the resident before you throw anything away.
- Adjust lighting to the resident's liking, such as raising window shades in the morning and closing them in the evening.
- If possible, adjust the room temperature and ventilation for the resident's comfort.
- Help care for residents' plants and flowers, if needed.
- Carefully dust pictures and other mementos.

- Display postcards and greeting cards if the resident wants them in view.

Call System

You cannot be with every resident all the time. To make sure residents get help when they need it, facilities have **call systems** for all residents.

A *call button* on a cord plugs into an outlet over or near the resident's bed, and the resident pushes the button when help is needed. The cord has a clip that can be attached to the pillow or sheet to keep the button from falling on the floor out of reach. A light outside the resident's door comes on when the call button is activated (Figure 7-16). Many facilities have a call board or monitor at the nurses' station. When a resident pushes the call button, the resident's room number lights up or is shown on the screen. Some facilities also have an intercom system from the station to residents' rooms.

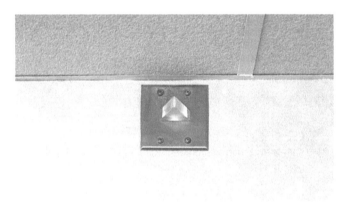

Figure 7-16   The call light outside the resident's room is activated when the resident pushes the call button.

It is your job to help residents learn how to use the call system. You must explain the purpose of the call system and demonstrate how to use the call button. Then have the resident show that they can use the call button. If a resident does not understand the call system or cannot pull the cord or push the button, work with the charge nurse to find another way for them to call for help.

As you go about your duties, watch for call lights and answer quickly when you see one, even for residents you are not caring for that day. Turn off the call light when you enter the room so that another staff member does not also come to help.

Make sure that each resident's call button is always plugged in, working properly, and within reach when they are in bed or sitting near the bed. If a resident's call light is not working, report it to the charge nurse immediately. A bell can be used until the light is repaired.

Transferring a Resident

Residents may be transferred to a different unit or wing in a facility for various reasons. The resident, family, and physician decide this in consultation with other team members. Residents are often transferred because of a change in their needs or level of care. Even though a person who is being transferred is already a resident in the facility, the transition can still be difficult. The change can raise many questions and concerns and cause anxiety. You can help minimize any negative effects with good communication and a caring attitude.

Interdisciplinary Approach to Resident Transfer

Transferring a resident can be an involved procedure. Nursing has a role along with other departments in the facility. Everyone works together to coordinate the process. The social worker gets permission from the resident and family before a transfer or a room move takes place. The social worker also communicates with other departments and staff, such as the dietary department, front office, medical records, etc.

Housekeeping cleans the new room to prepare it for the resident. Sometimes housekeeping staff assist nursing staff in packing the resident's belongings and moving them to the new room. Nurse assistants may help, as well.

The charge nurse helps staff in the new unit or wing get to know the resident. The nurse records information about the resident's mental and physical condition at the time of the transfer. The nurse helps transfer the resident and takes all treatments and medications to the new wing or unit.

When transferring a resident to another unit, wing, or room, keep these things in mind:

- Transfer procedures are usually routine for staff, but we must remember that they are very stressful for residents.
- A resident may be upset and concerned about the move. The resident may be comfortable with and attached to the former staff, other residents, and even the environment. The resident may not want to leave their roommate. These changes can create a sense of loss.
- A resident may be concerned that they will not like the new unit or wing as much as the former one.
- It can be very confusing to switch environments.

Preparing for the Transfer

Just as nurses in the two units communicate about the resident being transferred, nurse assistants of the two units must communicate, as well. Share information about a resident's likes and dislikes. Pass on ideas and techniques that have proven helpful in caring for them. Try to think of any information that would make the transition to the new unit easier.

Before the transfer, make sure that the transfer has been approved by the appropriate members of the facility staff and that permission has been obtained from the resident and family. Verify that the new room is ready the same way you would for a new admission. It often helps to call ahead and ask staff on the new unit to come meet the resident before the transfer.

The Transfer Process

The transfer should be handled professionally and warmly. If you are doing the transfer, reassure the resident. Help them resolve any fears or concerns.

If you are receiving the resident on the new unit, offer a warm, sincere greeting. Be sure to ask how the resident wants to be addressed and introduce yourself. Introduce the resident to their new roommate and help both residents feel more comfortable (Figure 7-17).

Treat the resident like a new admission. Help them unpack and orient them to the new room, again, in the same manner as for a new admission. Orient a resident to the areas and features in the room they need to know about. Also provide an orientation to important areas in the unit or wing, even if they cannot presently leave the room or bed, because they may be able to in the future. Make sure that all personal belongings and medical records are transferred.

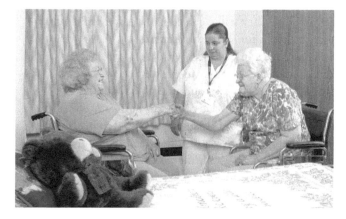

Figure 7-17 You can make a transfer easier on residents by orienting them to their new surroundings and introducing them to staff and their new roommate.

Discharging a Resident

Discharge is the process that occurs when a resident leaves the facility. Many team members are involved in discharge planning. For some residents, discharge planning begins the day of admission to the facility. This commonly happens when residents are admitted for rehabilitation and subacute care.

Residents being discharged may feel many different emotions. Often the discharge is a joyful occasion, as when a resident's condition has improved enough to go home or to a less-restrictive facility. But sometimes a discharge is not a happy occasion. In all cases, do your best to help residents and family feel good about their decision. The most common reasons for discharge are:

- The resident's condition has changed, and a different setting is required.
- The resident has improved enough to go to a less-restrictive setting.
- The resident or family dislikes the facility and desires a move.
- The resident is moving to a facility closer to where family members are located.

Interdisciplinary Approach to Resident Discharge

A resident's discharge involves multiple departments within the facility. The social worker arranges a discharge planning meeting. For a resident going home, the social worker helps locate and arrange for community services that will meet the resident's needs. If a resident is moving to another facility, the social worker coordinates with the new facility to ensure a smooth transition. The social worker tells other staff when the discharge will take place.

Housekeeping staff may help pack up the resident's belongings. They will clean the room after the discharge and prepare it for the next resident.

The nurse works closely with the physician, resident, family, and social worker to ensure that the discharge proceeds correctly. The nurse obtains the necessary discharge order from the physician and communicates with the resident and family regarding care instructions. If a resident is moving to another facility, the nurse works closely with nursing staff there to ensure continuity of care. The nurse writes a discharge note, coordinates the discharge care plan, and sends the resident's medications and records to the new facility.

Helping Residents During the Discharge Process

If a resident is going home or to a less restrictive setting, you can let them know you are happy about their progress. If you have any negative feelings about the discharge, you cannot let these feelings show or affect your attitude or your assistance. Maintain your professionalism and your warmth in interacting with the resident and family.

Moving to a different place is a change that can be stressful or frightening, even when it's a positive move. A resident may be anxious and may demand more attention than usual. They may feel sad because of leaving residents and staff they have gotten to know or may feel angry about the change. To help a resident accept the change, you can:

- Acknowledge the resident's feelings such as sadness, anger, or fear.
- Keep a positive attitude. Even if a resident is leaving because they do not like the facility, you can say, "Another facility may be better able to meet your needs."
- Encourage the person being discharged to say goodbye to residents and staff.
- Ask the social worker to tell the resident about the new facility or residence if it is unfamiliar to them. He or she should share the name of the facility or residence, where it is located, how big it is, what it looks like, and what services are available there.

Day of Discharge

When it is time for a resident to leave, you should:

- Have a wheelchair available, if needed.
- Ask the resident for permission to pack their personal belongings unless they wish to do it themselves. Have a cart ready to transport belongings.
- Check the personal items inventory list, and account for each item.
- Check that the resident is appropriately dressed and groomed.
- Accompany the resident to the exit.
- Say goodbye to the resident and family and wish them well.

After a resident leaves, the room is prepared for the next resident. Usually housekeeping staff clean and disinfect the room and bathroom, but you may help with preparation, as well. Remove all linen from the bed and place it in a laundry bag. Remove unnecessary articles, including disposable personal care items. Throw away any trash. Take items such as the wash basin and bedpan to the service room.

Housekeeping staff remove the mattress, clean the bedsprings, and wash the bed frame and all furniture.

The mattress is replaced. After the room has been cleaned, you should make the bed with clean linen. Arrange the bedside table and store the items the next resident will need. The room is now ready for the next resident to be admitted.

Points to Remember

- Sources of information about residents include the residents themselves, family members, friends, the charge nurse and other staff, and the medical record.

- Objective information is factual information obtained through observation of a resident. Subjective information includes what residents say about symptoms and how they feel and your opinion about their condition or care.

- The resident's care plan lists the person's medical, nursing, and psychosocial needs. The plan also lists one or more objectives or goals related to each problem.

- Nurse assistants provide three main types of reports based on observations and interactions with residents: routine reports, immediate reports, and "by a certain time" reports.

- Each facility has established procedures for the nurse assistant's role in documentation. You must understand your facility's policies and procedures and be familiar with medical terminology and common abbreviations.

- The history and physical (H&P), usually performed by a physician, provides information about a resident's total physical, psychological, and social needs upon admission to the facility.

- Vital signs are the record of a person's temperature, pulse rate, respiration rate, and blood pressure.

- Vital signs are regularly monitored and recorded so the health care team can evaluate the significance of any changes or abnormalities.

- Height and weight measurements are taken upon admission and updated regularly. Weight loss or gain can indicate health problems.

- Your role includes welcoming new residents and helping them to feel at home in the facility.

- It is important to respect residents' privacy and to properly care for their personal belongings.

- Nurse assistants help with resident transfer and discharge by ensuring the residents' comfort and helping them deal with the changes associated with a new environment.

apnea — temporaty cessation of breathing, especially during sleep

assessment — evaluation of a patient or condition

auscultation — using a stethoscope to hear sounds produced by internal organs (such as heart, lungs, or bowels)

baseline — initial measurement or observation used for later comparison

blood pressure (BP) — measurement of the pressure of blood in the arteries

body mass index (BMI) — measurement that estimates the percentage of fat tissue in the body

bradycardia — slower than normal pulse rate

bradypnea — slower than normal respiratory rate

call system — system that enables residents to signal that they need assistance from staff

diastolic pressure — number that reflects the pressure when the heart is at rest between beats

documentation — written and/or digital reports maintained by the facility relating to a resident's care and condition

dyspnea — difficult or labored breathing

electronic medical record (EMR) — digital version of the patient chart and medical record

face sheet — one-page summary of important information about a patient/resident

fever — elevated body temperature

flow sheet — document used to record health and activity information about a resident over a period of time

history — information about a resident's previous health status, lifestyle, and medical treatment

history and physical (H&P) — patient/resident history combined with a physical exam

hypertension — high blood pressure

hypotension — low blood pressure

inspection — careful observation of the resident's body to determine health status

kiosk — centrally located electronic device used to input patient/resident data

objective information — factual information gathered through observation

palpation — physical examination conducted by touching the resident's body with the fingers and/or hands

percussion — tapping on a body area (chest, back, abdomen) to hear the sound produced; used to determine the status of internal tissues and organs

personal health record (PHR) — an individual health history kept by the patient, usually in electronic form

physical examination — an organized examination of the body to determine health status; includes visual inspection, auscultation, palpation, percussion, and smell.

policies and procedures (P&Ps) — guidelines and procedures established by a facility for daily operations and emergency/disaster situations

protocol — an official or standard way of doing something, usually put in writing

pulse — measure of heart rate taken by feeling the expansion of an artery as blood is pushed through when the heart contracts

radial pulse — pulse measurement taken by feeling the radial artery at the wrist

relocation stress syndrome — stress and anxiety experienced by a person relocating to a new environment, such as a resident entering a long term care facility

Resident Assessment Instrument (RAI) — assessment tool used in long term care facilities to document key information about residents, including care plans and outcomes

respiration — exchange of oxygen and carbon dioxide between the atmosphere and body cells; breathing

respiratory rate — measurement of the number of breaths per minute

subjective information — information based on an assumption, opinion, or on what the resident says about how they feel

systolic pressure — number that reflects the pressure in the artery when the heart is pumping

tachycardia — faster than normal pulse rate

tachypnea — faster than normal respiratory rate

temperature — measurement of the degree of heat in the body

vital signs — measurements of temperature, pulse, respiration, and blood pressure

1. **When should abnormal vital signs be reported to the charge nurse?**

   a. At the end of the shift
   b. As long as you have documented the vital signs, you do not have to report them to the nurse
   c. Immediately
   d. After your lunch break

2. **Why are vital signs monitored and recorded?**

   a. So the health care team can monitor and evaluate for any changes or abnormalities
   b. To make sure staff have interaction with the resident on a routine basis
   c. So the nurse assistants have data to document
   d. To provide to the physician on a yearly basis

3. **The blood pressure reading for the resident is a type of:**

   a. Objective information
   b. Subjective information
   c. Quality indicator
   d. Hearsay evidence

4. **To measure a radial pulse:**

   a. Place your thumb at the wrist and count for 30 seconds
   b. Place your first two fingers over the artery behind the knee
   c. Place your first two fingers over the artery at the resident's wrist and count for a full minute
   d. Place a blood pressure cuff over the upper arm and record the reading

5. **Subjective information is:**

   a. Factual data
   b. Obtained by touching or smelling
   c. Not important to the assessment process
   d. Your guess or opinion about what you observe

6. **One of the most important tasks when leaving a resident's room is:**

   a. Take the resident's vital signs
   b. Explain the meal schedule to the resident
   c. Hand the call light to the resident or make sure it is in reach
   d. Smile and wish them a good night

7. **A technique of listening through a stethoscope to sounds produced by organs, such as the heart, is called:**

   a. Palpation
   b. Auscultation
   c. Percussion
   d. Vital signs

8. **A possible reaction of an unprepared resident entering a long term care facility is:**

   a. Bipolar disorder
   b. Acquired immune deficiency
   c. Confusion and depression
   d. Schizophrenia

9. **A record of a person's background, including lifestyle and social information is called a/an:**

   a. Physical exam
   b. History
   c. Review of systems
   d. Autobiography

10. **A physical examination uses looking, listening, feeling, and:**

    a. Smelling
    b. Tasting
    c. Pinching
    d. Tickling

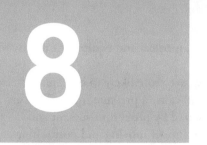

8

Positioning, Moving, and Restorative Care

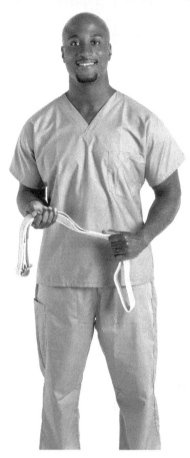

Helping a resident move and be comfortably positioned is one of the most important things you do. Moving about freely is a primary activity of daily living. As a nurse assistant, you work with the charge nurse and physical therapist to meet residents' mobility needs. Learning to move and position residents correctly ensures that you and the residents remain safe. According the U.S. Bureau of Labor Statistics, the leading cause of injury among long term care workers is incorrect body mechanics when moving and lifting. These injuries (most often to the back) often happen because of poor planning when moving or positioning a resident.

In this chapter, you will learn how to determine a resident's mobility in different situations and how to help them move safely and efficiently. You will also learn how to safely assist residents who cannot change positions on their own throughout the day. In addition, you will become familiar with the nurse assistant's role in restorative activities for residents.

OBJECTIVES:

- State the importance of moving and positioning residents correctly.

- List at least five questions to consider when preparing to move or position a resident.

- Demonstrate how to move a resident safely.

- Explain the correct way to assist a resident who has fallen.

- Describe your role in promoting residents' independence.

- List the types of equipment used to enhance mobility and promote independence and describe how each is used.

- Demonstrate range-of-motion exercises and assisted walking.

How Movement Affects Body Systems

The human body is designed for continual movement. When a person stops moving or has restricted movement, the body adapts and slows down to accommodate the reduction in movement. Because body systems are interconnected, even a small change in the level of mobility can affect all body systems. Aging slows down many body functions, so older adults are affected even more by movement restrictions. According to the National Institute of Aging (NIA), mobility is critical for functioning well and living independently. Mobility can improve muscular imbalances, improve posture, and prevent injuries.

Moving and positioning our bodies also has an emotional and psychological aspect. Without freedom of movement, residents have trouble meeting basic needs. In many cases, residents' self-esteem is connected to achieving at least some independence in mobility (Figure 8-1).

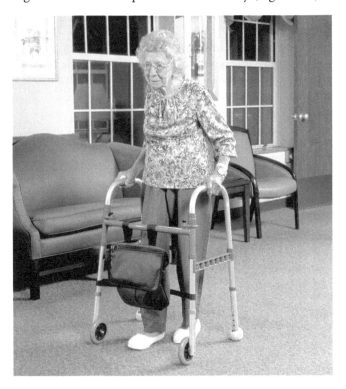

Figure 8-1 Walkers help residents with ambulation and promote independence.

Positioning is how you help residents sit, lie down, or change position when they cannot move independently. Even residents who can move on their own may need help with positioning. They may have trouble getting comfortable or have skin problems from not changing positions often enough. The best positions for an individual resident depend on the person's body type, health

status, skin condition, medical and equipment needs, and comfort.

Certain body areas are more likely to be damaged by pressure, which can cause a pressure injury. Pressure injuries can be prevented by proper movement and changing of position. Proper moving and positioning help residents by:

- Reducing swelling in a limb (arm or leg)
- Preventing stiffness of limbs and joints
- Preventing tubes or equipment lines from being pulled
- Keeping residents as comfortable as possible
- Preventing pain and discomfort from stiffness, pressure, and poor circulation

Preparing to Move or Position a Resident

Before you help move or position a resident, it is important to observe the resident's abilities and ask the charge nurse about the person's needs. You will work with the charge nurse and physical therapist to determine the best way to move or reposition a resident. When positioning a resident, you must observe and consider these factors:

- Spinal deformities (such as rounded back, forward head, leaning to one side)
- Areas of skin redness
- Bandaged areas, casts, or splints
- Stiffness or swelling in arms, legs, hands, or feet
- IV lines, oxygen, or other equipment in use
- Any recent surgery

Your next step is to ask yourself the following questions. You must know the answers to these questions before you move or position a resident:

Consider your capabilities and limitations:
1. Do you understand the physician's orders and the charge nurse's expectations?
2. Can you do what's needed?
3. Do you need help?

Consider the resident:
1. Can this resident understand what you are asking them to do?
2. Can this resident see and hear you? Do they need glasses or a hearing aid?
3. How large or heavy is this resident?

4. What tubes or equipment are connected, such as an IV or oxygen line?

5. Does this resident have any dressings or open wounds?

6. Does this resident have any special needs or behaviors to consider before you start the move?

7. Does this resident have any physical condition that affects moving, such as fragile skin or bones?

8. How much help does this resident need to move?

9. How much weight is the resident allowed to place on the limb?

10. How much limb motion is allowed?

11. Where are this resident's shoes and socks?

12. Does this resident use an assistive device such as a walker, cane, or brace?

13. What equipment do you need to most easily move this resident?

14. Can this resident tolerate all positions?

Consider the environment:

1. Could the lighting, noise level, or distractions such as family members or care of another resident affect moving and positioning?

2. Are any obstacles (such as medical equipment, linens, personal possessions, or furniture) in the way?

3. Is the bed at the proper height?

4. Is the bed in a locked position?

5. If transferring to a wheelchair, are the wheels locked?

6. Is everything needed close at hand?

7. Is it possible to move around any tubes or equipment near the resident?

8. Which chair or seating device does the resident use?

Safety First

Recall that in Chapter 6 you learned the importance of preventing on-the-job injuries and, that certain types of equipment can be used for safety when moving or positioning a resident. As a refresher, you can review Table 6-1 on page 111.

Before you move or position a resident, decide whether you need help. If you are not sure, then always get help. You may need help for many reasons. Always be safe and get help if you do not know the resident well, are not sure how he or she will respond to you, or if you are uncertain about your ability to lift the resident by yourself.

Clear communication with residents and coworkers is important. Serious injury can occur if someone does not understand how the move is to be done. Giving clear directions is important. Everyone must know what to do and when to do it. Be sure the resident understands their role. You can ask them to do things "on the count of three," such as to push off the bed to help you raise them to a standing position (Figure 8-2). The resident should be an active participant in the move to the degree that they are able. Unless contraindicated, always use a gait or transfer belt.

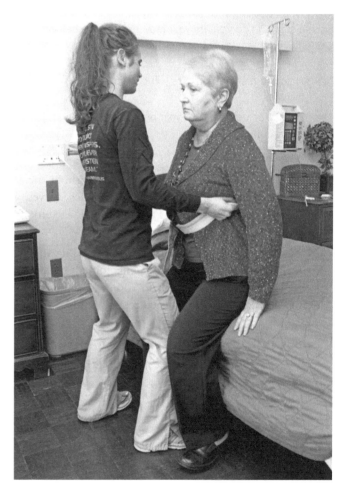

Figure 8-2 Some residents are able to push off the bed while the nurse assistant uses a gait belt to help them stand.

Tips to Promote Safety

Guidelines for proper body mechanics are outlined in Box 8-1. The tips listed below will make the process of moving a resident safer and easier:

- You can use the side rail of the bed during moving and positioning as long as it benefits the resident. But remember that side rails that restrict a resident's mobility are considered restraints and cannot be used without a physician's order except temporarily in moving and positioning.

Box 8-1

GUIDELINES FOR PROPER BODY MECHANICS

- Keep one foot slightly in front of the other, placed 10 to 12 inches apart.
- Always bend your knees when lifting to protect your back.
- When working with another helper, use counting as a signal to coordinate your movements. The helper moving the heaviest part of the resident's body does the counting.
- Hold the resident close to you body during a transfer.
- When transferring, turn your entire body as a unit. Do not lift and twist.

- Never move a resident by pulling on their arm or the skin under their arm. There are many arteries, nerves, and veins under the armpit. Pulling can damage blood vessels and nerves.
- Many older residents have osteoporosis. This means that their joints and bones are fragile; joints can be dislocated and bones easily broken. You must make sure that you support the joint when repositioning.
- Remember to first position the bed for the move. For example, put the bed in a flat position to move the resident up in bed, and raise the head of the bed when helping a resident out of bed.

Positioning

When residents cannot change positions by themselves, you need to do this for them. Make a positioning schedule that ensures that the resident is comfortable and has good blood flow to all body parts. Usually, you change their position every two hours. Some positions are better for individual residents than others. Some positions can potentially cause problems for a resident, depending on their condition. For example, a resident who is short of breath may have problems breathing when supine. Discuss all positions with the charge nurse to make sure that they are allowed for the resident.

You may be asked to assist the residents with the following positions:

- Supine— the resident is positioned on their back with the head of the bed flat.
- Side-lying or lateral — the resident is positioned on either side with their knees slightly bent.
- Sims — the resident is positioned on their left side with the hip and lower leg slightly bent and the right hip and knee is bent. This position can be used for administering an enema.
- Prone — the resident is positioned in a face down position on their abdomen. This position is typically used for resident's having difficulty breathing.

As previously noted, pay attention to proper body mechanics and always use available positioning devices to prevent injuries to you and the resident. Remove any wrinkles from the resident's clothing before positioning them because wrinkles can cause pressure injuries. Always make sure to protect the skin from shearing and tearing when assisting with position changes. When assisting a resident to move up in the bed, make sure that their skin is not rubbing against the bed linen as they are moved up. Use positioning devices to prevent shearing that can occur when a resident slides down in bed or in a chair.

Procedures 8-1 through 8-10 outline the steps for assisting residents in moving from one position to another. Before you focus on learning these procedures, be sure to review the common preparation steps shown in Table 5-3 (page 82) and common completion steps shown in Table 5-4 (page 82).

8-1: Moving Up in Bed When a Resident Can Help

PREPARATION STEPS

1. Check the care plan.
2. Knock, introduce yourself, and address resident by preferred name.
3. Perform hand hygiene.
4. Gather supplies and secure assistance if needed.
5. Explain procedure and ask about resident preferences.
6. Respect privacy and rights at all times.

1   With the resident lying supine, lower the head of the bed to a flat position (if the person can tolerate it). Move the pillows against the headboard to prevent the resident from injuring their head.

2   Help the resident bend their knees and place their feet flat on the bed. Place one arm under the resident's upper back behind the shoulders and the other arm under their upper thighs.

3   On the count of three, have the resident push down with their feet and lift their buttocks (creating a bridge) while you help move them toward the head of the bed. You may also have the resident help by holding on to the side rails. If side rails are used, be sure to lower the rails when you are done.

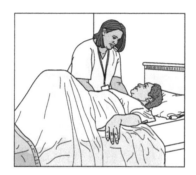

COMPLETION STEPS

1. Determine the resident's preferred position for comfort and ask them if they need anything else.
2. Examine the environment for safety and cleanliness.
3. Secure the call light and any other needed items within reach of the resident.
4. Perform hand hygiene.
5. Document the procedure and report any findings to the staff in charge.

PREPARATION STEPS

1. Check the care plan.
2. Knock, introduce yourself, and address resident by preferred name.
3. Perform hand hygiene.
4. Gather supplies and secure assistance if needed.
5. Explain procedure and ask about resident preferences.
6. Respect privacy and rights at all times.

1 Ask another staff person to assist you.

2 With the resident lying supine, lower the head of the bed to a flat position (if the person can tolerate it). Move the pillows against the headboard to prevent the resident from injuring their head.

3 Help the resident cross their arms over their chest.

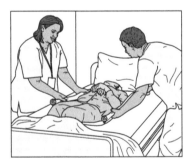

4 Roll the draw sheet up from the side toward the resident until you and your helper have a tight grip on it with both hands. Keep your palms up if that gives you more strength for moving. (If the linen is soiled, use a barrier to prevent contaminating your uniform.) You can place one knee on the bed to get as close to the resident as possible and to provide more leverage.

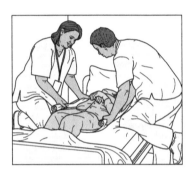

5 On the count of three, you and your helper lift the resident up to the head of the bed, using good body mechanics. You can do this in stages until the resident is in position. If the resident can lift their head off the bed, ask them to do this during the move.

6 Unroll the draw sheet and tuck it in.

COMPLETION STEPS

1. Determine the resident's preferred position for comfort and ask them if they need anything else.
2. Examine the environment for safety and cleanliness.
3. Secure the call light and any other needed items within reach of the resident.
4. Perform hand hygiene.
5. Document the procedure and report any findings to the staff in charge.

8-3: Moving to the Side of the Bed When a Resident Can Help

PREPARATION STEPS

1. Check the care plan.
2. Knock, introduce yourself, and address resident by preferred name.
3. Perform hand hygiene.
4. Gather supplies and secure assistance if needed.
5. Explain procedure and ask about resident preferences.
6. Respect privacy and rights at all times.

1 Stand on the side to which you plan to move the resident.

2 Help the resident bend their knees and place their feet flat on the bed.

3 Help the resident lift up their buttocks (creating a bridge), and move their buttocks to the side of the bed.

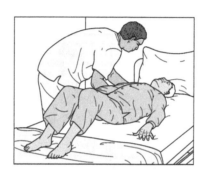

4 Help the resident move their legs over, followed by their head and upper body. Slide your arms underneath and glide them toward you if they need additional help.

5 You can do this in stages to reach the desired position.

COMPLETION STEPS

1. Determine the resident's preferred position for comfort and ask them if they need anything else.
2. Examine the environment for safety and cleanliness.
3. Secure the call light and any other needed items within reach of the resident.
4. Perform hand hygiene.
5. Document the procedure and report any findings to the staff in charge.

8-4: Moving to the Side of the Bed When a Resident is Unable to Help

PREPARATION STEPS

1. Check the care plan.
2. Knock, introduce yourself, and address resident by preferred name.
3. Perform hand hygiene.
4. Gather supplies and secure assistance if needed.
5. Explain procedure and ask about resident preferences.
6. Respect privacy and rights at all times.

1 Stand on the side to which you plan to move the resident.

2 Ask the resident to fold their arms across their chest or do this for them, if necessary.

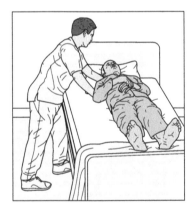

3 Slide both your hands under the resident's head, neck, and shoulders and glide the upper body toward you. Keep the resident's body in proper align¬-ment as you move them.

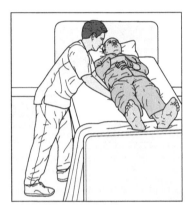

4 Slide your arms under the resident's hips and glide them toward you.

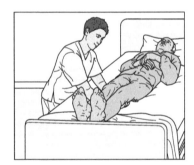

5 Slide your arms under their legs and glide them toward you.

COMPLETION STEPS

1. Determine the resident's preferred position for comfort and ask them if they need anything else.
2. Examine the environment for safety and cleanliness.
3. Secure the call light and any other needed items within reach of the resident.
4. Perform hand hygiene.
5. Document the procedure and report any findings to the staff in charge.

8-5: Moving a Resident to the Side of the Bed Using a Draw Sheet (Two Assist)

PREPARATION STEPS

1. Check the care plan.
2. Knock, introduce yourself, and address resident by preferred name.
3. Perform hand hygiene.
4. Gather supplies and secure assistance if needed.
5. Explain procedure and ask about resident preferences.
6. Respect privacy and rights at all times.

1 Ask another staff person to help you.

2 Help the resident place their arms across their chest.

3 Roll the draw sheet up from the side toward the resident until you and your helper have a tight grip on it with both hands. Keep your palms up if that gives you more strength for moving. (If the linen is soiled, use a barrier to prevent contaminating your uniform.)

The staff member who is moving the heaviest part of the resident's body may want to place one knee on the edge of the bed for more leverage.

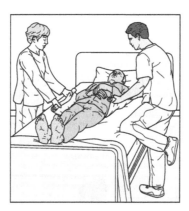

4 The person with the heaviest load leads the count to three. On three, you both lift the resident to the side of the bed. You can do this in stages until the desired position is reached.

5 Unroll the draw sheet and tuck it in.

COMPLETION STEPS

1. Determine the resident's preferred position for comfort and ask them if they need anything else.
2. Examine the environment for safety and cleanliness.
3. Secure the call light and any other needed items within reach of the resident.
4. Perform hand hygiene.
5. Document the procedure and report any findings to the staff in charge.

8-6: Turning a Resident from Supine to Side-Lying (Lateral) for Personal Care

PREPARATION STEPS

1. Check the care plan.
2. Knock, introduce yourself, and address resident by preferred name.
3. Perform hand hygiene.
4. Gather supplies and secure assistance if needed.
5. Explain procedure and ask about resident preferences.
6. Respect privacy and rights at all times.

1 Help the resident bend their knees and place their feet flat on the bed.

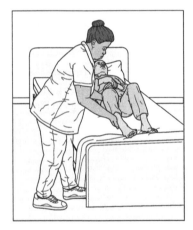

2 Place one hand on the resident's shoulder that is farthest from you.

3 Place your other hand on the hip farthest from you.

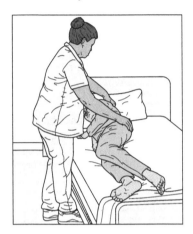

4 On the count of three, help the resident roll toward you. Some residents may be more comfortable guiding the turn by holding on to the side rails. Lower the side rails when done.

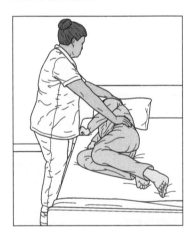

5 Continue personal care.

COMPLETION STEPS

1. Determine the resident's preferred position for comfort and ask them if they need anything else.
2. Examine the environment for safety and cleanliness.
3. Secure the call light and any other needed items within reach of the resident.
4. Perform hand hygiene.
5. Document the procedure and report any findings to the staff in charge.

8-7: Moving a Resident from Supine Position to Sitting (Dangling)

PREPARATION STEPS

1. Check the care plan.
2. Knock, introduce yourself, and address resident by preferred name.
3. Perform hand hygiene.
4. Gather supplies and secure assistance if needed.
5. Explain procedure and ask about resident preferences.
6. Respect privacy and rights at all times.

OPTION 1:

If a second person assists you, you both stand on the same side of the resident. One person lifts the head and upper body, and the other person lifts the legs and lower body.

1 The resident is lying in supine position. Help the resident roll onto their side facing you and raise the head of the bed.

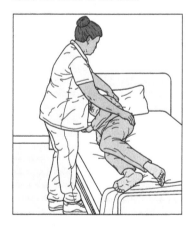

2 Using your arm that is closest to the head of the bed, reach under the resident's head and place your hand under their shoulder. The resident's head should be supported by and resting on your forearm.

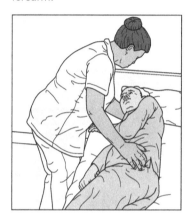

3 With your other hand, reach over and behind the resident's knee that is farthest from you.

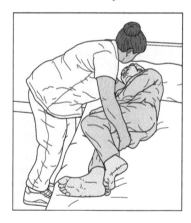

4 Bring the resident's head and trunk up as you swing their legs down to the sitting position. Keep one arm behind the resident to support them in the sitting position. With your other arm, support the resident's legs, with the back of their knees in the crook of your elbow. Stay close to their body to prevent rocking or a fall.

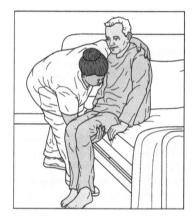

5 Help the resident get comfortable in the dangling or sitting position.

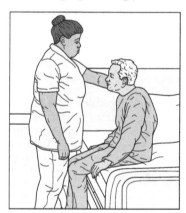

8-7: Moving a Resident from Supine Position to Sitting (continued)

OPTION 2:

1 Help the resident roll onto their side facing you and raise the head of the bed.

2 Slide their feet over the edge of the bed.

3 Using your arm that is closest to the head of the bed, reach under the resident's head and put your hand under their shoulder. The resident's head should be supported by and resting on your forearm.

4 Place your other hand on the resident's hip. As you help the resident sit up, place gentle but firm pressure on their hip (using leverage) and help raise the resident upward to a sitting position. Keep one arm behind the resident to support them in the sitting position. Stay close to their body to prevent rocking or a fall.

COMPLETION STEPS

1. Determine the resident's preferred position for comfort and ask them if they need anything else.
2. Examine the environment for safety and cleanliness.
3. Secure the call light and any other needed items within reach of the resident.
4. Perform hand hygiene.
5. Document the procedure and report any findings to the staff in charge.

8-8: Moving a Resident from Sitting to Supine Position

PREPARATION STEPS

1. Check the care plan.
2. Knock, introduce yourself, and address resident by preferred name.
3. Perform hand hygiene.
4. Gather supplies and secure assistance if needed.
5. Explain procedure and ask about resident preferences.
6. Respect privacy and rights at all times.

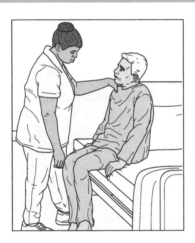
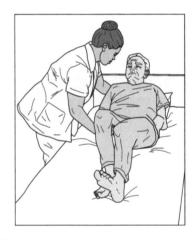

1 Before beginning the move, make sure that the resident is centered in the bed with the backs of the knees against the mattress. You may want to elevate the head of the bed.

2 Place one hand behind the resident's shoulder, and let their head and neck rest on your forearm. Place your other arm under their knees, and let their legs rest in the crook of your elbow.

3 Use your legs to lift and breathe out as you help the resident lift their legs up onto the bed. Gently lower their trunk and head onto the bed. If the resident is able, they can push down on the bed with their hands to help move their body back onto the bed.

4 Lower the head of the bed, if necessary, for the resident's comfort.

COMPLETION STEPS

1. Determine the resident's preferred position for comfort and ask them if they need anything else.
2. Examine the environment for safety and cleanliness.
3. Secure the call light and any other needed items within reach of the resident.
4. Perform hand hygiene.
5. Document the procedure and report any findings to the staff in charge.

8-9: Positioning a Resident on Their Back (Supine)

PREPARATION STEPS

1. Check the care plan.
2. Knock, introduce yourself, and address resident by preferred name.
3. Perform hand hygiene.
4. Gather supplies and secure assistance if needed.
5. Explain procedure and ask about resident preferences.
6. Respect privacy and rights at all times.

1 First, move the resident's trunk and lower body so that their spine is in a neutral position. Do the positioning from the top of the body to the bottom.

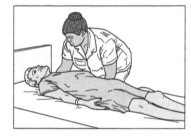

2 Position the resident's head and neck. Place a pillow under the resident's head, neck, and the tops of their shoulders. Do not elevate the head too high. Keep it as close to even with the chest as possible or as is comfortable.

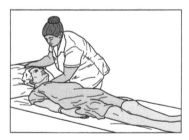

3 Position the resident's arms. The backs of the shoulders and elbows are common places for pressure injuries in residents who cannot change position by themselves. Vary their arm positions to prevent this. Keep the arms straight and resting on the mattress away from their sides, or bend the arms slightly at the elbow with a pillow between the inner arm and their side so that their arm rests on the pillow and their hand on top of the abdomen. Always support the arms in two places when moving them, and move them gently.

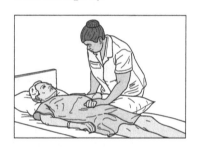

4 Position the resident's legs. The hips, buttocks, sacrum, and coccyx (the tip of the spine at the buttocks, or "tailbone"), and the backs of the heels are common places for pressure injuries. If a resident has pressure injuries on a hip, place a towel roll along the hip between the hip and the mattress on the affected side. For redness or pressure injuries under the heels, support the legs by placing a pillow lengthwise to raise the heels above the bed, or place a towel roll under the legs. Position the resident's legs straight and slightly apart. Always support the legs in two places when moving them, and move them gently. For those residents who tend to keep their legs tightly together or crossed, you may place a pillow between the legs.

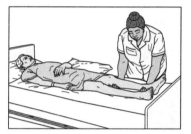

5 If a resident has a cast or splint on a limb, hand, or foot or a swollen arm or leg, you can place a pillow lengthwise to support the affected limb, hand, or foot.

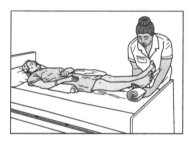

COMPLETION STEPS

1. Determine the resident's preferred position for comfort and ask them if they need anything else.
2. Examine the environment for safety and cleanliness.
3. Secure the call light and any other needed items within reach of the resident.
4. Perform hand hygiene.
5. Document the procedure and report any findings to the staff in charge.

8-10: Positioning a Resident on Their Side (Side-Lying Position)

PREPARATION STEPS

1. Check the care plan.
2. Knock, introduce yourself, and address resident by preferred name.
3. Perform hand hygiene.
4. Gather supplies and secure assistance if needed.
5. Explain procedure and ask about resident preferences.
6. Respect privacy and rights at all times.

Note that the positions described may be modified for the resident's comfort and to prevent pressure injuries.

1 Begin with the resident in supine position. Stand on the side to which the resident will be turning.

2 Help the resident bend their knees.

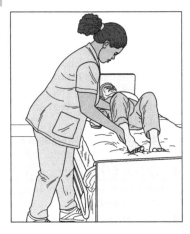

3 Place one hand on the resident's shoulder that is farthest from you. Place your other hand on the hip farthest from you. On the count of three, help the resident roll toward you. Position the resident comfortably with proper body alignment.

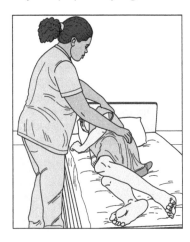

4 Position the resident's head and neck. Place a pillow under their head so that the neck is properly aligned and comfortable.

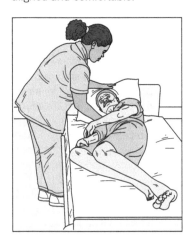

5 Fold a pillow lengthwise and place it behind the resident's back. Gently push the top edge of the pillow under their side and hip.

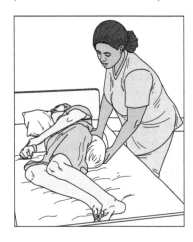

6 Position the resident's arms. Gently pull the arm against the mattress out from under the resident's body if it is not already in front of the body. Place a pillow diagonally under the top arm between the arm and the resident's side. Bend the top arm at the elbow and shoulder to rest the arm comfortably on the pillow.

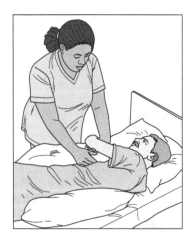

7 Position the resident's legs. Bend the top hip up and rotate it slightly forward. Place a pillow lengthwise between the resident's knees to separate their legs down to their ankles.

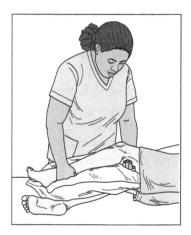

COMPLETION STEPS

1. Determine the resident's preferred position for comfort and ask them if they need anything else.

2. Examine the environment for safety and cleanliness.

3. Secure the call light and any other needed items within reach of the resident.

4. Perform hand hygiene.

5. Document the procedure and report any findings to the staff in charge.

Fowler's Position

Some residents have breathing problems due to obesity, pulmonary disease, heart disease, or other causes. For these residents, the physician or charge nurse may order the **Fowler's position**. In this position, the resident lies on their back, and the head of the bed is raised 45 to 60 degrees. The most common angle is about 45 degrees. Sometimes the knees are bent slightly (Figure 8-3). A high-Fowler's position has the head of the bed from 60 to 90 degrees and a semi-Fowler's position has the head of the bed raised 30 to 45 degrees.

This position is also used when feeding a resident or helping them with personal care tasks. It is also used when the resident wants to sit in bed to read, watch television, or converse with visitors.

When you elevate the head of the bed, this raises the resident's head, neck, and body. You can place the resident in Fowler's position by elevating the head of the bed or by placing pillows under the back, head, and neck. Be careful to keep the resident's head and neck in alignment to prevent neck pain or injury.

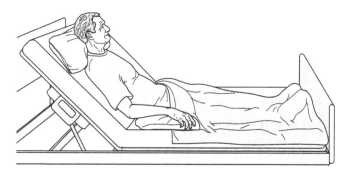

Figure 8-3 Fowler's position is often used for residents with breathing problems or respiratory diseases.

Moving a Resident from One Place to Another

In Chapter 6, we used the term *transfer* to refer to a resident moving to a new unit or wing in the facility. This term is also used to describe physically moving a resident from one place to another. When transferring a resident, safety must be your top priority. You must make sure that both you and the resident remain safe and avoid injury.

Many facilities require using a **gait belt** (also called a safety belt, guard, or transfer belt) and other safety equipment (Figure 8-4). Refer to chapter 6, Procedure 1 for how to apply (page 112) and use a gait belt.

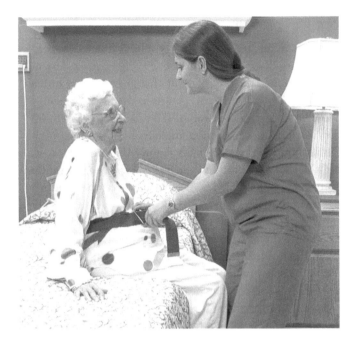

Figure 8-4 A guard belt (gait belt) is often used to help prevent injuries while transferring residents.

There are various types of transfers:

- Stand-pivot transfer
- Transfer with an assistive device
- Sliding board and seated transfers (less common)
- Mechanical lift transfers
- Dependent lift using two or more staff

The stand-pivot transfer and assisted transfer with an assistive device are the methods most commonly used. See Procedures 8-11 through 8-16 for detailed steps for all transfer procedures.

Considerations in transferring a resident:

- *For all residents* – Determine their weight bearing status. Some residents may not be able to be full weight bearing (FWB) on a particular extremity. Some residents may be partial weight bearing (PWB) or non-weight bearing (NWB).
- *Residents getting out of bed* — The bed usually should be at its lowest position or raised, if needed, for a tall resident. When transferring a resident out of bed, allow them to dangle their legs over the edge of the bed for a few minutes before standing. This helps to prevent dizziness due to a sudden change in posture. If the resident complains of dizziness, help them lie down and call the charge nurse. Do not leave a resident unattended unless they are secure.

- *Residents who use wheelchairs* — The wheelchair should be locked and set alongside the bed with the arm of the chair next to the bed. The chair should be on the resident's stronger side. For example, if the resident has a weakened left side due to a stroke, put the chair on their right side.
- *Residents who use assistive devices* — A resident's walker or cane should be next to or in front of them. A brace or other special equipment should be correctly in place.
- *When using a mechanical lift* — Only operate lifts that you have had training on how to use. Check your facility policy on how many assistants are needed to safely operate the lift as well as the age requirements. Use the correct size and type of sling for the transfer.
- *Transferring to or from a stretcher* — If possible, make sure that the resident is in a supine position and the stretcher, bed or shower chair the resident is being transferred to are at the about the same height or slightly lower for proper body mechanics.

Before you can transfer a resident from bed to a chair, the resident must first roll onto their side or have them in a Fowler's position and then sit up. When starting to transfer a resident from bed to chair, watch for any problems that may occur. Table 8-1 summarizes common problems and how to deal with them.

Table 8-1 Problems and Solutions in Transferring a Resident from Bed to a Chair

Problem	Solution
You lose your grip on the resident.	Help the resident sit back on the bed. Change your position so you have a better grip and can provide better support.
The resident's legs cannot support their weight.	If a resident's legs start to collapse once you are moving, place your legs in front of theirs and help them sit back on the bed. You may need to get help to complete the transfer.
The resident gets dizzy when they change position.	Changes in position can cause dizziness because blood pools in the extremities, and for a brief time less blood reaches the brain (postural hypotension). Wait a few minutes and begin again.
The resident becomes weak, unsteady, or starts to faint.	Help the resident sit back on the bed. Lower them to supine position, if necessary. Call the charge nurse immediately.

PREPARATION STEPS

1. Check the care plan.
2. Knock, introduce yourself, and address resident by preferred name.
3. Perform hand hygiene.
4. Gather supplies and secure assistance if needed.
5. Explain procedure and ask about resident preferences.
6. Respect privacy and rights at all times.

These steps are used to transfer a resident from bed to a chair or wheelchair.

1 Stand in front of the resident. If a wheelchair is the target, make sure that its wheels are locked and the leg rests are out of the way or removed. Ensure that the resident has on non slip footwear. Apply gait belt unless contraindicated.

2 Place one of your legs between the resident's legs and the other close to the chair or wheelchair. (This gives you better control over the speed and the direction of the movement.)

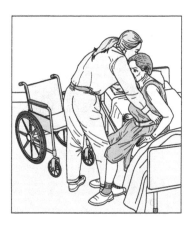

3 Hold onto the gait belt at the resident's back, slightly to one side. If you are not using a gait belt, wrap your arms around the resident's waist.

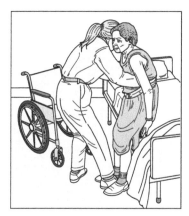

4 Ask the resident to push down on the bed with their hands, lean forward, and stand up. If the person cannot push off the bed, you can have them hold onto your waist during the transfer. Do not let the resident hold you around your neck because this places you at risk for injury.

5 On the count of three, help the resident stand by leaning your body back and up, bringing the resident's body forward. Ask them to lean forward and stand up.

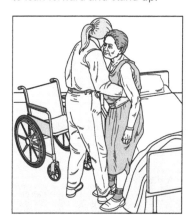

6 Once the resident is standing, keep your back neutral and body facing forward. Pivot (turning your feet or taking small steps) to turn them until the backs of their knees are against the chair.

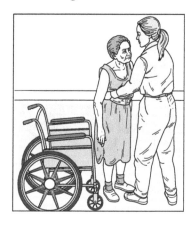

7 Ask the resident to reach back for the arm of the chair with one or both hands, if possible.

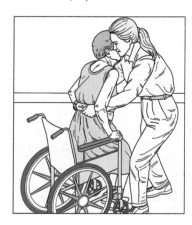

8 Help the resident bend their knees and sit.

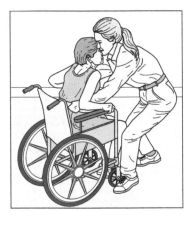

9 Once the resident is seated, ask them to push back in the chair by pushing down with their feet on the floor and arms on the armrests. If they cannot do this, you will need to help them move back in the chair. Remove gait belt and position feet on leg rests.

COMPLETION STEPS

1. Determine the resident's preferred position for comfort and ask them if they need anything else.
2. Examine the environment for safety and cleanliness.
3. Secure the call light and any other needed items within reach of the resident.
4. Perform hand hygiene.
5. Document the procedure and report any findings to the staff in charge.

PREPARATION STEPS

1. Check the care plan.
2. Knock, introduce yourself, and address resident by preferred name.
3. Perform hand hygiene.
4. Gather supplies and secure assistance if needed.
5. Explain procedure and ask about resident preferences.
6. Respect privacy and rights at all times.

These steps are used to transfer a resident from bed to a chair or wheelchair.

1 Once the resident is sitting on the side of the bed, place the assistive device in their hand (cane) or in front of them (walker). If transferring to wheelchair make sure the brakes are locked and the leg rests are out of the way or removed. Ensure that the resident has on non slip footwear. Apply gait belt unless contraindicated.

2 If a cane is being used, stand to the side of the resident that is opposite the hand holding the cane. If a walker is being used, you can stand to either side.

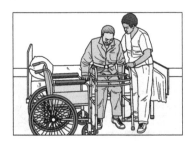

3 Ask the resident to push down on the bed with their hands and stand on the count of three. If they cannot do this, you can help by pulling up and forward on the back of the gait belt with one hand while pushing down on the walker or cane to keep it stable while the resident stands. Encourage a resident using a walker to stand before grabbing hold of the assistive device.

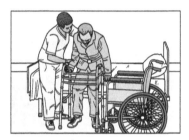

4 For residents using a walker, once they are standing, help them place both hands securely on the walker. The resident may need to stand still for a few minutes before moving to prevent dizziness or to allow it to pass.

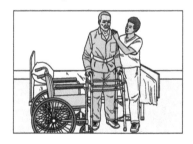

5 Help the resident move toward the chair or wheelchair. Guide them with statements such as: "Turn, turn, take a step toward me, now back up."

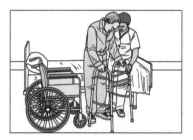

6 If a wheelchair is the target, make sure that its wheels are locked. Help the resident back up to the chair. Ask if they can feel the chair against the back of their legs. Explain that they should not sit until they can feel the chair behind their legs.

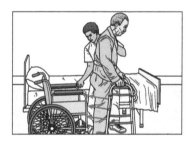

7 With the resident in front of the chair, ask them to reach back and put one hand on the armrest.

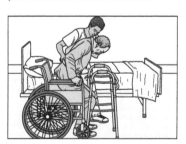

8 Help the resident reach back with the other hand for the arm of the chair and slowly sit down.

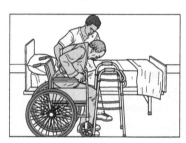

COMPLETION STEPS

1. Determine the resident's preferred position for comfort and ask them if they need anything else.
2. Examine the environment for safety and cleanliness.
3. Secure the call light and any other needed items within reach of the resident.
4. Perform hand hygiene.
5. Document the procedure and report any findings to the staff in charge.

8-13: Transfer from a Chair to Bed, Commode, or Toilet

PREPARATION STEPS

1. Check the care plan.
2. Knock, introduce yourself, and address resident by preferred name.
3. Perform hand hygiene.
4. Gather supplies and secure assistance if needed.
5. Explain procedure and ask about resident preferences.
6. Respect privacy and rights at all times.

If a resident is capable of helping with the transfer, use the stand-pivot or assistive-device transfer method. If a resident cannot help, use the mechanical lift (described in Procedure 8-14) or have a coworker assist with the transfer.

1 Position the chair or wheelchair with the resident's stronger side closer to the bed, commode, or toilet. Ensure that the resident has on non slip footwear. Apply gait belt unless contraindicated.

2 If the resident is in a wheelchair, make sure the wheels are locked. Ask them to move their feet off the footrests. Raise the footrests or move them out of the way.

3 Ask the resident to slide forward to the edge of the chair. If this movement is difficult for the resident, you may need to assist.

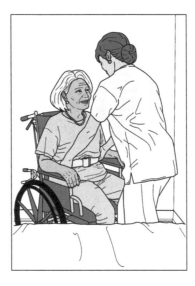

4 Use either the stand-pivot or assistive-device transfer procedure in reverse to move the resident from the chair to the bed, commode, or toilet.

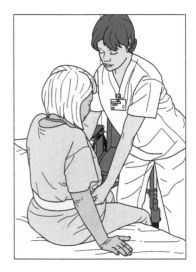

COMPLETION STEPS

1. Determine the resident's preferred position for comfort and ask them if they need anything else.
2. Examine the environment for safety and cleanliness.
3. Secure the call light and any other needed items within reach of the resident.
4. Perform hand hygiene.
5. Document the procedure and report any findings to the staff in charge.

8-14: Moving a Resident with a Mechanical Lift (Two Assist)

PREPARATION STEPS

1. Check the care plan.
2. Knock, introduce yourself, and address resident by preferred name.
3. Perform hand hygiene.
4. Gather supplies and secure assistance if needed.
5. Explain procedure and ask about resident preferences.
6. Respect privacy and rights at all times.

1 One helper stands on each side of the bed.

2 Adjust the head of the bed as flat as possible if the resident can tolerate it. Make sure you have to correct size and type of sling for the transfer.

3 To place the sling under the resident, first turn the resident toward you. Help them move toward you while your helper pushes the fan-folded sling under the resident as far as possible. Then help the resident back toward the other side and pull the sling under them. The sling should be placed from under the shoulders to the back of the knees. For stability, the resident should be centered within the sling.

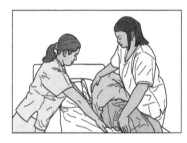

4 Place the lift frame facing the bed with its legs under the bed. Lock the wheels on the base.

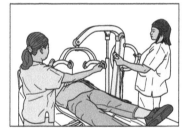

5 Elevate the head of the bed so the resident is partially sitting up.

6 Attach the sling to the lift following the manufacturer's directions.

7 Ask the resident to cross their arms over their chest before operating the lift. If they cannot achieve this position, ask them to hold onto an object such as a towel to keep their arms near their body.

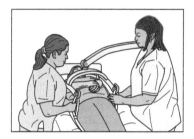

8 Follow the manufacturer's directions and use the lift to raise the resident to a sitting position. While you operate the lift, your helper should help guide the resident. As you move the resident, ask several times to confirm that they are okay. Being lifted by machine can be frightening, especially the first time.

9 Once the resident is sitting upright, keep raising the lift until they are six to 12 inches above the bed and chair height.

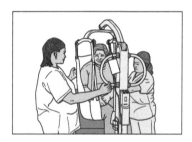

10 Unlock the swivel, if the lift has one, or use the steering handle to move the resident directly over the chair. You may need to guide the resident's legs.

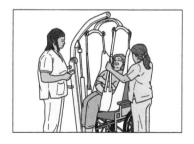

11 Tell the resident that you are now going to lower them slowly into the chair. Your helper guides the resident into the chair by moving the sling. Press the release button to slowly lower them down.

12 Once the resident is securely in the chair, unhook the sling and remove the lift frame.

13 Position the resident in the chair, leaving the sling underneath them (unless the sling is removable) until it is time to return to bed. Pull the metal bars of the sling out so that the resident does not lean against or sit on them.

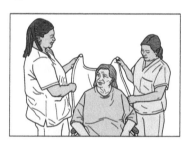

COMPLETION STEPS

1. Determine the resident's preferred position for comfort and ask them if they need anything else.
2. Examine the environment for safety and cleanliness.
3. Secure the call light and any other needed items within reach of the resident.
4. Perform hand hygiene.
5. Document the procedure and report any findings to the staff in charge.

PREPARATION STEPS

1. Check the care plan.
2. Knock, introduce yourself, and address resident by preferred name.
3. Perform hand hygiene.
4. Gather supplies and secure assistance if needed.
5. Explain procedure and ask about resident preferences.
6. Respect privacy and rights at all times.

The following steps are used to move a resident up in a chair or wheelchair after a transfer to the chair.

1 Place the gait belt on the resident.

2 With one helper on each side of the resident, you each grasp the gait belt with one hand and place the other hand under the resident's knee. Ask the resident to cross their arms in front of their chest.

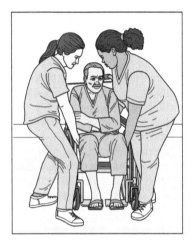

3 On the count of three, exhale, lift, and move the resident so that their back is against the back of the chair. Be sure to bend your knees and use proper body mechanics. Remove gait belt and if positioning in a wheelchair place feet on footrests.

COMPLETION STEPS

1. Determine the resident's preferred position for comfort and ask them if they need anything else.
2. Examine the environment for safety and cleanliness.
3. Secure the call light and any other needed items within reach of the resident.
4. Perform hand hygiene.
5. Document the procedure and report any findings to the staff in charge.

8-16: Returning a Resident to Bed Using a Mechanical Lift (Two Assist)

PREPARATION STEPS

1. Check the care plan.
2. Knock, introduce yourself, and address resident by preferred name.
3. Perform hand hygiene.
4. Gather supplies and secure assistance if needed.
5. Explain procedure and ask about resident preferences.
6. Respect privacy and rights at all times.

The following steps for returning a resident to bed reverse those used to transfer a resident from the bed.

1 One helper stands on each side of the chair.

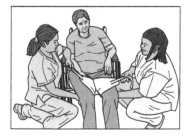

2 Position the lift facing the chair.

3 Attach the sling to the lift following the manufacturer's directions.

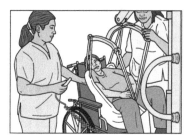

4 Again, following the manufacturer's directions, raise the resident using the lift. Your helper guides the resident by holding the sling.

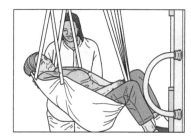

5 Swing the frame of the lift over the bed and slowly lower the resident down onto the bed.

6 Unless the resident will spend only a short time in bed, roll them from side to side to remove the sling. (The sling can cause skin irritation if left under the resident.)

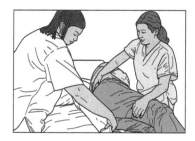

7 Position the resident as preferred.

COMPLETION STEPS

1. Determine the resident's preferred position for comfort and ask them if they need anything else.
2. Examine the environment for safety and cleanliness.
3. Secure the call light and any other needed items within reach of the resident.
4. Perform hand hygiene.
5. Document the procedure and report any findings to the staff in charge.

Assisting a Falling Resident

If you are moving or walking with a resident and they start to fall, what do you do? This can be a frightening experience for both of you. Always be prepared for a possible fall. If the resident starts to fall, use the steps shown in Procedure 8-17 to help them.

If a resident seems to be injured, or if you are not sure of their status, do not move them. Leave the resident on the floor until a nurse or physician examines them. Call for help. Do not leave the person alone unless absolutely necessary, as when you believe that their condition is serious, and no one is answering your call for help. When help arrives and the nurse or physician determines that it is safe to move the resident, use the steps shown in Procedure 8-18 to lift the resident from the floor.

8-17: Assisting a Falling Resident

If a resident starts to fall, use these steps to help them:

1 First, pull up on the gait belt, and ask the resident to try to stand up.

2 If you cannot completely stop the fall, move behind the resident, hold onto the gait belt with both hands or gently hold the person around the chest, and support them against your knee. Use good body mechanics, and call for help immediately.

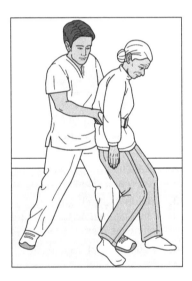

If you cannot support the weight of a resident until help arrives:

1 Gently and slowly lower the person to the floor by sliding the resident down your leg to prevent injury to both of you.

2 Once the person is in a safe, stable position, such as sitting or lying on the floor, call for help again. Ask if the resident is all right, and reassure them that help is on the way. Do not leave the resident, because he or she is likely to be frightened and feeling helpless.

3 If you absolutely must leave a resident to get help, first confirm that the person is okay. Help them lie down on the floor with their head supported (you can use a pillow or folded sheet, towel, or clothing). Explain that you must leave to get help and that you will be right back.

4 As you seek help, try to keep an eye on the resident. In a busy area, be sure the person is not in anyone's path, or ask someone else to get help so you can stay with the resident.

5 If the resident seems to be hurt or you are unsure if they are okay, do not move them. Leave the resident on the floor until a nurse or physician examines them.

COMPLETION STEPS

1. Determine the resident's preferred position for comfort and ask them if they need anything else.
2. Examine the environment for safety and cleanliness.
3. Secure the call light and any other needed items within reach of the resident.
4. Perform hand hygiene.
5. Document the procedure and report any findings to the staff in charge.

8-18: Lifting a Resident After a Fall

PREPARATION STEPS

1. Check the care plan.
2. Knock, introduce yourself, and address resident by preferred name.
3. Perform hand hygiene.
4. Gather supplies and secure assistance if needed.
5. Explain procedure and ask about resident preferences.
6. Respect privacy and rights at all times.

Once a nurse or physician has examined the resident and determined that they can be moved, use the following steps.

1 Help the person to a sitting position on the floor.

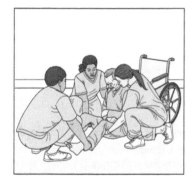

2 If the person can walk, apply a gait belt. You and another staff member can help them stand. Place one of you on each side and pull up on both sides of the gait belt.

3 If a resident needs to be moved onto a stretcher or into a chair, use a mechanical lift or other device the facility has for this purpose.

4 If a mechanical lift or other device is not available, get as many staff members to help as needed. Once the resident is in a seated position on the floor, apply a gait belt, gently bend their knees and place their feet flat on the floor. Ask the resident to fold their arms across their chest.

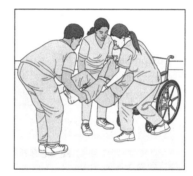

5 Before lifting, one person kneels on each side of the resident and holds on to the gait belt with one hand while placing the other hand under the resident's thigh. A third person kneels in front of the resident, supporting the resident's legs. A fourth person may hold the chair or stretcher to keep it stable.

6 The team leader asks if everyone has a good grip and is ready. The leader says, "On the count of three, lift. Ready? One, two, three, lift." This process may be done in two steps, first lifting the resident to a standing position and then into the chair or onto the stretcher.

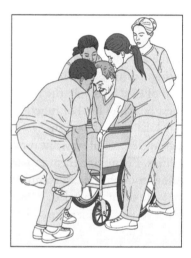

COMPLETION STEPS

1. Determine the resident's preferred position for comfort and ask them if they need anything else.
2. Examine the environment for safety and cleanliness.
3. Secure the call light and any other needed items within reach of the resident.
4. Perform hand hygiene.
5. Document the procedure and report any findings to the staff in charge.

Restorative Activities

Rehabilitation and **restorative** activities are used to help residents improve their abilities such as getting up, walking, moving, dressing, and bathing. Rehabilitative care focuses on restoring, improving, or maintaining these abilities. Residents in rehab develop new skills or work on existing skills to live as independently as possible.

Restorative activities involve teaching, prompting, and encouraging residents to care for themselves. You can help residents by using restorative activities as often as possible in your caregiving. It is part of your job to help residents retain their abilities and improve whenever they can. Always ask yourself, "What can I do to help this person regain or maintain their independence?"

Restorative activities promote a person's independence in the activities of daily living. These activities include eating, bathing, dressing, toileting, and mobility. The goal of care is to help the resident achieve their optimal (best possible) level of functioning.

Make sure you ask the resident to perform activities in a clear, respectful way, always keeping in mind their capabilities. Encourage them to participate as fully as possible. Allow enough time to complete each task. Prompt, teach, and cue them as needed, being patient with each step. How you ask residents to do something, how patient you are, and how you encourage them makes a big difference in their ability to do a given task.

You may need to teach simple everyday activities such as how to get out of bed, get dressed, and use a walker (Figure 8-5) or wheelchair. As you support residents in their daily routine, be sure not to perform tasks for residents that they can do themselves.

Restorative programs include these key elements:

- Short- and long-term goals
- Teaching, prompting, and encouraging
- The use of assistive devices
- Exercises designed to increase function and mobility

In the following sections, we discuss each of these elements. You can design your caregiving around these key elements. If you do not understand how any activity in a resident's care plan will be of help in achieving the specified goals, speak with the charge nurse or the physical therapist.

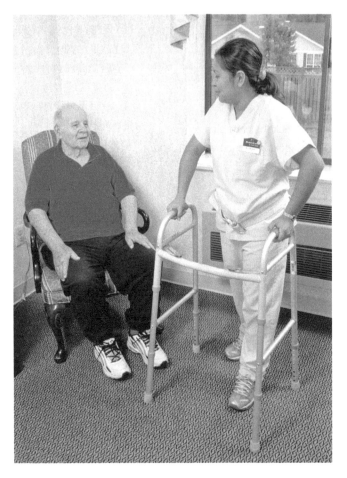

Figure 8-5 An important part of your job is helping residents learn to safely use assistive devices such as walkers.

Short- and Long-Term Goals

A **goal** is something that a person wants to accomplish. Goals help us plan specific ways to make improvements. To help residents optimize their independence, the interdisciplinary team and resident set goals. You should be involved in helping to set these goals because you spend the most time with residents.

Once you know a resident's goals, desires, and preferences, be creative in finding ways to help them meet their goals and to feel good about their progress. Once the resident shows improvement, goals can be changed. The staff can revise the goals as often as needed to keep pace with the resident's condition and progress. Your ideas for helping a resident achieve their goals must fit with the care plan and should be realistic for the resident. Discuss your ideas with the nurse or physical therapist before you try any new activities with a resident.

Cuing, Prompting, and Encouraging

In your role as the daily caregiver, take the time to cue and encourage residents to do tasks more independently. **Cuing** means that you prompt a resident to get them started. You do this by telling, teaching, or showing them part or all of the steps to take. Use common sense and your knowledge to teach using clear, simple steps:

- *Explain* what you want to help them do. If they do not understand at first, say it in a different way. If a resident has hearing difficulties, speak clearly while facing the person. If hearing is better on one side, speak to that side. Write things down if needed.

- Always give a resident *time* to respond to your request. The person may be trying to move but have trouble getting started or they may move slowly

- If a resident looks puzzled or appears to be confused by what you said, *break down the activity into simple steps*.

- If a resident continues to have difficulty, you may need to *show them what to do* or even start each step for them. If a resident does not want to participate, try some gentle encouragement before you do a task for them.

Assistive Devices

Many kinds of devices are used to improve a resident's ability to function. These include braces, walking devices, splints, a **trapeze**, and dressing aids. Often the therapist assigns this equipment to the resident to help them function safely. You must become familiar with each piece of equipment and understand how and why it is used so you can best help the resident. Residents may forget to use equipment or resist using it, even if it helps keep them safe from injury. Types of assistive devices that help with walking are described in Table 8-2.

Table 8-2   Assistive Devices that Help with Walking

Device	How the Device is Used
Canes: - *Straight cane* (J cane) is typically made of wood or metal. Metal canes may be adjustable for height. - *Quad cane* has a four-pronged base for additional stability. Made of metal and other materials.	- Used to support a weaker leg: The resident should hold the cane in the hand opposite the weaker leg. - Used for balance: The cane can be used on either side; people usually prefer to hold the cane in their dominant hand. - Top of the cane should be at the level of the resident's wrist so the person does not have to bend forward when using it.
Walkers: - *Standard walker* has four nonskid rubber-tipped legs. Provides balance support and help with walking. - *Two-wheeled walker* has wheels on the two front legs. Provides balance support and help with walking. - *Four-wheeled walker* has wheels on all four legs. This type is used for walking assistance but not for balance support because it isn't as stable as the other types.	- When using a walker to support a weaker leg, the resident moves the walker first, then the weaker leg, and then the stronger leg. - If legs are of equal strength, the resident walks forward moving the walker first, then stepping with one leg and then the other. - Rolling (wheeled) walkers allow a person to walk with a more normal gait and at a faster pace than with a standard walker. - Top of the walker should be at the height of the resident's hips for proper use without bending forward too much while walking. - When turning, both of the resident's feet should remain between the walker's legs.

Prosthetic and Orthotic Devices

A **prosthesis** is an artificial body part. These devices are also called *prosthetic devices*. They are custom made for residents to replace a body part that is missing or not fully functioning. Artificial limbs and artificial eyes are common prosthetic devices. The most common artificial limbs are artificial legs (Figure 8-6). A resident may need your help in attaching the artificial leg onto the leg stump. Use stump socks and prosthesis liners to protect the resident's skin. Inspect their skin daily during application and removal of the prosthesis. If the stump skin is red or bruised, report this promptly to the charge nurse.

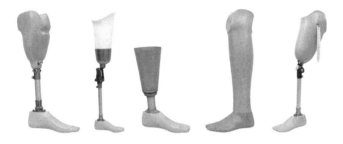

Figure 8-6 Prosthetic devices are custom made for each resident.

An **orthosis**, also called *orthotic device*, is an external apparatus used to support or align a body part to prevent or assist with movement. These devices include braces, splints, and shoe inserts. They improve or help restore the function of a limb or body part. Most often they are custom made.

Many residents use a leg, neck, or back **brace**. Braces provide support for a body part that is not strong enough to provide support on its own. They are often used during transfers and walking. Some residents use braces permanently for an injured, chronically painful, or weak joint. Others use braces temporarily during recovery from a stroke, injury, or surgery. Rigid brace material is used for weaker or more severely injured body parts. Some braces are worn only out of bed, and others are worn all the time. You must learn how to put on and remove braces correctly and know when the resident should wear it.

A knee brace may be made of elastic, which provides less support, or a more rigid material. The brace may have metal strips on both sides of the knee.

An ankle-foot orthosis (AFO) provides support for a weak ankle or to correct foot drop. *Foot drop* is an inability to flex or bend the ankle without assistance. One type of AFO is a shoe with metal uprights that are attached to a calf band. Another type is a plastic shoe insert extending from the back of the calf to the bottom of the foot. Residents who have lost use of their leg above the knee may use a knee-ankle-foot orthosis (KAFO), which supports both the knee and the ankle.

A common type of back brace is an elastic brace like a corset that closes in front with Velcro or straps. More rigid materials may be used to support any part of the back. Usually, the brace supports only the lower back.

After surgery or a spinal cord injury, a resident may have a body jacket brace extending from the lower back to the armpits. A resident wearing this type of brace generally has a very severe back problem.

Residents may wear soft or hard neck collars to support their neck. These devices may be used only in or out of bed, and some people need them all the time.

Splints are used to immobilize a joint or body part or restrict its movement in a certain way. Splints are commonly used on the hand, finger, wrist, knee, ankle, or foot. Splints keep joints in a correct position or restrict movements that may cause pain or injury. A resting splint keeps a body part at rest in the splint. A dynamic splint allows some motion of the joint but restricts undesirable movement.

Residents should use their prosthetic or orthotic devices as intended. The physical therapist will provide instructions about when and how the devices should be used. To be safe and effective, you must understand the use and care of each of these devices. Before helping a resident with a prosthetic or orthotic device, you should be instructed by the therapist or nurse. Inspect devices daily for any damage or wear and tear.

Positioning and Seating Devices

These devices include a variety of cushions, supportive chairs, pillows, towel rolls, and heel and elbow protectors. They are used to position a resident with limited independent movement in the best functional position while lying or sitting. These devices also help prevent problems such as skin breakdown and contractures. A **contracture** is an abnormal shortening of muscle tissue that occurs due to lack of movement or improper positioning. The resident's arm or leg joint may become stuck in a certain position and cannot move through its full range of motion (ROM). Heel and elbow protectors are cloth sleeves that cover the elbows and heels to protect the skin from pressure sores. Reclining chairs (also called recliners or geri-chairs) are large chairs with additional padding on the seat and back. They can be positioned for sitting upright or reclined at various angles. They are used for residents who are unable to move or sit comfortably upright, who sit for long periods throughout the day, or who may be likely to tip over a wheelchair.

Wheelchairs

Wheelchairs are available in many configurations:

- Standard, narrow, or wide width
- High back or regular back
- Lightweight or regular weight
- Standard upright or reclining

- Removable, stationary, or swing-away arm and leg rests

Most residents who use a wheelchair daily have one assigned to them. The physical therapist adjusts the wheelchair for proper positioning. A special cushion may be used for pressure relief, comfort, or seat height.

Each chair should have leg rests, which are adjusted to the correct length for proper positioning of the resident's ankle, knee, and hip joints. There are several types of leg rests. All have footplates that swing away or remain stationary. Some elevate with calf pads for support. Elevating leg rests are usually used for residents with significant edema (swelling) in their legs or feet. The physical therapist or charge nurse will instruct you when and how to elevate the leg rests. Remove or swing leg rests out of the way (if possible) during all transfers for safety and convenience. Learn how to remove and elevate them quickly and easily.

Correct positioning of a resident in a wheelchair is very important for their overall health and well-being. It helps protect skin integrity, promote good posture and comfort, and limit or prevent contractures in certain joints.

You can help residents learn about their wheelchair and its use. Show the locations of the brakes below the armrests in front of each wheel. Teach residents to lock the chair at all times when it is not being moved. Make sure the brakes are locked securely before starting any transfer. The armrests may or may not be removable or swing out of the way. You might want to remove them or swing them out of the way when transferring a resident to or from the chair. Inspect the wheelchair daily. Report any broken, loose, or nonfunctioning mechanical parts, especially brakes, to the maintenance department or the charge nurse.

Aids for Activities of Daily Living

Many types of assistive equipment are available to help with the activities of daily living (ADLs). If you notice that a resident is having difficulty with activities such as bathing, dressing, toileting, or eating, you can talk to the nurse or physical therapist to find a solution that will make these tasks easier and allow more independence.

Some assistive devices help residents dress and bathe without having to bend down as far. These include dressing sticks, long-handled shoehorns, long-handled sponges, sock donners, elastic shoelaces, and reachers.

A raised toilet seat is used by residents who have difficulty getting on or off a standard-height toilet. It is also used by residents recovering from hip replacement

surgery. A raised toilet seat may be attached to the floor or temporarily placed over the toilet. Grab bars on the walls of bathrooms, tubs, and showers are used for safety and convenience. They provide a hand-hold for support during toilet activities, showering, and bathing.

Expanded grips on any item or device can help a resident with a weak grip hold it better. For example, raised grips may be added to eating or writing utensils or even a toothbrush. The grip may include a strap that wraps around the hand for more support.

Preventing Equipment-Related Injuries

Most equipment-related injuries are caused by improper use or because the equipment itself is broken, damaged, or not working properly. You can help prevent these injuries by being observant and sharing your observations with other staff.

You can help prevent injuries to residents by following these guidelines:

- Notice if a resident is using a piece of equipment improperly. If so, help the resident learn the correct way to use it.
- Keep an eye out for broken or faulty equipment. If you notice that any equipment has broken, missing, or wobbly parts, report the problem to your supervisor and/or notify the therapist. Follow your facility's protocol for requesting repairs or replacement. Address even minor equipment problems immediately to prevent injuries.

Exercise

Exercise is important for health and mobility and should be part of a resident's routine. All residents benefit from exercise that is tailored to their abilities. An exercise program can greatly increase muscle strength and flexibility and is a key factor for residents to improve or regain mobility. Many facilities offer regular group exercise programs for residents. Encourage your residents to participate in such programs.

How Joints Move

The motion of each joint in the body depends on its structure. The specific movements of major joints in the body are shown in Box 8-2. There are three basic types of joints (Figure 8-7):

- Ball-and-socket joint — as in the shoulder and hip
- Hinge joint — as in the knee and elbow

- Pivot joint — as in the forearm or joint between the first and second vertebra

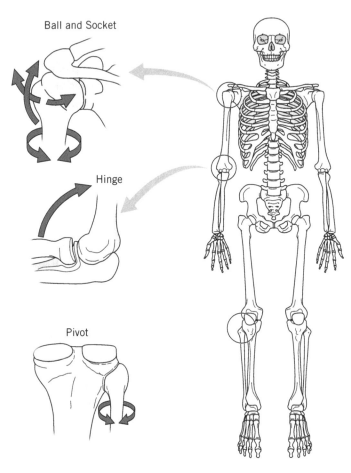

Ball and Socket

Hinge

Pivot

Figure 8-7 There are three basic types of joints in the body: ball-and-socket, hinge, and pivot joints.

Range-of-Motion Exercises

Range-of-motion (ROM) exercises are one of the most common restorative programs used with long term care residents. Each joint in the body is moved through its full range of motion. The resident's physician, along with the physical therapist and nurse, determines an appropriate ROM exercise program depending on the resident's needs, capabilities, and motivation.

Many residents perform different types of ROM exercises. A person may be able to move some parts of their body better than others, while not being able to move other parts at all. For example, you may need to help a resident move their right arm (active assisted ROM exercise), yet they can move the left arm independently (AROM exercise). Various types of ROM exercise are described in the following sections.

Box 8-2

MOVEMENTS OF MAJOR JOINTS

SHOULDER

Flexion: bringing the whole arm up toward the resident's head in front of the body

Extension: bringing the arm straight back to their side

Abduction: moving the arm away from the body out to the side

Adduction: bringing the arm back toward the side

Internal rotation: turning the shoulder in

External rotation: turning the shoulder out

ELBOW

Flexion: bending the elbow

Extension: straightening the elbow

Supination: turning the palm up

Pronation: turning the palm down

WRIST

Flexion: bending the wrist up

Extension: bending the wrist back

Ulnar deviation: with the hand held at the same level as the forearm, moving the hand toward the little finger side

Radial deviation: with the hand as above, moving the hand toward the thumb side

HAND

Finger abduction/adduction: spreading fingers apart and then together

Finger flexion: bending the fingers at each of the finger joints (three on each finger, two on the thumb)

Finger extension: straightening the fingers out at the finger joints

Opposition: touching each finger-tip to the thumb

HIP

Flexion: bringing the knee toward the chest

Extension: lay the leg down flat

Abduction: bringing the hip out to the side by moving the leg

Adduction: bringing the hip back toward the side by moving the leg

Internal rotation: turning the hip inward by moving the leg

External rotation: turning the hip outward by moving the leg

KNEE

Flexion: bending the knee

Extension: straightening the knee

ANKLE

Dorsiflexion: bending the top of the foot up toward the face

Plantarflexion: pointing the foot down, like stepping on a gas pedal

Inversion: turning the bottom of the foot inward

Eversion: turning the bottom of the foot outward

FOOT

Toe flexion: bending the toes down

Toe extension: straightening the toes back up

Active Range of Motion Exercise

In active ROM (AROM) exercises, the person moves the body part using their own muscle power. Exercise is active when the resident can do it independently. Based on the resident's needs, you still might help in some way. You might simply need to provide a reminder to do the exercises. You may need to read the exercise program aloud to guide the resident through the exercises. Or the resident may need you to cue them for how to move each body part correctly.

Active Assistive Range of Motion Exercise

In active assistive ROM (AAROM) exercises, you help move the body part. Some residents need you to help them physically with some or all parts of the exercise. Doing active exercise may be too strenuous for an injured body part that is healing, or a resident may simply need your help to move a certain part of their body.

Passive Range of Motion Exercise

With passive ROM (PROM) exercises, you move the resident's body part to perform the exercise, usually because they cannot move it at all or enough to help with the exercise. Some residents may be recovering from an injury or surgery but have limited movement during recovery. Always ask the charge nurse or therapist if you are not sure about a resident's condition or capabilities.

Guidelines for ROM Exercises

A general ROM program exercises most joints of the body, including the shoulder, elbow, wrist, hand (fingers), hip, knee, ankle, and foot (toes). You can complete an entire ROM exercise program with a resident in about 15 minutes when you use a system that works every major joint in a specific sequence (Procedure 8-19). With this system, use the same order of exercises. You may have to change specific exercises depending on each resident's needs.

If there are no restrictions on the resident's movement, move each joint through its full available range at least once a day. Based on his or her ability, the resident may move some joints actively, some actively with your assistance, and some passively with you doing the motion. Let the resident do as much as possible and help them with the rest. Give the resident time to respond to what you are asking them to do.

Following are general guidelines for ROM exercise:

- Know what type of exercise a resident needs for each body part, the position they should be in during each

exercise, and the amount of assistance required. If a written plan has been provided by the physical therapist, follow the plan.

- Remove any obstacles in the immediate environment such as pillows, sheets, blankets, and personal items.

- Explain to the resident what you would like to do and why (Figure 8-8).

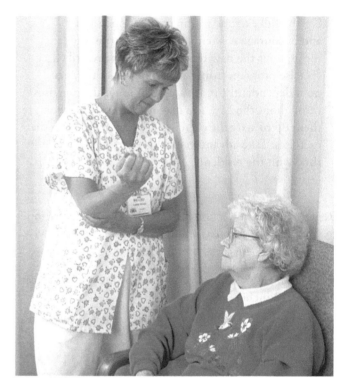

Figure 8-8 A nurse assistant demonstrates how she will perform passive ROM exercise.

- If assistance is needed, help the resident into the correct position for each exercise.

- If possible, keep both hands on the person's limb (arm or leg) during each exercise for the best support and guidance.

- When moving a joint, place one hand above and the other hand below the joint. Generally, the hand above the joint stabilizes the limb (holds it in place), and the hand below the joint guides the body part through the range of motion.

- When moving a resident's arm or leg, be gentle and never force the joint. Pushing or pulling can cause severe damage. You could cause pain or swelling, rupture a tendon, pull a muscle, tear the skin, or even break a bone. Many residents have osteoporosis or other conditions that cause weakened bones, muscles, tendons, or ligaments. They may have fragile skin or unstable joints. The most easily damaged joints are in the neck, hands, wrists, and feet.

- Make sure to tell the resident what you are doing before each movement. During exercise, ask the resident often how they are doing, if they feel any pain, and if your level of pressure on their arm or leg is okay. Watch the person's facial expressions because they may not always tell you when they are uncomfortable.

- Do the full exercise routine at least once a day and encourage residents to use their arms and legs throughout the day. If a resident has a prescribed exercise program from the therapist that they can do independently, motivate them to do the exercises throughout the day. You may need to remind them, set them up to start the exercise, or cue them during the exercises. Take advantage of this time to spend quality time with the resident.

Proper Body Mechanics

Remember your own body mechanics and pay attention to your body position as you help residents with ROM exercises. Here are some useful pointers:

- Maintain a broad base of support by keeping your feet 10 to 12 inches apart.

- Keep your back in a neutral position, and always bend your knees when lifting and moving to protect your back.

- Turn your whole body as a unit instead of twisting at the waist.

- Experiment with different standing positions, hand placement, and bed heights to find the best position to avoid straining your back.

- For stability, it may help to stand on one leg and place your other knee on the bed. If you want to work in this position, first ask the resident's permission. If this is okay, put down a bed protector before placing your knee on the bed.

Walking with a Resident

Walking (ambulation) is an important restorative activity that helps the resident maintain their independence. It is an effective exercise and helps to maintain optimal function. The term *gait* refers to how someone walks. If a resident needs assistance or supervision when walking, use a gait belt around their waist.

Before you begin walking with a resident, you need to know the following:

- Do they use an assistive device?

- Do they need a brace, prosthesis, or other equipment?

- How much weight can they place on their legs while walking?

- How much help do they need to walk, if any?

- Do you need another staff person to help?

- How much cuing do they need to stay safe?

- How far can they walk safely?

Once you have determined a resident's needs and abilities, you can help them walk (Figure 8-9). Combine short walks with other activities such as getting out of bed, walking to and from the bathroom, and walking to meals and other activities (Procedure 8-20) Encourage residents who can walk on their own to do so throughout the day.

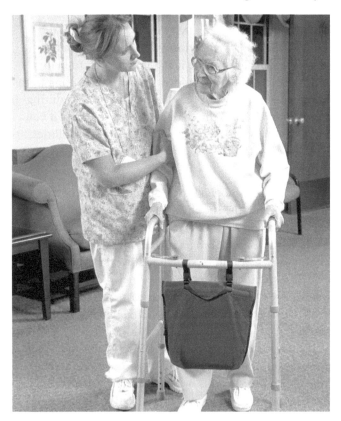

Figure 8-9 Nurse assistants learn each resident's capabilities and provide the specific help needed when walking.

Each exercise should be performed five to 10 times, depending on the resident's comfort level and ability.

PREPARATION STEPS

1. Check the care plan.
2. Knock, introduce yourself, and address resident by preferred name.
3. Perform hand hygiene.
4. Gather supplies and secure assistance if needed.
5. Explain procedure and ask about resident preferences.
6. Respect privacy and rights at all times.

SHOULDER, ARM, AND HAND

Start with the shoulder and work your way down to the hand. For each exercise, help the resident move the joint or move it yourself, depending on how much they can do independently.

SHOULDER

1 Place one hand under the resident's elbow and the other under their wrist. Allow the resident's forearm to rest on your body as you move the arm. If the resident is on their back, stand close to the side of the arm you are moving.

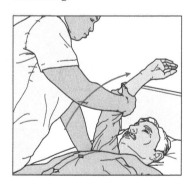

2 Help the resident to lift their arm up toward the head of the bed with the elbow straight (flexion).

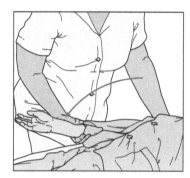

3 Bring the arm back down to the bed (extension).

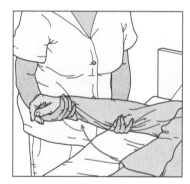

4 Help the resident lift their arm out to the side with the elbow straight (abduction).

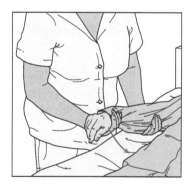

5 Bring the arm back toward the side (adduction)

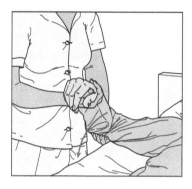

6 Help the resident lift their arm halfway out to the side. With the elbow bent, rotate the arm down (internal rotation) and up (external rotation).

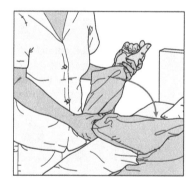

ELBOW

1 Place one hand above the resident's elbow, and use your other hand to support the wrist. The wrist position should be neutral, not bent forward or backward.

2 Help the resident bend the elbow by bringing the hand toward the upper arm with the palm facing up (flexion).

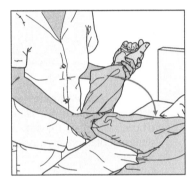

3 Help the resident straighten the elbow by bringing the hand down toward the bed until the elbow is as straight as possible (extension).

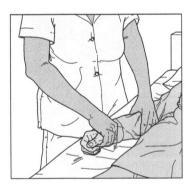

4 Help the resident turn the palm over with the elbow fairly straight and the wrist neutral (pronation).

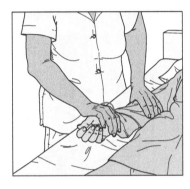

5 Help the resident turn the palm back up with the elbow fairly straight and the wrist neutral (supination).

WRIST

1 Place one hand around the resident's forearm just above the wrist and your other hand in their hand.

2 Help the resident bend their wrist down (flexion)

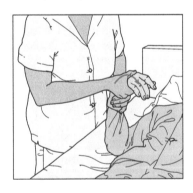

3 Help the resident bend their wrist back (extension).

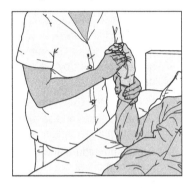

4 Help the resident move their hand toward the little finger side of the wrist (ulnar deviation).

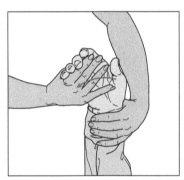

5 Help the resident move their hand toward the thumb side of the wrist (radial deviation).

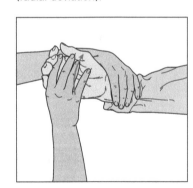

1 Using your fingers, help the resident move their fingers one by one. Bend and straighten each finger at each of the creases (joints).

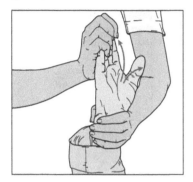

2 Curl the hand into a fist, then straighten the fingers back out (flexion and extension).

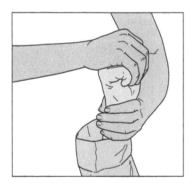

3 Spread the fingers away from each other one at a time (abduction) and then back together one at a time (adduction).

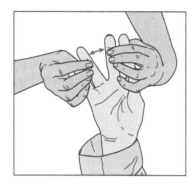

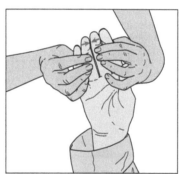

4 Bring each finger across the palm to the thumb and back out (opposition).

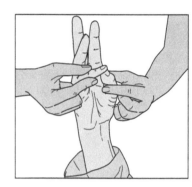

HIP, LEG, AND FOOT

Start with the hip and work your way down to the foot.

HIP

1 Place one hand under the thigh and the other hand below the knee around the calf. Adjust your hand placement as needed to be comfortable for both you and the resident.

2 Help the resident bring their leg up toward the chest with the knee bent (flexion).

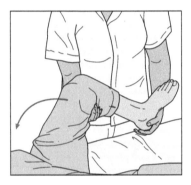

3 Bring the leg back down toward the bed (extension)

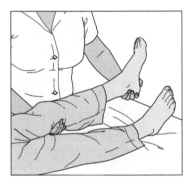

4 Help the resident move their leg out to the side (abduction).

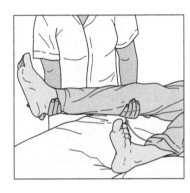

5 Bring the leg back toward the other leg (adduction).

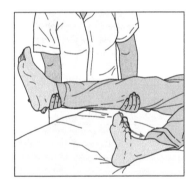

6 Help the resident bring the leg partly up toward the chest with the knee bent. Now gently turn the leg in (internal rotation) and out (external rotation).

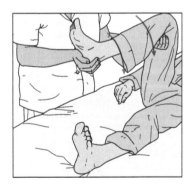

KNEE

1 Place one hand above the resident's knee, under or on their thigh. Place the other hand below their knee around the calf.

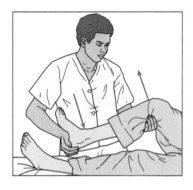

2 Help the resident bend the leg up toward the chest slightly. From this position, help them bend the knee (flexion).

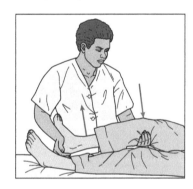

3 With the hip in the same position as described above, help the resident straighten the knee (extension).

ANKLE

1 Place one hand above the resident's ankle around the lower part of the calf. Place the other hand around the bottom of their foot.

2 Help the resident bend the foot up toward the head while the knee is held straight (dorsiflexion), and then point the foot downward (plantarflexion).

3 Help the resident turn the bottom of the foot outward (eversion) and then inward (inversion).

FOOT

1 Place your fingers around each of the resident's toes and gently bend (flexion) and straighten each toe at each of the joints (extension).

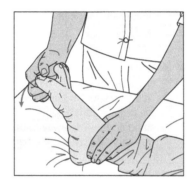

2 You can also bend and straighten all the toes at once.

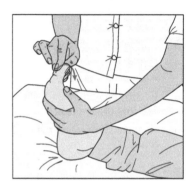

COMPLETION STEPS

1. Determine the resident's preferred position for comfort and ask them if they need anything else.

2. Examine the environment for safety and cleanliness.

3. Secure the call light and any other needed items within reach of the resident.

4. Perform hand hygiene.

5. Document the procedure and report any findings to the staff in charge.

If a resident questions why they have to walk, you can explain that walking will help them get stronger or stay strong. If a resident who usually walks regularly does not feel well, you must respect the person's need to rest or recover. Encourage walking at a later time when they feel better.

You'll need to ask the nurse or therapist if a resident on oxygen can safely walk. Find out if they need oxygen when they walk and how much. Ask the nurse to put this resident on a portable tank for the walk. You may need another staff person if they need help to walk. The second person pulls the oxygen tank and brings along a wheelchair in case it is needed, while you walk holding onto the gait belt and resident's walker (if used).

Sometimes, a resident may act unpredictably when walking. Their legs may get tired and give out easily. They may become confused and simply sit down. Place a gait belt securely (not too tight or too loose) around their waist, and position your hand on the belt, usually at their back. Try to avoid holding onto their arm so you don't risk injury to fragile joints. In such cases, have another staff member follow you with a wheelchair as you walk with the resident so the chair is available if they suddenly need to sit.

8-20: Assisting with Walking

PREPARATION STEPS

1. Check the care plan.
2. Knock, introduce yourself, and address resident by preferred name.
3. Perform hand hygiene.
4. Gather supplies and secure assistance if needed.
5. Explain procedure and ask about resident preferences.
6. Respect privacy and rights at all times.

1 Ensure that the resident is wearing non slip shoes that fit properly before assisting with walking.

2 Place the gait belt on the resident.

3 If the resident walks without any type of assistive device, stand at their side so you can see their face as you hold onto the gait belt from behind.

4 If the resident needs help using a cane, stand on the same side as the hand holding the cane, with one hand on the back of the belt and the other on the cane. Most residents who use a cane can hold it by themselves, so with them, you can stand on the opposite side. Make sure that the resident holds the cane in the correct hand.

5 If the resident uses a walker, stand at their side, with one hand on the walker if the resident needs help with the walker.

6 Walk with the resident. Have them take small steps and slowly progress to larger steps, if possible.

7 When walking in hallways, encourage residents not using a walker to use the safety bars along the wall for added support. Always stand on the side away from the wall so they may use the bars.

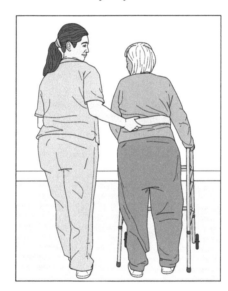

8 When the resident has finished walking, remove the gait belt.

COMPLETION STEPS

1. Determine the resident's preferred position for comfort and ask them if they need anything else.
2. Examine the environment for safety and cleanliness.
3. Secure the call light and any other needed items within reach of the resident.
4. Perform hand hygiene.
5. Document the procedure and report any findings to the staff in charge.

Points to Remember

- Nurse assistants help with restorative activities to assist residents in regaining or maintaining the highest possible level of independent functioning.

- You must learn to help move and position residents correctly to ensure their safety and your own.

- You must know how to assist a resident who has fallen and how to prevent falls.

- Various types of assistive devices are available to promote residents' mobility and independence.

- Restorative activities include range-of-motion exercises designed to maintain flexibility and mobility.

Key Terms

brace — device that supports and strengthens a body part

contracture — abnormal shortening of muscle tissue due to lack of movement or improper positioning

cuing — prompting a resident to begin a task or activity by telling or showing

Fowler's position — lying on the back with the head of the bed raised 45 to 60 degrees

goal — a desired result or outcome

mobility — ability to move freely

orthosis — equipment or device, such as a brace or splint, used to provide support to a weak or injured part of the body

positioning — assisting a resident in changing position

prone position — lying in a face down position on the abdomen

prosthesis — an artificial body part

rehabilitation — process of regaining a former state of health or function

restorative — activities designed to help a person be as independent and functional as possible

side-lying position — (lateral) positioned on either side with knees slightly bent

sims position — the resident is positioned on their left side with the hip and lower leg slightly bent and the right hip and knee bent

splint — device to use to support or immobilize a body part

supine — lying on the back

trapeze — suspended horizontal bar used to help position a person in bed

1. What device is used to support or immobilize a body part?
   a. Splint
   b. Prosthesis
   c. Trapeze bar
   d. Foot cradle

2. When preparing to move a resident, you need to think about the resident, the environment and:
   a. How much time it will take
   b. Your own capabilities and limitations
   c. If this is in your job description
   d. Not bothering the charge nurse

3. Principles of body mechanics include keeping a broad base with feet about 10-12 inches apart and one foot slightly in front of the other, and:
   a. Always bend your knees when lifting to protect your back
   b. Keeping your knees straight and your back bent
   c. Twisting from the waist
   d. Holding the resident away from your body

4. Placing a resident on their back with the head of the bed flat would be considered what position?
   a. Side-lying
   b. Fowler's
   c. Supine
   d. Prone

5. A gait belt can help to move the resident safely and prevent injury. It is placed:
   a. Under the arms
   b. Around the hips
   c. Around the waist
   d. Across the chest

6. Activities designed to help residents regain or maintain their ability to take care of themselves are called:
   a. Palliative
   b. Recreation
   c. Restorative activities
   d. Patients Choice

7. Devices used to improve a resident's ability to function such as braces, walking devices and splints and are called:
   a. Orthotic devices
   b. Prescribed devices
   c. Prosthetic devices
   d. Resistive devices

8. A device made to replace a missing body part or function such as an artificial eye or limb is called a/an:
   a. Orthotic device
   b. Prescribed device
   c. Prosthetic device
   d. Resistive device

9. In range-of-motion (ROM) exercises, each joint is moved through the resident's full range of motion. When the resident uses their own muscle power, it is called:
   a. Passive range of motion
   b. Active range of motion
   c. Assistive range of motion
   d. None of these

10. The goal of restorative activities is to:
    a. Help the resident look better
    b. Help the residents and staff get along better
    c. Help the resident to regain function and independence
    d. Help the staff avoid injuring themselves

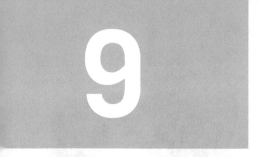

9 Nutrition

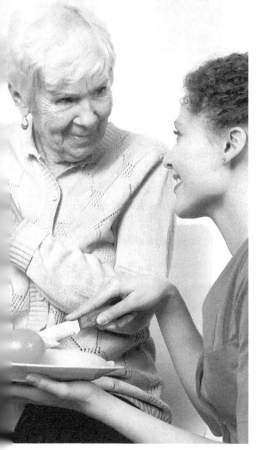

Obtaining nutrition from food is an important part of life. When people age or become ill, their appetite and patterns often change. This can create a challenge for their care. Some residents have chronic diseases that lead to loss of appetite or weight loss. These illnesses may affect their ability to chew, swallow, or eat on their own. Many residents take medications that can alter their appetite. Memory loss due to dementia can cause some residents to forget to eat or question why they are being fed. All of these problems can lead to weight loss and deteriorating health.

Poor nutritional status has negative effects on residents' health. It can lower their resistance to infection and can contribute to pressure injuries and other conditions that can affect their quality of life.

The goal is to prevent health declines through timely interventions. As a nurse assistant, you play an important role in maintaining and improving residents' nutritional status while maintaining their dignity and supporting their independence to the degree possible.

OBJECTIVES:

- Explain the role of the facility food service department.
- List ways to provide and encourage good nutrition for residents.
- Name the five food groups.
- Provide examples of ways to make dining a pleasant experience.

- Demonstrate how to properly record residents' food and fluid intake and output.
- Explain why some residents need enteral nutrition or total parenteral nutrition and the methods used to provide it.

- Describe your role in caring for a person receiving enteral feedings or total parenteral nutrition.

Assisting with Nutrition

Think about what food means to you. You've heard the saying "You are what you eat." This means that what you put in your body affects how you look and feel (Figure 9-1). **Nutrition** is the nourishment that we obtain from food. Poor nutritional status negatively affects residents by lowering their resistance to infection, which can contribute to pressure injuries and other diseases. It significantly reduces their quality of life.

Consider how our culture emphasizes food on television and in magazines. Most people associate food with pleasant activities such as being with friends and family. We all have our own food preferences and customs. The following factors affect our eating habits:

- **Cognitive abilities**: to recognize food and remember how to eat
- **Taste:** a person's individual likes and dislikes
- **Culture:** traditions rooted in family and cultural background
- **State of health:** people often eat less when they feel ill or they may have a physical disability that prevents them from being able to prepare or feed themselves
- **Emotional state:** people tend to enjoy food more when they are happy and enjoy it less when depressed or anxious
- **Ability to chew and swallow:** a person's appetite or ability to eat may change after dental work, or due to an infection or a stroke
- **Social situation:** people often eat differently when they are alone than with friends and family
- **Economic situation:** people may not have the financial resources to purchase adequate amounts of food

Everyone is affected by these factors in different ways. Keeping these factors in mind can help you understand how residents' eating may be affected.

Dietary Requirements

The U.S. Department of Agriculture (USDA) and the U.S. Department of Health and Human Services (HHS) publish an updated version of the Dietary Guidelines for Americans, every five years. This guideline provides advice on healthy eating to promote a healthy lifestyle and prevent chronic disease.

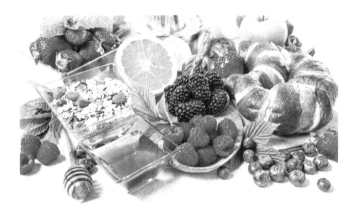

Figure 9-1 Eating a variety of nutrient-dense foods helps residents stay healthy.

To help plan meals and provide nutritional information the USDA created MyPlate, an online tool. This tool emphasizes the importance of healthy eating and helps plan well-balanced meals, incorporating food from all food groups.

The five food groups are Fruits, Vegetables, Grains, Protein Foods, and Dairy.

- **Fruits** — most fruits are naturally low in fat, sodium, and calories. Eating a healthy diet that is rich in fruits may reduce the risk for heart disease, including heart attack and stroke and may protect against certain types of cancers.
- **Vegetables** — Provide nutrients that are vital for health and maintenance of body functions. Most vegetables are low in fat and calories. Eating a healthy diet that is rich in vegetables may reduce the risk for heart disease, including heart attack and stroke and may protect against certain types of cancers.
- **Beans, peas,** and **lentils** belong to the vegetable group (but could be counted as protein group as well). They are an excellent source of fiber and provide nutrients such as folate, potassium, iron, and zinc. They are a great sources of plant protein.
- **Grains** — Provide nutrients such as, complex carbohydrates, dietary fiber, some several B vitamins and minerals. Eating whole grains as part of a healthy diet may reduce the risk of heart disease and can support digestion.
- **Protein Foods** — Meat, poultry, seafood, beans, lentils, peas, nuts, eggs, seeds, and soy products provide many nutrients, such as B vitamins, vitamin E, iron, zinc, and magnesium. Proteins are the building blocks for bones, muscle, skin, and blood.

- **Dairy** — provides nutrients such as, calcium, phosphorus, vitamin A, vitamin D, potassium, and protein. Dairy products can promote bone health and prevent the onset of osteoporosis.

Food Service Department

The food service department in a long term care facility has many functions. It provides residents with food that is safe, nourishing, and appealing. This department must also ensure that each resident receives the correct diet ordered by the physician in a form that meets their needs.

Many facilities allow residents to select from a menu based on their individual preferences. Most provide therapeutic diets (special diets designed to meet health goals) that offer choices based on residents' preferences. This is important because residents on therapeutic diets often do not enjoy all the foods they are allowed. If they do not enjoy their food, they may not eat enough and may lose weight, leading to negative health effects. In addition to preparing food that is appropriate for therapeutic diets, the food service department also provides alternate food choices for residents with food allergies, food intolerances, or other special needs or preferences.

Residents' Food Preferences

Like you, residents have food preferences. These may be based on personal, religious, regional, or ethnic factors. The best way to learn residents' likes and dislikes is to ask them and/or family members. Personal preferences may involve the appearance, familiarity, or taste of a food. Ask questions such as:

- What foods do you like?
- What do you dislike?
- What does an appropriate portion size look like to you?
- How often do you eat and at what times?

All of these factors play a role in what residents want to eat, how they like their food to be prepared, and when they prefer to eat. Work with the resident, family members, and the food service to meet each resident's preferences.

Special Diets

While many residents eat a regular diet that includes a wide range of food choices, some require a special diet for health reasons, known as a therapeutic diet. A therapeutic diet is ordered by the resident's physician as part of treatment for a specific condition such as obesity, diabetes, or

heart disease. A therapeutic diet can sometimes reduce or eliminate the need for medication.

Diets may also be modified in regard to the consistency or texture of foods to meet the resident's needs. Food may be chopped, ground, or pureed for residents who have problems chewing. Problems with chewing may result from ill-fitting dentures, missing teeth, or a tooth or gum condition. Chewing or swallowing problems caused by a stroke or digestive difficulties may also require changes in food consistency. The consistency of liquids can be modified for those who are at risk for aspirating liquids into their lungs. Liquids can be thickened to a nectar, honey or pudding thick consistency. The facility usually tries to liberalize the resident's diet, in order to increase quality of life and enjoyment of meals. Discussing dietary needs and food preferences with residents can help in finding a balance.

Commonly ordered therapeutic diets include:

- **Calorie-restricted diets.** These diets usually range from 1,200 to 1,800 calories per day and are generally ordered for weight reduction.

- **Consistent carbohydrate (CCD or CCHO) diet.** This diet focuses on eating the same amount of carbohydrates every day.

- **No-added-salt or sodium restricted diets.** These diets are usually ordered for residents with fluid retention or high blood pressure (hypertension). These residents do not receive salt on their trays and do not receive foods containing high amounts of sodium, such as canned soups, salted crackers, and cured meats such as ham, bacon, and corned beef.

- **Fat-restricted and/or cholesterol-restricted diets.** Fat-restricted diets may be ordered for residents with diseases of the liver, gallbladder, pancreas, or cardiovascular system or for residents who have a mal absorption syndrome (difficulty absorbing nutrients) and cannot tolerate fat. Low-cholesterol diets are used to reduce blood fat levels. Foods high in fat, such as bacon, sausage, cream, margarine, gravy, whole milk, and high-fat desserts, are restricted.

- **Renal diets.** These diets are ordered for residents with kidney or liver disease and may make it possible to postpone dialysis or transplant surgery. Sometimes there are protein, sodium, phosphorus, and potassium restrictions as well. These diets can be difficult for a resident to follow if the restriction is severe. Restricted foods may include meat, eggs, dairy products, some breads, and other foods that contain small amounts of protein. The specific components of a renal diet must be calculated by the dietician.

- **Gluten free diet.** This diet is ordered for residents with celiac disease or an allergy to wheat. This diet eliminates gluten. Gluten is a protein found in barley, rye and triticale.

- **Clear liquid diet.** This diet is frequently ordered for residents scheduled for a test that requires the stomach and intestine to be empty, such as a colonoscopy or to rest the intestine for digestive problems. Clear liquids are considered transparent, such as broth, Jello or apple juice.

- **Full liquid diet.** This diet is usually ordered for a resident transitioning to a soft diet. It includes any liquid or any foods that will turn into a liquid at room temperature.

Some residents choose alternate diets such vegetarian or vegan options. These diets can be chosen for religious or other beliefs, health issues, or concerns over animal rights or the environment. Vegetarians do not eat meat, including poultry and fish. Vegans do not eat meat or any meat products like eggs or dairy products.

Making the Dining Experience Pleasant

A meal is much more than simply consuming food. Mealtimes should be pleasurable and enhance the resident's well-being (Figure 9-2). Many factors influence how residents feel about the experience, and these factors affect their food intake. Environmental, service, and social factors are all important.

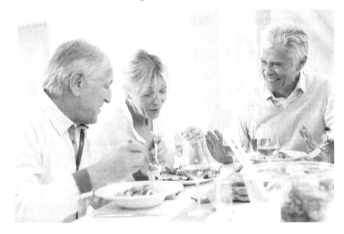

Figure 9-2   Meal times should be a positive experience for residents.

Environmental factors involve the physical surroundings. Residents have a right to expect the following:

- A dining area that is clean, uncluttered, and free of unpleasant odors.
- Table linens (if used) that are clean and pressed.
- A comfortable room temperature.
- Soft lighting without glare. Window coverings should be adjusted so the sun does not shine directly in anyone's eyes.
- A table height that is appropriate for residents' comfort. Residents in wheelchairs should sit at tables high enough to allow the wheelchair arms to fit under the table.
- Tables arranged so that residents can come and go freely while using walkers or wheelchairs.
- Soft music playing.
- Flowers and attractive dishes on the table. Dishes should be clean and free of chips and cracks.
- An environment free of distractions such as a loud TV or radio.

Service factors involve the residents' interactions with staff:

- Speak to residents in a polite, pleasant voice. Your caring, patient attitude adds to their enjoyment of the meal.
- Encourage residents to take their time to finish. Do not hurry or rush them.
- Describe the food in a positive way as you encourage them to eat.
- Do not begin to cleanup or scrape dishes while residents are still eating.

Social factors involve the interactions of residents while dining:

- Encourage residents to sit with their friends. If a resident is new to the facility and has not yet developed friendships with other resident, direct them to a table of residents of similar mental status.
- Try to sit residents together that have similar interests.
- Serve all residents at a table before moving on to the next one.
- Try to create a pleasant, home-like atmosphere where residents will look forward to meals and enjoy the experience.

To prevent residents from feeling isolated, encourage those who are physically able to come to the dining room for meals. Some residents must eat in their rooms, and you can make meals a pleasant experience by following these guidelines:

- Remove any clutter from the over-bed table and adjust the table height to an appropriate level.
- Clean to eliminate any unpleasant odors before serving food.
- Remove food from the tray and position it properly on the plate.
- Do not carry out nursing tasks, such as taking vital signs, during meals.

Assisting Residents with Meals

One of your most important duties as a nurse assistant is to help residents with meals. Although you might think this is a simple task, it requires a lot of attention (Figure 9-3). Your ability to do it well directly affects residents' nutritional status and overall health. Procedure 9-1 describes the steps involved in assisting residents with meals.

Preparing Residents for Meals

Residents more fully enjoy their meals when they are properly prepared for them. Before meals, some residents may need assistance combing or brushing their hair.

Some female residents may need help with their makeup. If needed, help the resident with toileting before taking them to the dining room. Encourage residents to use their dentures, glasses, and hearing aids. These devices improve residents' functional abilities and help them be more independent. Help residents with hand hygiene and oral care as needed. Oral care before meals may improve residents' taste sensitivity to some food flavors.

If a resident is eating in bed, elevate the head of the bed to at least 30 degrees. Make each resident as comfortable as possible. Use clothing protectors or napkins to protect their clothing if the resident requests.

Assisting with Feeding

Many residents can eat independently or with a little help from a staff member. Other residents must be fed. These residents totally depend on you and your coworkers to meet their nutritional needs. Guidelines for feeding residents are outlined in Procedure 9-2. An occupational therapist may assess residents who are difficult to feed or who have special problems. The therapist will train you to use special feeding techniques if needed.

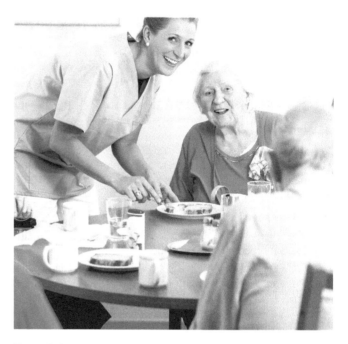

Figure 9-3   Some residents may need help cutting their food.

When you feed a resident, imagine how it would feel to be in his or her situation. Before leaving the resident, ask yourself:

- Have I done all I can to encourage this resident to eat?
- Have I provided the best nutrition possible?

Special Devices for Eating

Residents who have difficulty feeding themselves may benefit from using specially designed utensils, cups, and plates (Figure 9-4). Residents need to be taught to use these devices. Usually, the occupational therapist teaches the resident and staff how to use them.

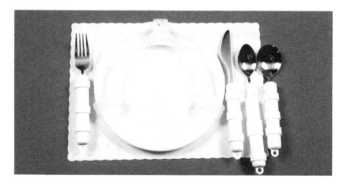

Figure 9-4   Special utensils, cups, and plates may be used by some residents to help them eat independently.

PREPARATION STEPS

1. Check the care plan.
2. Knock, introduce yourself, and address resident by preferred name.
3. Perform hand hygiene.
4. Gather supplies and secure assistance if needed.
5. Explain procedure and ask about resident preferences.
6. Respect privacy and rights at all times.

1 Prepare the resident before the meal by helping with grooming, hand hygiene, and oral care as needed.

2 Help the resident to the dining room or make him/her comfortable in their own room.

3 In the dining room, transfer the resident from a wheelchair to a dining room chair, if possible.

4 Perform hand hygiene. This is an important part of infection control.

5 Position napkins and clothing protectors if requested by the resident.

6 Deliver trays as quickly as possible to keep foods at the correct temperature.

7 When you remove the tray from the cart, first check the tray card. Confirm that you have the correct tray for the person you are serving and that the food is correct for the resident's diet. Check if there are any special feeding instructions.

8 Remove the food from the tray, and place plates and bowls directly on the table. When the resident is ready to eat, remove any covers, liners, and wrappings and open condiments and cartons. Place covers and wrappings back on the tray and return the tray to the service cart or to another cart.

9 Place plates and bowls within the resident's easy reach. Review the meal items with residents who may not see well or who may be unfamiliar with some foods. Describe the foods positively so the resident looks forward to eating.

10 Once you have served the first resident at the table, move on to others at the same table. Serve all residents at a table before moving to the next table.

11 Ask residents if they need help cutting food or if they would like seasoning (if permitted). Encourage residents to be as independent as possible, but watch for those who need help. Cut food into small pieces to prevent choking.

12 Check with residents often to offer help as needed or to encourage them to eat.

13 Give all residents enough time to finish their meal. Some residents eat much more slowly than others.

14 If a resident does not eat well or rejects a food, offer to get a substitute, especially if the resident is underweight or poorly nourished. A resident should never leave the dining room hungry or be given food they cannot eat. Residents should not take food from the dining room to eat later. Unrefrigerated food increases the risk of foodborne illness.

COMPLETION STEPS

1. Determine the resident's preferred position for comfort and ask them if they need anything else.
2. Examine the environment for safety and cleanliness.
3. Secure the call light and any other needed items within reach of the resident.
4. Perform hand hygiene.
5. Document the procedure and report any findings to the staff in charge.

PREPARATION STEPS

1. Check the care plan.
2. Knock, introduce yourself, and address resident by preferred name.
3. Perform hand hygiene.
4. Gather supplies and secure assistance if needed.
5. Explain procedure and ask about resident preferences.
6. Respect privacy and rights at all times.

1 Prepare each resident for the meal. Provide oral care, wash the resident's hands, and make him/her comfortable. Check the resident's positioning. Elevate the head of the bed to at least 75 to 90 degrees. Cover the resident with a clothing protector or a large napkin, if requested by the resident.

2 Make sure to check the tray card to ensure the accuracy of the meal being served.

3 Remove foods from the tray, place them on the table in front of the resident, and describe each one. Encourage residents to help themselves eat in any way possible, such as by holding their own cup.

4 Sit next to the resident while feeding them, making eye contact. Use a spoon from which the resident can easily remove the food. Usually a teaspoon is better than a larger soup spoon. Fill the spoon no more than half full. Offer small bites, making sure the resident swallows each bite before offering another. Feed residents in a manner as close to normal as possible to preserve their dignity. Speak softly and maintain eye contact. Let the resident decide what to eat and in what order.

5 Check the food temperature. If the food seems too hot, give it time to cool. Do not mix foods together unless the resident requests this.

6 Encourage the resident to eat more nutritious foods first (meats, fish, eggs, vegetables, and fresh fruits). Save dessert until last, if possible. Do not rush the resident. Offer liquids between bites to keep their mouth moist.

7 Maintain a caring attitude, and encourage residents to eat all of their meal. Offer to get a substitute if they are not eating or refuse a certain food.

8 When the resident is finished eating, remove the clothing protector, any remaining food, and the tray.

9 Give oral care.

10 Report to the charge nurse any changes that occur with feeding, such as the resident experiencing nausea, stomach pain or discomfort, choking, or decreased appetite.

COMPLETION STEPS

1. Determine the resident's preferred position for comfort and ask them if they need anything else.
2. Examine the environment for safety and cleanliness.
3. Secure the call light and any other needed items within reach of the resident.
4. Perform hand hygiene.
5. Document the procedure and report any findings to the staff in charge.

Assisting Residents with Dysphagia

Some residents may have difficulty swallowing. This condition, called dysphagia, can be caused by a stroke, brain or spinal cord injury, certain diseases (such as Parkinson's disease), and certain immune, muscular, and digestive problems.

Residents with dysphagia may choke or aspirate some of their food. Aspiration means that food that enters the mouth is misdirected into the airway instead of passing through the esophagus into the stomach. Pneumonia or a lung infection may result, which can be fatal. Residents may be reluctant to eat if they are afraid of choking. Thus, they may not eat enough and may lose weight.

Many problems caused by dysphagia can be corrected with proper diagnosis and treatment. The therapist or nurse may give you special instructions for feeding a resident in a way that prevents problems. Positioning the resident is very important. If possible, the resident should be sitting upright during and at least 30 minutes after meals. Follow the therapist's instructions carefully to help the resident swallow without choking.

The therapist may also recommend a modified diet. A pureed diet or thickened liquids may make swallowing easier. A powdered product may be used as a thickening agent. Often, liquids continue to thicken for some time after the powder is added. To get the desired consistency, wait a minute or two before adding more thickener; you may not need it. Some residents tolerate thick liquids better than thin liquids. Thickeners can also be added to water, coffee, and other beverages. Many facilities offer prethickened liquids. As discussed earlier, liquids can be thickened to a nectar, honey, or pudding consistency.

How do you recognize dysphagia? Observe residents for symptoms such as the following. Report any of these to the charge nurse:

- Hoarse, breathy voice
- Gurgling breathing
- Drooling
- Feeling that something is caught in the throat
- Repeatedly clearing the throat
- Repetitive rocking motion of the tongue from front to back
- Coughing before, during, or after swallowing food, liquid, or medication
- Needing to swallow three or four times after each bite
- Pocketing food in the side of the mouth

A resident may also be a "silent aspirator." This means that dysphagia may be present even though the resident does not have obvious symptoms. Silent aspiration may be indicated by unexplained weight loss, decreased appetite, or a long-lasting low-grade fever. If you observe one or more of these symptoms, discuss your observations with the charge nurse.

Observation is Important

Your duties include helping residents with meals and monitoring their intake. If a resident avoids any major food group, ask why. Food and fluid intake is usually documented after observing the resident's tray in the dining room or in their room after a meal (not at the end of the day). Report any of the following observations to the nurse:

- Weight loss
- Avoidance of any major food group, such as not eating meats or vegetables
- Sudden change in the amount of food eaten
- Consistently eats less than 75% (3/4) of meals or snacks, especially if the resident is underweight or losing weight
- Complains of food tasting funny or receiving food they do not like and will not eat
- Experiences a changed status, such as needing more help with meals due to trembling hands or other problems
- Change in behavior, such as playing with food or taking food from the trays of other residents
- Change in attitude, such as becoming depressed, agitated, or lethargic or withdrawing from others
- Any swallowing problems, (including coughing or choking while eating)
- Any chewing problems
- Confusion, wandering, or pacing or leaving the dining room without eating

You play an important role in helping the interdisciplinary team identify residents at risk for nutritional problems. Upon admission, residents are assessed for nutritional risk. Later, you may be asked about your observations of residents' eating habits. You have a responsibility to help prevent unintended weight loss and other health problems by observing and reporting changes. If you notice any change in the resident, report this information immediately. Even small changes in a resident's eating habits can signal a change in health status. Your reported observations allow the interdisciplinary team to intervene early on and prevent significant problems from occurring.

Dietary Supplements

Many residents cannot eat enough food to supply the calories and protein they need. In these cases, dietary supplements are used to provide concentrated nutrition. Many different supplement products are available. Some provide just calories and protein, while others are fortified with vitamins and minerals. Supplement products include shakes, puddings, and frozen bars or "pudding pops." Adding supplements to a resident's diet is often called "calorie packing" or "power packing." The goal of calorie packing is to provide large amounts of calories and/or protein in the smallest amount of food.

Extra meals or snacks may be used as supplemental feedings. For example, a small sandwich may be offered between meals. The food service department will guide you.

Residents who benefit from supplements include those who:

- Accept liquids better than solid food
- Cannot consume large amounts of food
- Have an altered sense of taste and/or smell
- Are very thin and underweight

Although supplements often play an important role in maintaining a resident's nutritional status, you should think of the supplement as an addition to meals. Getting the resident to eat their meals is the priority. Except in extreme cases, supplements do not replace the meal but are given in addition to it. Encourage residents to consume as much of the meal as possible before offering a supplement.

If a resident who is supposed to receive a supplement refuses it, report this to the nurse so that another supplement can be offered.

Food and Fluid Intake

Nutrition and hydration affect residents' quality of life and quality of care in many ways. Good nutrition and hydration contribute to maintaining skin integrity, helping the body fight infections and disease, maintaining overall strength, and preserving functional abilities. It also helps in maintaining normal weight and energy stores and normal bowel and bladder function.

If a resident does not want the meal that was initially served or requests a different choice, they should be offered an option of similar nutritional value.

A person's nutritional and fluid needs sometimes change. Needs can change when a resident has a fever, persistent vomiting or diarrhea, pressure ulcers, urinary tract infection, or has fractured a bone or undergone surgery. Hot weather also increases residents' fluid needs because they lose fluid through perspiration.

Because adequate food and fluid intake are essential for residents' health and well-being, accurate intake measurements are important. These measurements help determine if a resident needs nutritional intervention.

Evaluating Food Intake

Reporting the amount of food a resident eats is your responsibility. This can sometimes be a challenge because

you must estimate how much the resident ate based on what is left on their plate. Facilities have various ways of recording the amounts of food the resident eats. During your orientation, you will learn the proper way to record this information.

Recording intake usually involves observing the meal and judging the percentage of food that has been consumed. Take the time to evaluate each resident's intake carefully and to record the percentage eaten immediately after the meal or snack. If a calorie count is ordered for a particular resident, you will need to record the percentage for each item of food they consumed. This allows the dietitian to calculate the number of calories or amount of protein consumed and to adjust the resident's diet, if necessary. Follow your facility guidelines for documentation.

Evaluating Fluid Intake

Like food intake, adequate fluid intake is vital. Exact fluid needs depend on the person's age, size, physical condition, and level of activity. Most residents need 1,500 to 2,000 cc of fluid per day (Figure 9-5). Residents with diseases such as congestive heart failure or renal disease may be restricted to less fluid. In these residents, too much fluid can negatively affect their overall health.

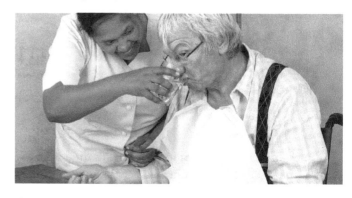

Figure 9-5 Residents who are not on any fluid restriction should consume 1,500 to 2,000 cc of fluid per day.

The physician determines each resident's proper intake and gives instructions about how much fluid to allow. Unless a resident is on a fluid restriction, offer fluids often and encourage the resident to drink.

To record fluid intake, you need to be familiar with how much fluid is in commonly used containers. Table 9-1 shows the fluid capacity of various types of cups and containers.

Since intake is usually recorded in cc's or ml's there may be times where you will need to convert ounces to cc's or ml's. Refer to Appendix E for information on converting from ounces to cc's or ml's.

Table 9-1   Capacities of Common Containers

Container Sizes and Examples	Contents (cc) [Note: 1 fluid ounce (oz) = 30 cubic centimeters (cc)]
3 ounces: ■ Small ice cream container	■ 90 cc
4 ounces (1/2 cup): ■ Juice glass ■ Small sherbet container ■ Small container of pudding or gelatin dessert	■ 120 cc
6 ounces: ■ Styrofoam or plastic cup (3 inches high) ■ Small can of juice ■ Small soup bowl	■ 180 cc
8 ounces (1 cup): ■ Standard cereal or soup bowl ■ Standard water tumbler or beverage glass ■ Individual carton of milk ■ Individual coffee pot ■ Individual pot of broth	■ 240 cc
12 ounces (1-1/2 cup): ■ Large water tumbler or beverage glass	■ 360 cc

Fluid Intake and Output

At times, it is critical to monitor a resident's fluid intake and output (called I&O). You will learn about monitoring output in chapter 10.

When recording intake, you should:

■ Know how much fluid is in the glasses and cups in your facility (see Table 9-1)

■ Count any liquids given throughout the day.

■ Accurately record all fluid intake for your shift.

Dehydration

If someone does not drink enough, even if they are healthy, they may experience a very serious condition called **dehydration**. Dehydration can be devastating and even cause death. Many factors can contribute to dehydration, including:

■ Medications such as laxatives and diuretics

■ Resident's reduced ability to recognize thirst or inability to communicate the need for fluid due to mental status

■ The kidneys' reduced ability to retain fluid when needed

Dehydration can occur quickly in an elderly resident. The signs and symptoms of dehydration include:

■ Dry or cracked lips and/or dry mouth

■ Sunken eyes and/or dry eyes

■ Dark urine

■ Decreased or excessive urine output

■ Constipation

■ Sudden confusion

■ Excess sleepiness

■ Reduced ability to do tasks

■ Sudden weight loss

■ Frequent falls

■ Frequent urinary tract infections

■ Skin on the chest or forehead is easily "tented" (you can pull up skin between your thumb and forefinger to form a "tent" that does not immediately smooth out)

If you notice any of these, report it right away. This is an emergency that requires immediate treatment. Providing residents with fluids is a key part of your daily tasks. Carefully monitor all residents to ensure that they are getting enough fluid.

To help ensure adequate fluid intake, you should:

■ Ask the resident what they like to drink and have these beverages on hand in the refrigerator. Plain water is always better than beverages containing sugar or artificial sweeteners.

■ Make sure every resident has a water pitcher. Place the pitcher within easy reach and pass fresh ice water every shift. Make sure the water in the pitcher is changed at least once each shift. Make sure there is a clean cup next to the water pitcher.

■ Place a clean flexible straw next to the cup for residents who may have difficulty drinking from a cup.

■ Encourage the resident to drink every time you interact with them, helping as needed.

■ Tell the charge nurse immediately about any resident who refuses your offering of fluid.

Residents with Feeding Tubes

Some residents cannot eat any food at all or enough food to keep them alive. The resident or responsible family member may then decide that tube feeding is appropriate. A feeding tube is placed either directly into the stomach or into the stomach through the nose and is used to deliver liquid nourishment.

Residents with tube feedings may have a doctor's order stating that they are NPO, meaning that they cannot have anything by mouth. Residents receiving tube feeding may still crave food or fluids. Some doctors may order pleasure feedings, where the resident can have minimum oral intake.

The nurse will administer the tube feeding according to the doctor's orders, which can be continuous feeding or at intervals throughout the day.

There are times when a resident may be unable to eat normally. These can be due to:

- Swallowing difficulties
- Choking problems
- Persistent vomiting
- Confusion
- Anorexia (eating disorder)
- Bowel infection or disease
- Semi-consciousness or unconsciousness
- Recent surgery of the mouth, throat, or digestive tract

In these situations, the physician will decide the best way to provide nourishment for the resident. The most common alternative routes are enteral nutrition or intravenous total parenteral nutrition (TPN).

Enteral Nutrition

Enteral nutrition or feeding is liquid nourishment passed through a nasogastric tube (NGT), which passes through the nose to the stomach (Figure 9-6). Or the tube may be inserted surgically through the abdomen into the stomach (gastrostomy tube; G-tube). Residents receiving enteral feedings may or may not be restricted from eating food and drinking liquid (NPO). You must know why the person has the enteral tube and you must follow the physician's orders regarding the type and amount of nutrition to be provided.

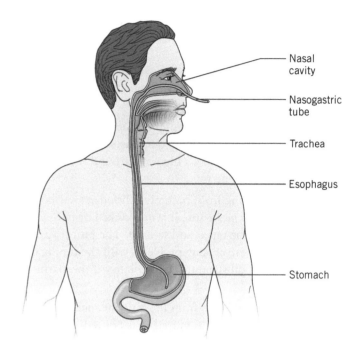

Figure 9-6   Placement of a nasogastric tube.

The nutrition bottle is connected to a pump hooked to the NGT or G-tube. The pump is used to control the amount of nutrition so it is delivered over the correct period of time. Your role is to monitor the resident during the feeding process. You must always make sure that the head of the bed is elevated at least 30 degrees during and for at least 30 minutes after feedings to prevent aspiration of liquid nutrition into the lungs (Figure 9-7). You can position the person carefully from side to side slightly, while the head of the bed is elevated, to prevent skin breakdown.

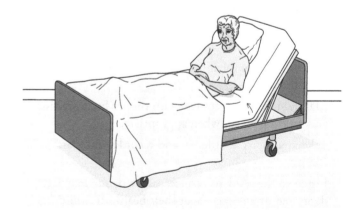

Figure 9-7   For the resident's safety, the head of the bed should be elevated during and after feedings.

Important guidelines in caring for a person receiving enteral feedings include:

- Monitor the skin at the insertion site of the G-tube for signs of infection (redness, swelling, and/or drainage) and keep the skin clean and dry.

- Monitor and report any respiratory problems such as shortness of breath, choking, gurgling sounds, or skin color changes, especially a blue tint around the lips and mouth (cyanosis).

- Prevent the tubing from becoming dislodged. Always check tubing to make sure it is not kinked or twisted. Tubing should be taped and secured. The pump alarm will go off if there are any problems with the tubing or the infusion. Call the nurse immediately if the alarm sounds.

- Report any complaints from the resident such as feeling that the tube has moved or is twisted. It is important that the nurse checks to be sure that the tube remains in the proper place.

- Provide comfort measures such as back rubs to increase circulation and prevent skin breakdown. Always provide good mouth care for a person who is NPO, especially if an NGT is in place. Often a person with an NGT will mouth-breathe, which causes the mouth to become dry and the lips to crack. Inspect the nose area for any sores or signs of infection.

- Monitor the person's intake and output. Note any loose watery stools. Always report and record the amount, color, and consistency of bowel movements. The physician may change the strength or rate of the feeding if diarrhea persists. Assist with cleaning the area after voiding or bowel movements.

- Monitor the person's weight every day. Weights should be taken each day at the same time, preferably wearing the same amount of clothing. Report any gain or loss.

- Monitor and report any abdominal swelling.

- Monitor for complaints of discomfort or dryness in their throat.

- Maintain infection control with proper handwashing and wearing gloves when appropriate.

- Take vital signs as ordered, and record and report changes.

- Listen to the resident's concerns. He or she may feel depressed or anxious about their health. It is important to listen and be supportive.

Total Parenteral Nutrition

Total parenteral nutrition (TPN), sometimes called hyper-alimentation, involves providing nutrients through a vein. TPN is used when a person cannot tolerate enteral nutrition or digestion must stop to allow the bowel to rest and heal. The nutrients in TPN include carbohydrates for energy, protein for muscle strength, lipids for essential fats, electrolytes, and trace minerals. It is administered intravenously through a large central vein. The IV line is connected to a pump machine programmed to administer the amount ordered by the physician for the specified time.

A person receiving TPN must be weighed every day at the same time wearing the same amount of clothing to obtain an accurate weight. Ensure that the tubing does not get dislodged. A clamp must be placed in a visible location at all times in case the tubing is dislodged. If the tubing is dislodged, it is extremely important to clamp the tubing close to the person's body so no air can enter the tubing. Notify the nurse immediately should this occur. If air gets into the line, it could be fatal.

Important guidelines in caring for a person on TPN nutrition include:

- Monitor the skin at the IV insertion site for signs of infection such as redness, swelling, and drainage (pus). Watch for swelling or redness near the collarbone area. The nurse will use sterile technique to change the dressings. It is important to keep the skin clean and dry around the infusion site.

- Always check the tubing to make sure it is not kinked or twisted. Tubing should be taped and secured. The pump alarm will go off if there are any problems with the tubing or the infusion. Call the nurse immediately if the alarm sounds.

- Provide comfort measures such as back rubs to increase circulation and prevent skin breakdown. Always provide good mouth care for a person who is NPO.

- Monitor the person's intake and output. Note any issues with loose watery stools. Always report and record the amount, color, and consistency of bowel movements. Assist with cleaning the area after voiding or bowel movements.

- Maintain infection control with proper hand hygiene and wearing gloves when appropriate.

- Observe for pain in the neck or chest area, recording and reporting any changes immediately.

- Take vital signs as ordered, recording and reporting changes.

- Listen to the resident's concerns. He or she may feel depressed or anxious about their health. It is important to listen and be supportive.

Points to Remember

- Assisting residents with meals is one of the most important parts of your job. You must provide and encourage good nutrition for residents. How you help residents eat and drink is critical to ensuring that they receive proper nutrition and have adequate fluid intake.

- Observing and reporting changes related to nutrition and elimination is important in maintaining residents' health.

- Most facilities provide therapeutic diets to address certain health conditions that also try to accommodate residents' food preferences.

- You have a responsibility to make residents' experiences with eating as pleasant as possible. Environmental, service, and social factors all play a role in a resident's dining experience and food intake.

- You must follow your facility's procedures for proper recording of residents' intake.

- Adequate fluid intake is vital. Most residents need 1,500 to 2,000 cc of fluid per day to prevent dehydration.

- Nurse assistants must develop the skills that allow them to care for residents who need enteral or total parenteral nutrition.

Key Terms

dehydration — serious condition that results from excessive loss of water from the body; can occur due to inadequate fluid intake

dysphagia — difficulty swallowing food, liquid, or medication

enteral nutrition — providing liquid nourishment using a nasogastric tube or a tube surgically inserted through the abdominal wall into the stomach

hydration — supplying water to the body to maintain fluid balance

nutrition — nourishment obtained from food

therapeutic diet — special diet used as a treatment for a disease or condition

total parenteral nutrition (TPN) — nutrition administered intravenously

1. **Providing residents with food that is safe, nutritional, and appealing is the role of the:**

   a. Activities department
   b. Nursing staff
   c. Occupational therapy department
   d. Food service department

2. **Aspiration occurs when:**

   a. Food or liquids enter the airway instead of passing through the esophagus into the stomach
   b. The resident falls, hitting their head
   c. Food enters the stomach
   d. The resident does not like the food they were offered

3. **The signs and symptoms of dehydration may include:**

   a. Rosy pink skin color
   b. Elevated blood pressure
   c. Decreased urine output
   d. Blurred vision

4. **How can you make a resident's dining experience more enjoyable?**

   a. Seat residents at a different table every meal
   b. Turns the television up loud so everyone can hear it
   c. Try to create a pleasant, homelike environment
   d. Turn the dining room lights on a brightly as possible

5. **In some cases, a resident's fluid intake must be monitored and recorded accurately. To do this:**

   a. Give the resident a piece of paper to write it down
   b. Know the capacity of glasses and cups in your facility
   c. Ask the resident's roommate to write down everything the resident drinks
   d. Never take your eyes off the resident

6. **When a person cannot or should not eat food, another way to feed them with liquid nourishment passed through a tube through the nose to the stomach is called:**

   a. Total parenteral nutrition
   b. Gastric lavage
   c. Peritoneal dialysis
   d. Enteral nutrition

7. **What is the best position to reduce the risk of aspiration with a resident who is receiving tube feeding?**

   a. Prone position
   b. Fowler's position, with the head of the bed elevated at least 30 degrees
   c. Sims position
   d. Supine position

8. **What diet would be best for a resident with cardiovascular disease and high cholesterol?**

   a. A restricted fat diet
   b. A renal diet
   c. A full liquid diet
   d. A pureed diet

9. **Which of the following would be considered an overall healthy diet?**

   a. A diet consisting of any fruits and vegetables
   b. A diet consisting of food from all five food groups
   c. A diet consisting of only foods from the dairy group
   d. A diet consisting of only foods from the protein group

10. **If a resident doesn't like the meal that was served or requests something else, the nurse assistant should:**

    a. Do nothing and chart they refused their meal
    b. Offer an alternative that is of similar nutritional value
    c. Offer them two desserts
    d. Tell them that they must eat what was served

10

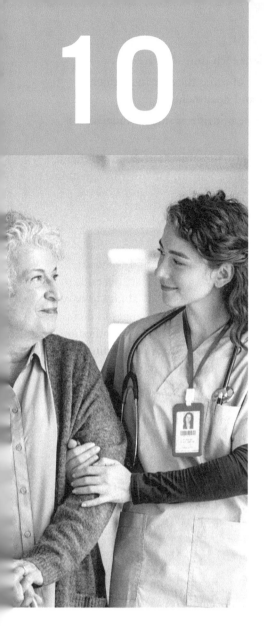

Elimination

Elimination refers to how the body gets rid of waste products. Urine is the liquid waste and stool or feces is the solid waste. Eliminating waste products are an important part of life. When people age or become ill, their elimination patterns often change. This can create a challenge for their care. Some residents have chronic diseases that lead to changes in elimination patterns. Many residents take medications that can alter elimination. Other residents may have mobility issues that make getting to the bathroom very difficult.

The goal is to prevent health declines through timely interventions. As a nurse assistant, you play an important role in maintaining and improving residents' elimination status while maintaining their dignity and supporting their independence to the degree possible.

OBJECTIVES:

- Demonstrate how to properly record residents' output.

- List ways to help residents maintain their dignity when you help them with elimination.

- Name and describe equipment used to help with elimination.

- Demonstrate correct ways to help a resident use a bedpan, urinal, and portable commode.

- State how to identify changes in residents' elimination patterns.

- Demonstrate specimen collection techniques.

- Describe your role in ostomy care.

Fluid Output

A person's output — the amount of their urine — depends on how much fluid they take in. Most people produce about 1,500 cc of urine per day. Output is usually recorded after meals and immediately after serving fluids and assisting with toileting. If a resident has an indwelling Foley catheter, the amount of urine is measured in the collecting bag at the end of each shift or when the bag is full. Procedure 10-1 describes steps involved in measuring output.

When recording output, you should:

- Pour urine into a measuring container to measure, if a bedpan is used.
- Read container at eye level for an accurate measurement.
- Record the output for your shift.

If a resident has incontinence, you should:

- Check the resident frequently for wetness.
- Change the resident each time they are wet.
- Count the number of times they are incontinent during your shift and document.
- Estimate the volume of urine as small, moderate, or large.
- If a resident is incontinent with diarrhea, it is difficult to determine their urine output. Discuss this situation with the charge nurse.

Assisting with Elimination

Elimination is the process of ridding the body of waste products. Urine is the liquid waste, and stool (feces) is the solid waste. Many things affect a person's ability to have normal bowel and bladder functions. Changes in diet or fluid intake can upset a resident's normal elimination pattern. Age-related changes can also affect elimination. As we age, food passes through our digestive tract more slowly, and digestion slows. This results in a slowed bowel pattern and decreased absorption of nutrients. You will learn more about common age-related changes or the urinary and digestive system in chapter 11.

PROCEDURE

10-1: Measuring Output

PREPARATION STEPS

1. Check the care plan.
2. Knock, introduce yourself, and address resident by preferred name.
3. Perform hand hygiene.
4. Gather supplies and secure assistance if needed.
5. Explain procedure and ask about resident preferences.
6. Respect privacy and rights at all times.

ITEMS NEEDED

- Paper towel or barrier
- Measuring container
- Gloves
- Output record

1. Perform hand hygiene.
2. Put on gloves.
3. Transfer urine to a measuring container.
4. Place measuring container at eye level on a flat surface, the container should be placed on a barrier, such as a paper towel.
5. Read the output.
6. Observe for urine for: sediment, mucus, dark color, signs of blood, or a change in odor.
7. Empty urine in the toilet and rinse out or clean measuring container according to facility policy.
8. Remove glove and perform hand hygiene.
9. Record output and report any abnormal findings to the charge nurse.

COMPLETION STEPS

1. Determine the resident's preferred position for comfort and ask them if they need anything else.
2. Examine the environment for safety and cleanliness.
3. Secure the call light and any other needed items within reach of the resident.
4. Perform hand hygiene.
5. Document the procedure and report any findings to the staff in charge.

The inability to eliminate without assistance and *incontinence* — the inability to voluntarily control elimination — are upsetting for residents. This affects their quality of life. You need to understand how to support residents with their elimination needs while maintaining their dignity.

Determining Elimination Patterns

Each resident has their own pattern of elimination. This pattern involves their frequency of elimination and usual amounts of urine and stool. Some residents urinate more often than others. Some residents have bowel movements daily, while others have them every other or every third day. You learn a resident's normal pattern so that you can base your care on their needs. This enables you to recognize when a problem occurs or illness changes their pattern. A change in elimination can result from changes in food or fluid intake or from a serious condition.

In addition to your own observations, you can gather information from the resident, family members, and the resident's chart. This information is part of the resident's bowel and bladder assessment. The nurse typically gathers this information, but you may be asked to assist. Be sure you understand what information the nurse needs.

Residents use many different words to refer to urine and stool elimination. Get to know what words they are most comfortable with as you care for them. You may ask the resident or family what words they prefer to use.

Although residents may use many different words, you must always be professional when you communicate with the resident and family members.

When you gather information about elimination, remember that talking about this subject is often uncomfortable for people. Help ease this situation by asking questions only in private. When you cannot obtain enough information from the resident, you will need to speak with a family member.

Ask these questions about the resident's elimination habits:

- How often do you have a bowel movement?
- What time of day do you normally have a bowel movement?
- Is there anything I should know that will help you keep your normal schedule?
- How often do you urinate?
- Do you usually urinate in large or small amounts?
- Do you have a pattern of urinating at specific times of day?

- Do you wake up at night needing to urinate?
- Do you ever urinate and then find you have to go again soon after?
- Do you currently use products to absorb your urine? If yes, what types of products are you using?

Review a resident's chart to learn their elimination patterns. This information is collected starting on the day of admission. If the resident has any problems with elimination, the care plan has information about how to care for them. The chart usually contains the following information:

- How often the person has a bowel movement
- The shift during which a resident usually has a bowel movement
- The amount, color, and consistency of the resident's stool
- The resident's urination pattern
- The amount and color of urine
- Any odor or pain with urination
- If the resident has urinary or bowel incontinence

Promoting Regular Elimination Patterns

To support regular elimination, you must respond to call signals promptly and help residents to the bathroom as soon as you are asked. If a resident cannot ask, help them to the bathroom. When they awake in the morning, before and after meals, before and after activities, at bedtime, when they wake at night, and any other time you think they may have to go. Make sure residents eat a balanced diet and drink plenty of fluids, especially water. You can also do all you can to ensure that residents get enough rest and exercise.

Maintaining Residents' Dignity When Helping with Elimination

Elimination is a very private act. Like bathing or grooming, this is something the resident has always done in private. Residents have the right to dignity, respect, and privacy even when they need your help. Help maintain their dignity in these ways:

- Ask questions about elimination only in private.
- Maintain a professional attitude.
- Never use nicknames, slang, or unprofessional gestures to refer to elimination.
- Help residents in private. Close the door, pull the bedside curtains around the bed, and cover the person.

- Ask others to leave the room, if possible.

- Explain that you wear gloves as an important part of infection control and that this practice protects them as well as you.

- Empty bedpans and commodes and flush toilets immediately after elimination.

- Use an odor-control spray if needed. Control your reaction to any odors and remain professional as you provide care.

- When changing disposable incontinent products, place them in a bag, secure bag by tying and remove from the room when you leave.

Equipment for Elimination

Some residents may need to use special equipment to help with elimination. Depending on their care plan, mobility, and health status, they may use the toilet, bedpan, urinal, or bedside commode. Using the bathroom toilet is easiest and the most familiar. A resident who cannot get to the bathroom may use a bedpan, urinal, or portable commode. With any of these, try to create an environment that feels as private as possible. Procedure 10-2 describes the steps used to help a resident use a bedpan, and Procedure 10-3 describes how to assist a male resident in using a urinal.

PROCEDURE

10-2: Helping a Resident Use a Bedpan

PREPARATION STEPS

1. Check the care plan.
2. Knock, introduce yourself, and address resident by preferred name.
3. Perform hand hygiene.
4. Gather supplies and secure assistance if needed.
5. Explain procedure and ask about resident preferences.
6. Respect privacy and rights at all times.

ITEMS NEEDED

- Bedpan with cover
- Wash basin
- Two towels
- Two washcloths
- Soap
- Toilet paper
- At least three pairs of gloves
- Two plastic-covered pads or protective covers
- Body powder or cornstarch
- Disposable trash bag

Remember — if you contaminate your gloves in any way during the procedure, you must change to a new pair.

1 Put on gloves.

2 Put a pad or cover on the surface where you will put the bedpan after it is used.

3 Fold the bedspread and blanket down to the bottom of the bed, leaving the top sheet in place to cover the resident's lower legs. Help the resident lift their nightgown or remove pajama bottoms or underpants.

4 Put a protective cover under the resident's buttocks to protect the bed linen.

5 Ask the resident to bend both knees and lift their buttocks up while you slide the bedpan underneath them. Adjust it for the resident's comfort. Using powder or cornstarch on the bedpan prevents the resident's skin from sticking when the bedpan is removed. If the resident cannot lift their buttocks on their own, you can help them turn onto one side. Hold the bedpan flush against the buttocks. Have the resident turn back onto the bedpan or help them move back onto the bedpan. (You may need another staff member to help with moving the resident.)

6 Remove your gloves and dispose of them in the trash bag. Wash your hands.

7 Cover the resident with the top sheet for privacy.

8 Elevate the head of the bed slowly until the resident is in a sitting position. Ask the resident if they are as comfortable as they can be. Change the position of the bedpan if needed to make them comfortable.

9 Provide toilet paper and position the call light button so the resident can reach it. Tell them to call you when finished. If a resident cannot tell you they are finished, check on them every five minutes. Because a bedpan puts pressure on the skin, do not leave a resident on a bedpan longer than necessary.

10 Once the resident has finished with elimination, put on gloves.

11 Lower the head of the bed. Ask the resident to lift their buttocks up while you slide the bedpan out. If needed, help them roll onto one side while you hold the bedpan to prevent a spill. Move the bedpan to the covered surface.

12 If needed, help with wiping the perineal area. Put the used toilet tissue in the bedpan. You may need to wash the perineal area for some residents. Remember to wash, rinse, and dry thoroughly. (Some facilities may use premoistened disposable washcloths for this purpose. Others use a cleansing solution that is squeezed from a bottle over the perineal area.) Wash or wipe from front to back. Remove and dispose of the protective pad on the bed.

13 Remove your gloves and dispose of them in the trash bag. Perform hand hygiene, and put on clean gloves.

14 Help the resident perform hand hygiene. If perineal washing was done, change the water in the basin and use a fresh washcloth and towel for hand hygiene.

15 Remove your gloves and dispose of them in the trash bag. Perform hand hygiene, and put on clean gloves.

16 Help the resident get dressed.

17 Put the bedpan cover on the bedpan and dispose of the contents in the resident's toilet. Clean the bedpan and return it to the bedside table. Remove and dispose of the protective pad on which you placed the bedpan. Most facilities have a water sprayer attached to the toilet for cleaning bedpans and urinals. Follow your facility's procedures for using this equipment. When you empty and clean the bedpan, be careful not to splash the contents.

18 Remove your gloves and place them in the disposable trash bag. Properly dispose of the trash bag, and perform hand hygiene.

COMPLETION STEPS

1. Determine the resident's preferred position for comfort and ask them if they need anything else.

2. Examine the environment for safety and cleanliness.

3. Secure the call light and any other needed items within reach of the resident.

4. Perform hand hygiene.

5. Document the procedure and report any findings to the staff in charge.

10-3: Helping a Male Resident Use a Urinal

PREPARATION STEPS

1. Check the care plan.
2. Knock, introduce yourself, and address resident by preferred name.
3. Perform hand hygiene.
4. Gather supplies and secure assistance if needed.
5. Explain procedure and ask about resident preferences.
6. Respect privacy and rights at all times.

ITEMS NEEDED

- Urinal
- Wash basin
- Towel
- Soap
- Toilet paper
- At least three pairs of gloves
- Plastic-covered pad or protective cover
- Disposable trash bag

Remember — if you contaminate your gloves in any way during the procedure, you must change to a new pair.

1. Put on gloves.

2. Put a pad or cover on the surface where you will put the urinal after use.

3. If the resident can stand beside the bed to use the urinal, help him to stand, and provide privacy. Put the call button within reach so he can call you when finished

4. If the resident must use the urinal while in bed, fold the bedspread and blanket down to the bottom of the bed, leaving the top sheet over the resident. Help the resident lower his bottom clothing.

5. Place the urinal between the resident's legs at an angle to avoid urine spillage. Gently place the penis into the urinal.

6. Remove your gloves and put them in the trash bag. Perform hand hygiene. Cover the resident with the top sheet. Put the call button within reach so he can call you when finished. Check in a few minutes if he does not call you.

7. Perform hand hygiene and put on new gloves.

8. When the resident is finished, remove the urinal and place it on the pad or protective cover.

9. If needed, help the resident wipe off excess urine with toilet tissue.

10. Perform hand hygiene and put on new gloves.

11. Help the resident perform hand hygiene.

12. Empty and clean the urinal, and replace it in the bedside table. Most facilities have a water sprayer attached to the toilet for cleaning bedpans and urinals. Follow your facility's procedures for using this equipment. When you empty and clean the urinal, be careful not to splash the contents.

13. Remove your gloves and place them in the disposable trash bag. Dispose of tissue and your gloves in the trash bag. Properly dispose of the trash bag, and perform hand hygiene.

COMPLETION STEPS

1. Determine the resident's preferred position for comfort and ask them if they need anything else.
2. Examine the environment for safety and cleanliness.
3. Secure the call light and any other needed items within reach of the resident.
4. Perform hand hygiene.
5. Document the procedure and report any findings to the staff in charge.

Bedpans are used by both male and female residents. A smaller fracture pan is often used for residents with hip or back problems (Figure 10-1). The bedside commode is a portable toilet. It is positioned beside the bed so the resident needs only to move from the bed to it. Most commodes are like a chair with a toilet seat cover and a container under the seat that catches the urine and stool (Figure 10-2). Procedure 10-4 outlines how to help a resident use a portable commode.

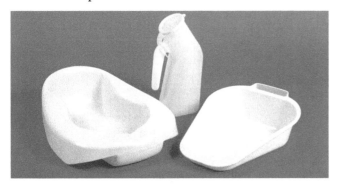

Figure 10-1 Examples of bedpan, fracture pan, and urinal.

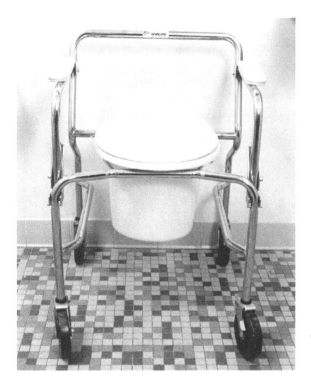

Figure 10-2 Example of a portable commode.

Problems with Elimination

When you help a resident with elimination, watch for anything unusual. Listen to any problems a resident describes. Any changes or even a minor complaint could mean something serious that you should report to the charge nurse. Some problems might be easily resolved. Others require immediate medical attention. Box 10-1 lists specific problems that must be reported.

Residents that have incontinence will usually wear disposable incontinent products (Procedure 10-5 provides steps on applying a disposable incontinent brief). Disposable incontinence products are available in many types, sizes, and levels of absorbency. Depending on the assessment and the type of incontinence, the nurse and resident will determine what type of incontinence products to use. The selection of incontinent products should be a person-centered approach. Using this approach to incontinent care means taking into consideration the resident's level of leakage, mobility status, and individual preferences. Choosing the right type of product is essential to maintain the residents skin health, dignity, and comfort. Types of products include: (Figure 10-3, p. 233)

- Bladder control pads
- Pant liners
- Protective underwear (adult style pull-up)
- Briefs

Once the type of product is selected, determining the correct size is very important to prevent discomfort, skin issues, and leakage. Size of products can be typically determined based on the resident's height and weight or waist measurements. It is a key point to remember when selecting the size of product is to follow the manufacturer's guidelines. Residents that wear a product that is too large may experience leaking. Larger products do not indicate more absorbency.

Nurse Assistant's Role in Observation and Intervention

- Identify residents at risk for incontinence.
- Support the assessment process.
- Closely monitor the resident's urinary pattern and report any changes.
- Report any abnormal signs or symptoms, including any skin issues.

Goals for Caring for an Incontinent Resident

- Help the resident regain as much control over urinary function as possible. Interventions may include a toileting program.

10-4: Helping a Resident Use a Portable Commode

PREPARATION STEPS

1. Check the care plan.
2. Knock, introduce yourself, and address resident by preferred name.
3. Perform hand hygiene.
4. Gather supplies and secure assistance if needed.
5. Explain procedure and ask about resident preferences.
6. Respect privacy and rights at all times.

ITEMS NEEDED

- Wash basin
- Towel
- Soap
- Toilet paper
- At least two pairs of gloves
- Disposable trash bag

Remember — if you contaminate your gloves in any way during the procedure, you must change to a new pair.

1 Position the commode by the bed. Place it so it will not move when you help the resident out of bed. You can place it against the wall or against the bedside table to keep it from moving.

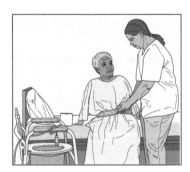

2 Put on gloves.

3 Help the resident out of bed or out of a chair to a standing position. Help pull down the resident's lower clothing, and help them sit on the commode.

4 Provide toilet paper and put the call button within reach. Remove gloves and perform hand hygiene.

5 If the resident needs help with wiping when finished, first put on gloves. Help with wiping, and throw the tissue into the commode or place in the trash bag.

6 Remove your gloves and dispose of them in the trash bag. Perform hand hygiene.

7 Help the resident with their clothing and to get back into the bed or chair.

8 Put on new gloves.

9 Help the resident perform hand hygiene.

10 Remove the container from the commode and empty its contents into the resident's toilet. Most facilities have a water sprayer attached to the toilet. Follow your facility's procedures for using this equipment. When you empty and clean the commode container, be careful not to splash the contents.

11 Clean and dry the container and replace it in the commode.

12 Remove your gloves and place them in the disposable trash bag. Properly dispose of the trash bag, and perform hand hygiene.

COMPLETION STEPS

1. Determine the resident's preferred position for comfort and ask them if they need anything else.
2. Examine the environment for safety and cleanliness.
3. Secure the call light and any other needed items within reach of the resident.
4. Perform hand hygiene.
5. Document the procedure and report any findings to the staff in charge.

BOX 10-1

PROBLEMS WITH ELIMINATION

Report any of the following to the charge nurse

URINATION CONCERNS

- Pain or burning sensation when urinating
- Foul-smelling urine
- Blood in the urine
- More frequent trips to the bathroom
- Voiding small amounts of urine
- Cloudy urine
- Lower abdominal discomfort or back pain
- A resident has not urinated during your shift
- A resident who usually is not incontinent becomes incontinent
- A resident who has never been incontinent has an accident
- The urine is not a light amber color but is dark and concentrated

BOWEL ELIMINATION CONCERNS

- A resident has difficulty moving their bowels
- A resident strains more while having a bowel movement
- Blood in a resident's stool, either bright red or black
- Frequent, watery stools
- Foul-smelling stool
- Stool is not brown and soft but greenish, black, hard, or watery
- A resident's abdomen is bloated or swollen and they have not had a bowel movement recently
- Swollen, bleeding tissue around the anus
- A resident has more difficulty getting to the bathroom
- A resident is not eating

- Maintain the resident's dignity by responding promptly and calmly providing assistance after incontinence episodes, as discussed earlier in this chapter.

- Prevent skin breakdown. Give routine personal care any time a resident is incontinent to prevent skin rashes and breakdown. Residents with incontinence are at risk for developing skin damage. The incontinent resident is at risk for developing Incontinence Associated Dermatitis (IAD). This is a form of dermatitis caused by frequent exposure from urine and/or stool.

IAD can be very painful, difficult to treat, and can lead to the development of a pressure injury, so prevention is critical. IAD can occur in different levels: mild, moderate and severe. The skin will appear burned or scalded and it may be open or closed (intact). The nurse assistant can assist in preventing IAD by changing incontinent products timely and providing perineal care after each incontinent episode (Figure 10-4).

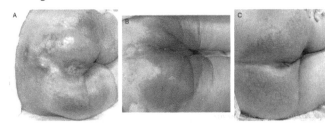

Figure 10-4   A. IAD in person with a light skin tone; B, IAD in a person with a light yellow skin tone with yeast; C, IAD in a person with a brown skin tone with yeast. Images copyright Ayello, used with permission.

- Prevent urinary tract infections. Urinary Tract Infections (UTI's) are one of the most common infections in nursing homes and the elderly. As a nurse assistant you have a very important role in the prevention of urinary tract infections. One of the most important prevention interventions is providing proper perineal care (as you learned earlier, in chapter 5) for the incontinent resident. Perineal care should be performed after each incontinent episode. You will learn more about UTI's in chapter 11.

Urinary Incontinence

Urinary incontinence refers to a condition in which a person cannot voluntarily control urination. In most cases, urinary incontinence can be treated or improved. The key to successful treatment is a proper assessment of the resident. This assessment is done by the primary care physician, a urologist, or a nurse. You help with the assessment by observing and recording the frequency and timing of incontinence, the resident's reaction, and related environmental factors, such as if incontinence occurs in the activity room because a bathroom is too far away. The goals of the assessment are to:

- Determine the resident's usual pattern of urination.
- Identify and treat causes of incontinence.
- Determine the care plan needed for the resident.

10-5: Applying a Disposable Incontinence Brief

PREPARATION STEPS

1. Check the care plan.
2. Knock, introduce yourself, and address resident by preferred name.
3. Perform hand hygiene.
4. Gather supplies and secure assistance if needed.
5. Explain procedure and ask about resident preferences.
6. Respect privacy and rights at all times.

ITEMS NEEDED

- Disposable incontinence pads
- Disposable briefs
- Plastic trash bag
- Underpants (if resident wears underpants over the brief)
- Three pairs of gloves
- Two washcloths
- Towel
- Soap or perineal wash

Incontinence briefs are available in various types and sizes. Make sure to use the correct size for the resident.

1. Place an incontinence pad on the bed to protect clean linen.

2. Help the resident onto their back.

3. Put on gloves.

4. Help remove garments below the waist.

5. Discard the soiled incontinence brief in the plastic trash bag.

6. Remove and dispose of your soiled gloves. Perform hand hygiene.

7. Put on new gloves.

8. With the resident on their side, give perineal care, including cleaning the rectal area.

9. Remove and dispose of your soiled gloves. Perform hand hygiene.

10. Put on new gloves.

11. Fan-fold one-half of the brief under the resident's buttocks.

12. Help the resident move onto their back. Unfold the side that was fan-folded, and open the adhesive tabs on both sides. Place the brief upward between the resident's legs, and join the tab from the back of the brief to the tab in the front of the brief. Make sure to have the leg openings pulled securely into the resident's groin areas and not resting on their thighs.

13. If the resident wears underpants over the brief, put these on, and help the resident put on their clothing.

Note: If a panty liner is used instead of briefs, use the same procedure but instead, place the liner over their buttocks. Then have the resident move onto their back, and bring the front of the liner up between their legs. Put on their underpants and help with other clothing.

COMPLETION STEPS

1. Determine the resident's preferred position for comfort and ask them if they need anything else.
2. Examine the environment for safety and cleanliness.
3. Secure the call light and any other needed items within reach of the resident.
4. Perform hand hygiene.
5. Document the procedure and report any findings to the staff in charge.

Incontinence can be caused by a number of factors. The bladder may contract when it should not, causing an abrupt gush of urine. Or, the bladder does not contract when it should, causing the bladder to fill, and urine spills over. A blockage of the urethral opening can lead to an overly full bladder and urine spilling over or weakness of the urethral opening.

Other causes not related to urinary system function include:

- Medications
- Urinary tract infection or vaginitis
- Lack of access to a bathroom
- Fecal impaction

Disposable Incontinence Products

Choosing the correct incontinence product is one of the key components to manage individuals with incontinence. There are many varying styles, absorbencies and functions of incontinence products. This chart describes frequently used products along with an example of what types of individuals and situations they would be applied.

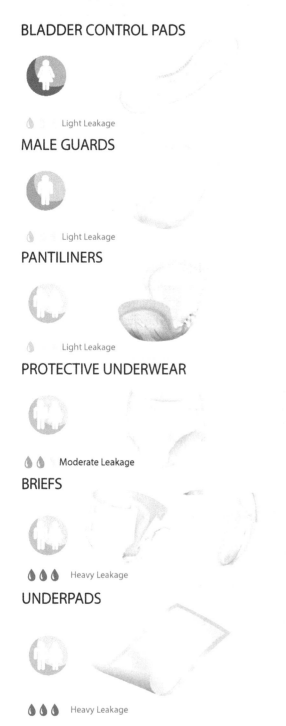

BLADDER CONTROL PADS

Light Leakage

Thin, smaller pad that is worn inside a females regular underwear secured with an adhesive strip. Ideal for light urinary incontinence and individuals that are able to use the toilet either independently or with assistance.

MALE GUARDS

Light Leakage

A product designed specifically for males with urinary incontinence. The design is provided to targeted the male anatomy for best absorption. It is secured in mens underwear with an adhesive strip.

PANTILINERS

Light Leakage

A product for light to moderate urinary leakage that can be used for both male and female. This comes in a variety of sizes and absorbencies. An adhesive strip secures the product into a mesh type style panty, or the resident's regular underwear.

PROTECTIVE UNDERWEAR

Moderate Leakage

Adult protective underwear may also be referred to as a "pull-up". This is an underwear style that pulls up and down when the individual needs to use the toilet. It is typically used for urinary incontinence and individuals that are able to use the toilet with or without assistance. It fits like regular underwear. This is available in male, female and unisex styles.

BRIEFS

Heavy Leakage

An adult brief should be used when the individual is completely incontinent of urine, stool or both. It is more absorbent than the other products and provides more protection. This product may come in a traditional 4 tab style or 2 tabs with stretchy side wings.

UNDERPADS

Heavy Leakage

Underpads are a product that is used underneath residents to absorb leakage while in bed, wheelchairs or furniture. They are available in a variety of absorbencies but do not provide protection like the other incontinent products. If a person is wearing a product that is the correct size and applied appropriately it should not leak and the underpad would not be needed. Underpads also add an extra layer in between the person and the support surface that could cause a build up of moisture and heat.

Figure 10-3   Disposable incontinence products. Copyright 2022, First Quality Products, Inc. Used with permission.

- Delirium
- Immobility
- Depression
- Diabetes mellitus
- Congestive heart failure
- Neurologic lesions

Types of Urinary Incontinence

There are five main types of urinary incontinence:

- **Stress incontinence** — occurs when pressure is put on the bladder like coughing, sneezing, laughing, lifting, or exercising. Small amounts of urine leak. The resident may be in a group activity and leaks urine when they lift an exercise ball.

- **Urge incontinence** — is a sudden strong urge to urinate, followed by urinary leakage. You may have a resident that rushes to the bathroom but doesn't make it on time and has an accident.

- **Mixed incontinence** — is a combination of stress and urge incontinence. Your resident may report that they feel a sudden urge to urinate and leaks when they laugh or sneeze.

- **Overflow incontinence** — occurs when the bladder doesn't fully empty causing constant or frequent dribbling. Your resident may report that they are "always wet" and requires frequent clothing changes.

- **Functional incontinence** — Occurs due to a physical or cognitive limitation. The resident may require assist to get to the bathroom due to a broken leg but doesn't get assistance in time. Someone with cognitive limitations may not realize that they are wet.

Toileting Programs

Toileting programs can help manage incontinence, regain bladder control or decrease the number of incontinent episodes. Some of these programs may include:

Bladder Retraining Program: The goal of this program is to regain control of the bladder by gradually lengthening the intervals between times the resident voids (urinates) and regain urinary continence. This program is successful with most residents with normal cognitive skills. Before initiating this program, a diary must be kept of the resident's voiding pattern, including the time between urinations, amount voided each time, and fluid intake. The charge nurse will set a schedule for expected voiding times based on the resident's voiding pattern. At the

chosen interval, you help the resident to the toilet. This interval is used for two days and the results documented.

If after two days the resident has not been incontinent, the interval is increased by 30 minutes. This cycle continues until the resident's voiding interval is four hours. Between times, encourage the resident to resist the urge to urinate.

It takes time, often several weeks, for an incontinent resident to regain control of their bladder. The resident needs continuous encouragement from staff. All staff must be attentive and consistent with the training schedule. Residents may also participate in a pelvic floor muscle exercise program (Kegel exercises). If so, remind the resident to perform the exercises.

Prompted Voiding: The goal of this program is to prompt the resident to void at intervals short enough to prevent leakage.

This program is frequently used for cognitively impaired residents. When initiated by charge nurse, you will ask the resident if they are wet or dry, every two hours. Then check for wetness and give feedback to the resident. Ask if the resident wants to go to the toilet. If they do, record the amount voided. If they don't, try to encourage the resident to go. If the resident still says no, come back in an hour. Repeat the check for wetness and the request to toilet. Increase the time between prompts if the resident's incontinence improves.

Habit Training: Involves documenting a resident's elimination patterns for at least three days to determine the resident's voiding habits. Using the data collected, the resident is placed on a toileting schedule to match the individual voiding habits or needs. The goal of this program is to decrease the number of incontinent episodes.

Preventing Urinary Tract Infections

Urinary Tract Infections (UTI's) are one of the most common infections in nursing homes and the elderly. As a nurse assistant you have a very important role in the prevention of urinary tract infections. One of the most important prevention interventions is providing proper perineal care (as you learned earlier, in chapter 5) for the incontinent resident. Perineal care should be performed after each incontinent episode. You will learn more about UTI's in chapter 11.

Urinary Catheters

Some residents may have an indwelling catheter (Figure 10-5). The catheter must be ordered by the physician for specific medical reasons. The nurse inserts the catheter using a sterile technique. The catheter passes through the urethra into the bladder, and a small balloon inflated with sterile water keeps the catheter in place. Urine passes from the bladder through the catheter tube and into a closed collection bag. Procedure 10-6 outlines the steps for urinary catheter care, and Procedure 10-7 describes how to empty a catheter drainage bag

A condom catheter, or external catheter, may be used for male residents. They are external urinary catheters that are worn on the outside of the penis like a condom. This type of catheter has a tube attached that allows urine out into a drainage bag. These may be used for male residents with urinary incontinence or those having physical limitations that prevent them from being able to get to the bathroom or use other devices such as a urinal.

Bowel Incontinence

Bowel or fecal incontinence is the inability to control bowel movement, causing leakage from the rectum. Bowel incontinence can be caused by factors such as, side effects of medications, diarrhea, constipation and muscle or nerve damage.

Bowel Retraining

The goal of bowel retraining is to help the resident maintain a regular pattern of bowel movements. Like bladder retraining, you will need to determine the resident's elimination habits in order to initiate a bowel retraining program. Once a pattern is established the nurse will develop an individualized program. As a nurse assistant it is important to:

- Follow the individualized retraining schedule, based off of the information collected about their elimination habits
- Encourage the resident to drink plenty of fluids, eight 8-ounce glasses every day (unless medically contraindicated)
- Encourage the resident to eat a diet high in fiber, such as bran cereals, fruit, and vegetables
- Provide privacy during elimination
- Report any changes in the residents' bowel habits to the charge nurse
- Assist with perineal care after each incontinent episode
- Encourage regular exercise, if possible, such as walking

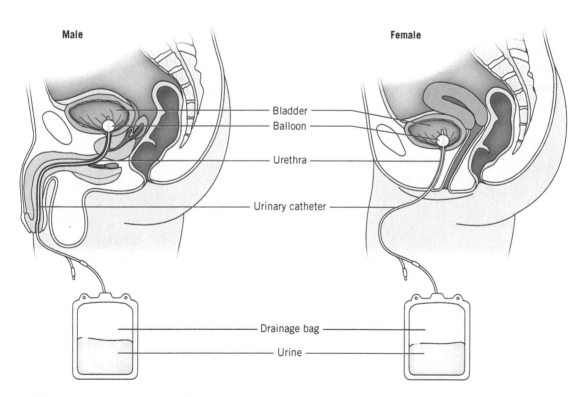

Male **Female**

Bladder
Balloon
Urethra
Urinary catheter
Drainage bag
Urine

Figure 10-5 Correct placement of a urinary catheter.

PREPARATION STEPS

1. Check the care plan.
2. Knock, introduce yourself, and address resident by preferred name.
3. Perform hand hygiene.
4. Gather supplies and secure assistance if needed.
5. Explain procedure and ask about resident preferences.
6. Respect privacy and rights at all times.

ITEMS NEEDED

- Gloves
- Soap and water
- At least 2 washcloths
- Towel

Your responsibility for a resident with a catheter is to give routine perineal care and position the external catheter tubing and drainage bag.

1 Put on gloves before giving perineal care. Pull back top sheet, only exposing area to be cleaned.

2 Always keep the external catheter tube as clean as possible.

3 Clean the tubing with soap and water and a washcloth. Clean the tube first at the urethral opening, and then cleanse downward and away from the opening. To prevent discomfort for the resident, do not pull on the catheter tube while cleaning it.

4 Use a clean area of the washcloth for each downward stroke.

5 Do the rest of perineal care as usual, cleansing with soap and water from front to back.

6 Check the tubing for kinks and leaks.

7 The urinary drainage bag is secured to the bed or chair below the resident's bladder, so that the urine flows downward into the bag by gravity. Never let the drainage bag touch the floor, which is considered an unclean area. Never lift the drainage bag above the resident because urine could flow back into the bladder, increasing the risk of infection.

8 When you help a resident with a catheter change position, follow these guidelines: The external part of the catheter tube can be secured with a strap to the resident's upper thigh to prevent pulling on the catheter when they move. The urinary catheter tube, connecting tube, and drainage bag should not be separated except by a nurse using a sterile technique to change the tubing or collect a specimen. The drainage system is kept closed to help prevent infection.

9 Remove gloves and cover resident. Perform hand hygiene.

COMPLETION STEPS

1. Determine the resident's preferred position for comfort and ask them if they need anything else.
2. Examine the environment for safety and cleanliness.
3. Secure the call light and any other needed items within reach of the resident.
4. Perform hand hygiene.
5. Document the procedure and report any findings to the staff in charge.

Ostomy Care

Normal urination and bowel elimination is not possible for everyone due to aging and certain disease or health conditions. Some residents may have had an **ostomy**, which is a surgical procedure that creates an opening in the body for the discharge of wastes. Ostomies can be done to divert a resident's urine (urostomy or ureterostomy) or stool (colostomy or ileostomy). The opening is called the **stoma**. The stoma is normally red and has a round shape. Immediately after surgery, the stoma may be swollen. After surgery, the stoma is measured for fitting the proper pouching system. In many cases, this is the resident's permanent method of elimination (Figure 10-6).

Many residents who have undergone ostomy procedures are very sensitive and concerned about how others perceive them. They may be afraid of being avoided or treated differently. Always maintain a positive attitude and treat the resident with respect and dignity. Be careful to avoid any facial expressions or comments that may be interpreted as offensive.

10-7: Emptying a Catheter Drainage Bag

PREPARATION STEPS

1. Check the care plan.
2. Knock, introduce yourself, and address resident by preferred name.
3. Perform hand hygiene.
4. Gather supplies and secure assistance if needed.
5. Explain procedure and ask about resident preferences.
6. Respect privacy and rights at all times.

ITEMS NEEDED

- Paper towels
- Gloves
- Measuring container
- I & O record

1 Put on gloves.

2 Place paper towels on the floor underneath the drainage bag.

3 Place the measuring container on the paper towels.

4 The drainage bag has a closed clamp that allows the urine to flow from the bag. Open the clamp and drain all the urine into the container, making sure not to touch the clamp to the sides of the container.

5 Close the clamp and secure it to the drainage bag immediately after it is completely drained.

6 Note the amount of urine and discard the urine in the resident's toilet.

7 Remove and discard your gloves, and perform hand hygiene.

8 Record the amount of urine on the intake and output record.

COMPLETION STEPS

1. Determine the resident's preferred position for comfort and ask them if they need anything else.
2. Examine the environment for safety and cleanliness.
3. Secure the call light and any other needed items within reach of the resident.
4. Perform hand hygiene.
5. Document the procedure and report any findings to the staff in charge.

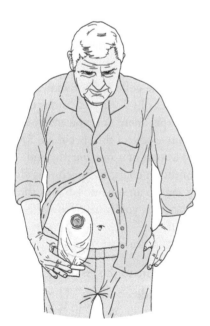

Figure 10-6 Following an ostomy procedure, a special bag (pouch) is used to collect waste excreted from the body.

Types of Ostomy Procedures

A *ureterostomy* is surgery that redirects both ureters to a stoma in the abdomen. This procedure may be done due to cancer or other diseases affecting urinary system function. The resident's urine is excreted through the stoma into a bag or pouch attached to their abdomen. A *urostomy* is a procedure that diverts urine due to a missing, defective, or diseased bladder.

A *colostomy* connects the colon (large intestine) to a stoma in the abdomen. This surgery is done for many reasons, such as colon cancer and other diseases that cause colon inflammation. Bowel elimination then occurs through this opening into an ostomy bag. A resident who has undergone a colostomy may have one or two stomas. Some colostomies are permanent, but others are temporary. An *ileostomy* connects the ileum (longest portion of the small intestine) to a stoma in the abdomen. This surgery is often permanent.

The main difference in postoperative care for residents who have had these intestinal procedures involves stool consistency. With colostomy, the feces eliminated may be semi-liquid or fairly well formed, depending on the site of the surgery. Ileostomy fecal contents are usually much more liquid. They also contain more digestive juices, which can irritate the skin.

Providing Ostomy Care

Follow your facility's policies and procedures for ostomy care. Many residents do their own care independently. They may only need you to provide supplies. How much support you give depends on the resident's level of independence.

As with all residents, pay attention to any changes in elimination patterns. Observe the stoma for changes. Because the stoma has a rich blood supply, it will bleed easily if irritated or injured. Even when injured, the resident will not feel pain or other sensations in the stoma because no nerve endings are present there. The skin around the stoma must be protected from digestive enzymes, which can cause irritation. Observe the skin around the stoma for any signs of irritation, and report any problems to the charge nurse. The exact care you give depends on the resident's needs, direction from the charge nurse, and the care plan.

Most residents with an ostomy use a bag device called an appliance or pouch. Your observations while providing care are very important. When helping a resident with dressing, undressing, or bathing, take time to observe the appliance and the resident's skin. Look for the following:

- Is the appliance leaking?
- Is the seal around the stoma secure?
- Is the ostomy draining well?
- Are the consistency and color of the stool or urine normal?
- Are the stoma and surrounding skin intact?
- Is there redness, bleeding, or other type of skin breakdown?

Emptying an Ostomy Bag

You may be asked to empty and measure the contents of a resident's ostomy bag (Figure 10-7). When emptying an ostomy bag, follow these guidelines:

- Always wear gloves.
- Measure the contents of the bag at least once during a shift.
- To empty the bag, undo the clip on the bottom of the bag, and empty the contents into a bedpan.

- Some bags do not have clips and must be changed after each use. Know the appliance your resident uses and how to empty it.
- Rinse out the bag each time you empty it. You may use a large irrigation syringe. Add a deodorizer if needed.
- Wipe off the end of the bag.
- Reseal the bag with the clip.

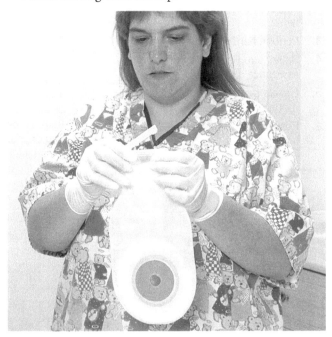

Figure 10-7 Be sure to read and follow the manufacturer's directions for emptying and changing an ostomy bag.

Collecting Specimens

A urine or stool sample collected for analysis is called a **specimen**. A resident's physician may order the collection of a urine or stool specimen, and you may be asked to help the charge nurse collect the specimen. Specimens may be collected as part of a routine physical exam or if the resident's condition changes. Specimens are analyzed at the facility or sent to an outside lab. For the specimen to be analyzed correctly, you must follow the proper collection procedure.

When collecting specimens:

- Explain the procedure to the resident.
- Specimens are considered "dirty." They should not be collected or stored in "clean" areas such as nurses' stations.

- Specimens can be collected in the resident's bathroom and stored per the facility's policy.
- Wear gloves and perform hand hygiene before and after obtaining a specimen.
- Never touch the inside of a specimen container.
- Most specimens must be as fresh as possible. Some need to be refrigerated if there will be any delay in getting them to the lab.

Specimens must be labeled correctly and promptly. Follow these guidelines for labeling:

- Put lids on specimen containers securely to prevent leakage.
- Include the resident's name, room number, and the date and time you collected the specimen.
- Follow your facility's protocol for labeling.

After collecting and labeling a specimen, follow your facility's protocol for how it is to be transported to the lab. Place the specimen in a plastic bag that is labeled as a biohazard. This bag creates an additional barrier to prevent contamination if the specimen cup or container leaks.

Urinalysis

A **urinalysis (UA)** is a laboratory analysis of a urine specimen. Urinalysis may reveal problems in the urinary system or other health problems. In most cases, the specimen should be as fresh as possible when analyzed.

When collecting a urine specimen, ask the charge nurse which container and method to use. Ask for help with the procedure if you are unsure how to do it. Procedure 10-8 describes the steps involved in collecting a urine specimen. Follow your facility's infection control policies. Sometimes you collect urine from a bedpan, urinal, or special device, such as a urine hat. Any equipment used must be as clean as possible.

Clean-Catch Urine Specimen

A *clean-catch urinalysis* is done to check for a urinary tract infection. It is called a clean-catch because the specimen is collected after the urethral opening is cleansed. This cleansing prevents organisms around the urethral opening from contaminating the sample. Procedure 10-9 describes the steps involved in collecting a clean-catch urine specimen.

24-Hour Urine Specimen

This test requires the collection of all urine a resident **voids** in a 24-hour period. The physician may order a 24-hour urine specimen to help diagnose a urinary system problem. Ask the charge nurse for directions on how to manage the specimen. A preservative may be added.

The bottle may be kept cool in a refrigerator or packed in ice in a bucket in the bathroom until the 24-hour period ends. Procedure 10-10 outlines how to collect and handle a 24-hour urine specimen.

Reagent Sticks/Test Strips

Reagent sticks (also called dipsticks or test strips) may be used to check the pH of the urine (whether the sample is acidic or alkaline) or to determine if blood, ketones (acetone), or proteins are present. These tests may reveal a disease or a need for additional tests.

These tests are easily performed using a paper dipstick that is dipped in the resident's urine. The dipstick then shows a change of color or other change to indicate the test result. Ask the nurse which substance(s) you are checking for. Read the instructions on the test strip container so you know how long to wait before you read the result. After you dip the strip in the urine and read the result, compare the result with the range of results in the chart on the container.

The urine of diabetic residents may need to be checked for **ketones** (acetone). This test may also be done for a resident with a change such as increased urine output. When the body burns fat, ketones may be present in the urine. This test is done early in the morning before the resident eats. After dipping the test strip in urine, you compare it to the color chart on the test strip container. Some strips use + and − symbols instead of color changes to show the presence or absence of ketones. Procedure 10-11 describes the steps involved in testing urine for ketones.

Stool Specimens

Stool specimens help physicians diagnose gastrointestinal problems. They may also be collected to check for **parasites** that can make a resident sick. Bleeding in the gastrointestinal tract may be visible or invisible. **Occult** blood is not visible to the human eye. Visible blood in the stool may be bright red or may make the stool look black and sticky (called tarry stool), depending on the source of the bleeding. Stool specimens may be tested for occult blood at the facility (Procedure 10-12) or may be sent to a lab for analysis.

10-8: Collecting a Urine Specimen

PREPARATION STEPS

1. Check the care plan.
2. Knock, introduce yourself, and address resident by preferred name.
3. Perform hand hygiene.
4. Gather supplies and secure assistance if needed.
5. Explain procedure and ask about resident preferences.
6. Respect privacy and rights at all times.

ITEMS NEEDED

- Bedpan, urinal, or toilet hat
- Specimen container
- Labels for container
- At least two pairs of gloves
- Biohazard specimen bag
- Disposable trash bag
- Cleaning solution (if needed)

Remember — if you contaminate your gloves in any way during the procedure, you must change to a new pair.

1. Have the resident urinate into a bedpan, urinal (if male), or clean collection hat in the toilet.

2. Put on gloves.

3. Pour about 60 cc of urine into the specimen container. Discard the remaining urine by emptying it into the toilet.

4. Close the container securely, and write the resident's name, room number, and date and time you collected the specimen on the container label.

5. Place the specimen container in a biohazard specimen bag and make sure the bag is properly sealed.

6. Remove your gloves and place them in the disposable trash bag. Properly dispose of the trash bag, and perform hand hygiene.

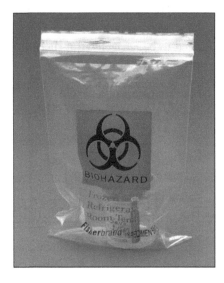

COMPLETION STEPS

1. Determine the resident's preferred position for comfort and ask them if they need anything else.
2. Examine the environment for safety and cleanliness.
3. Secure the call light and any other needed items within reach of the resident.
4. Perform hand hygiene.
5. Document the procedure and report any findings to the staff in charge.

10-9: Collecting a Clean-Catch Urine Specimen

PREPARATION STEPS

1. Check the care plan.
2. Knock, introduce yourself, and address resident by preferred name.
3. Perform hand hygiene.
4. Gather supplies and secure assistance if needed.
5. Explain procedure and ask about resident preferences.
6. Respect privacy and rights at all times.

ITEMS NEEDED

- Specimen container
- Labels for container
- At least two pairs of gloves
- Biohazard specimen bag
- Disposable wipes
- Disposable trash bag
- Cleaning solution (if needed)

Remember — if you contaminate your gloves in any way during the procedure, you must change to a new pair.

1 Put on gloves.

2 Clean the urethral opening. For a female, use one wipe to clean one side of the labia, a second wipe to clean the other side of the labia, and a third wipe to clean down the middle. Always clean in single strokes from front to back. Use each wipe only once and then dispose of it. For a male, clean the penis following the procedure used for perineal care. For an uncircumcised male, pull back the foreskin of the penis to clean it.

3 Have the resident begin to urinate and then stop if they can. Do not collect this first urine. (If the resident cannot stop the flow of urine, you must place the container under the stream before they finish.)

4 Hold the specimen container under the urethra, ask the resident to begin voiding again, and collect the remainder of the specimen.

5 Close the container securely, and write the resident's name, room number, and the date and time you collected the specimen on the container label.

6 Place the specimen container in a biohazard specimen bag and make sure the bag is properly sealed.

7 Remove your gloves and place them in the disposable trash bag. Properly dispose of the trash bag, and perform hand hygiene.

COMPLETION STEPS

1. Determine the resident's preferred position for comfort and ask them if they need anything else.
2. Examine the environment for safety and cleanliness.
3. Secure the call light and any other needed items within reach of the resident.
4. Perform hand hygiene.
5. Document the procedure and report any findings to the staff in charge.

PREPARATION STEPS

1. Check the care plan.
2. Knock, introduce yourself, and address resident by preferred name.
3. Perform hand hygiene.
4. Gather supplies and secure assistance if needed.
5. Explain procedure and ask about resident preferences.
6. Respect privacy and rights at all times.

ITEMS NEEDED

- Bedpan, urinal, or toilet hat
- 24-hour urine specimen container
- Labels for container
- At least two pairs of gloves
- Biohazard specimen bag
- Disposable trash bag
- Cleaning solution (if needed)

Remember — if you contaminate your gloves in any way during the procedure, you must change to a new pair.

1. Remind the resident not to discard any urine. Place a sign in the bathroom to alert other staff and family members. (Everyone involved needs to understand that if any urine is lost, the test may need to be restarted.) All urine must be collected in the same container.

2. Put on gloves.

3. Discard the first voided urine of the day. At this time, the 24-hour collection period begins. (The test would be inaccurate if the first voided urine was not discarded, because it contains urine that collected in the bladder before the starting period.) During the collection period the resident should use a bedpan, commode, urinal, or a collection hat on the toilet. Remind the resident to call you each time they urinate so you can be sure all urine is collected.

4. After handling each specimen, remove your gloves and place them in the disposable trash bag. Properly dispose of the trash bag, and wash your hands.

5. Once the 24 hours are up, put on a new pair of gloves.

6. Close the container securely, and write the resident's name, room number, and the date and the collection time period on the container label.

7. Place the specimen container in a biohazard specimen bag and make sure the bag is properly sealed.

8. Remove your gloves and place them in the disposable trash bag. Properly dispose of the trash bag, and perform hand hygiene.

COMPLETION STEPS

1. Determine the resident's preferred position for comfort and ask them if they need anything else.
2. Examine the environment for safety and cleanliness.
3. Secure the call light and any other needed items within reach of the resident.
4. Perform hand hygiene.
5. Document the procedure and report any findings to the staff in charge.

10-11: Testing Urine for Ketones

PREPARATION STEPS

1. Check the care plan.
2. Knock, introduce yourself, and address resident by preferred name.
3. Perform hand hygiene.
4. Gather supplies and secure assistance if needed.
5. Explain procedure and ask about resident preferences.
6. Respect privacy and rights at all times.

ITEMS NEEDED

- Bedpan, urinal, or toilet hat
- Test strips and instructions
- At least two pairs of gloves
- Watch with a second hand or digital timer
- Disposable trash bag

Remember — if you contaminate your gloves in any way during the procedure, you must change to a new pair.

1. Put on gloves.

2. Have the resident void in the bedpan, urinal, or collection hat on a toilet.

3. Either dip the end of the test strip in the fresh urine or pass it through the urine stream.

4. Pull the edge of the strip over the rim of the container you are collecting the urine in to get rid of excess urine.

5. Wait the number of seconds specified in the test kit directions, and compare the ketone portion of the test strip with the ketone color chart on the test strip container. (Or the strip may show a + or – symbol.)

6. Remove your gloves and place them in the disposable trash bag. Properly dispose of the trash bag, and perform hand hygiene.

COMPLETION STEPS

1. Determine the resident's preferred position for comfort and ask them if they need anything else.
2. Examine the environment for safety and cleanliness.
3. Secure the call light and any other needed items within reach of the resident.
4. Perform hand hygiene.
5. Document the procedure and report any findings to the staff in charge.

10-12: Testing a Stool Specimen for Occult Blood

PREPARATION STEPS

1. Check the care plan.
2. Knock, introduce yourself, and address resident by preferred name.
3. Perform hand hygiene.
4. Gather supplies and secure assistance if needed.
5. Explain procedure and ask about resident preferences.
6. Respect privacy and rights at all times.

ITEMS NEEDED

- Bedpan
- Toilet paper
- Specimen collection applicator
- Specimen collection container
- Test kit
- Watch with a second hand or digital timer
- At least two pairs of gloves
- Disposable trash bag

Note that testing is often done with three stools because bleeding may occur only at times (not continuously). Remember — if you contaminate your gloves in any way during the procedure, you must change to a new pair.

1. Put on gloves.

2. After the resident has a bowel movement, use an applicator to obtain a small sample of the fecal material.

3. Put a thin smear of the fecal material on the kit's test slide in the designated area. Some test slides have two sections so you can test smears from two different areas of the stool.

4. After putting the smear on the slide, remove your gloves and perform hand hygiene. Wait three to five minutes.

5. Put on gloves. Put two drops of the developer solution on the back of the slide directly behind the stool sample.

6. Read the results in 60 seconds (or follow the kit directions if the time differs). If any blue or blue-green color appears around the edge of the sample, the test is positive for occult blood.

7. After test results are obtained, dispose of the feces in the toilet or place soiled disposable brief in the trash bag. Clean bedpan per facility protocol.

8. Remove your gloves and place them in the trash bag. Properly dispose of the trash bag, and perform hand hygiene.

COMPLETION STEPS

1. Determine the resident's preferred position for comfort and ask them if they need anything else.
2. Examine the environment for safety and cleanliness.
3. Secure the call light and any other needed items within reach of the resident.
4. Perform hand hygiene.
5. Document the procedure and report any findings to the staff in charge.

Points to Remember

- Observing and reporting changes related to elimination is important in maintaining residents' health.

- You must follow your facility's procedures for proper recording of residents' output.

- It is important to determine a resident's normal elimination pattern so that you can base your care on their needs and recognize when a problem occurs.

- A key part of your job is maintaining residents' dignity when you assist with elimination by providing as much privacy as possible, treating residents with respect, and maintaining a professional attitude.

- You can support regular elimination by being attentive to residents' needs and ensuring that they get adequate rest and exercise.

- You must learn how to properly use equipment that helps residents with elimination.

- If your duties include the collection of specimens such as urine or stool samples, you must learn the correct procedures and ensure that samples are handled properly before being sent to a lab.

- Some residents may require ostomy care. Follow your facility's procedures for providing this care. The type of assistance you give depends on the resident's level of independence.

Key Terms

bowel or **fecal incontinence** — the inability to control bowel movement, causing leakage from the rectum

constipation — difficulty in emptying the bowels

elimination — process of ridding the body of waste products via urine and stool

functional incontinence — occurs when the bladder doesn't fully empty causing constant or frequent dribbling

incontinence — inability to voluntarily control urination or defecation

Incontinence Associated Dermatitis (IAD) — is a form of dermatitis caused by frequent exposure from urine and/or stool

ketones — substances made when the body breaks down fat for energy

mixed incontinence — is a combination of stress and urge incontinence

occult — hidden; not able to be seen

ostomy — surgical procedure that creates an opening from the intestine to outside the body for the discharge of wastes

overflow incontinence — occurs when the bladder doesn't fully empty causing constant or frequent dribbling

parasite — organism that lives in or on another organism

specimen — sample of fluid or tissue taken for examination and/or testing

stoma — surgically created opening that is kept open for drainage or the removal of waste

stool — feces; solid waste from the bowel

stress incontinence — occurs when pressure is put on the bladder like coughing, sneezing, laughing, lifting or exercising

urge incontinence — is a sudden strong urge to urinate, followed by urinary leakage

urinalysis — physical, chemical, and microscopic examination of a urine sample

urinary incontinence — condition in which a person cannot voluntarily control urination

urine — liquid waste produced by the kidneys and stored in the bladder

void — to empty the bladder; urinate

1. **Ketone testing is often used for residents with:**
   a. Diabetes
   b. Constipation
   c. An infection
   d. Alzheimer's disease

2. **After you collect a urine specimen, you should:**
   a. Leave it on the bedside table
   b. Label the specimen container promptly and accurately
   c. Take it to the medication room and leave it on the counter
   d. Place it in the refrigerator where food items are stored

3. **Why is it important to learn a resident's normal elimination pattern?**
   a. It enables you to recognize when a problem occurs or illness changes their pattern
   b. It is not necessary to learn each residents' elimination pattern
   c. It lets you know when they are hungry
   d. It enables you to know when they will need help from activities

4. **When a resident cannot physically go into the bathroom, what other methods may be used?**
   a. Using a bedpan, urinal or bedside/portable commode
   b. Always put briefs on a resident that cannot get to the bathroom
   c. Let the resident know that they can only go to the bathroom during therapy
   d. Let the nurse know so a catheter can be ordered

5. **Which toileting program is used to restore bladder function?**
   a. Habit training
   b. Prompting voiding
   c. Bladder Retraining
   d. Check and change

6. **What type of incontinence occurs when a resident has bladder leakage when they laugh or sneeze?**
   a. Stress incontinence
   b. Urge incontinence
   c. Fecal incontinence
   d. Mixed incontinence

7. **What is one important factor that a nurse assistant can do to prevent incontinence associated dermatitis?**
   a. Only change disposable incontinent care products once a shift
   b. Provide perineal care only with A.M. care
   c. Provide perineal care after each incontinent episode
   d. Toilet the resident every hour, even during the night

8. **When measuring output the nurse assistant should make sure to:**
   a. Estimate the urine from the bedpan
   b. Measure the container at eye level
   c. Always transfer the urine from a graduate to a bedpan to accurately measure output
   d. Record output once a week

9. **When providing catheter care, all of the following should be completed EXCEPT:**
   a. Check tubing for kinks and any signs of leakage
   b. Clean the catheter tubing from the urethral opening downward
   c. Use a clean area of the washcloth for each downward stroke
   d. Clean the catheter tubing from the drainage bag toward the urethral opening

10. **How can a nurse assistant support regular elimination?**
    a. Be attentive to the resident's needs
    b. Ensure that the resident is getting adequate sleep
    c. Ensure that the resident is getting adequate rest and exercise
    d. All of the above

11

Aging and Chronic Disease Management

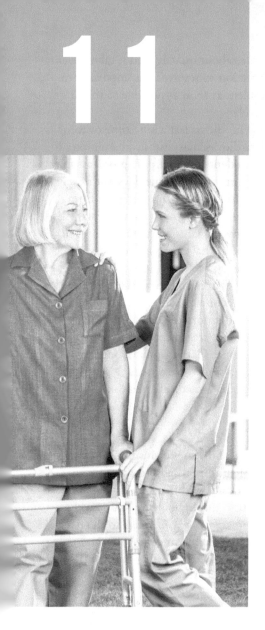

To provide quality care, you must understand changes that residents experience. Some changes may be part of normal aging, but others may indicate serious illness. You must learn to recognize what is normal and abnormal for each resident and know which signs point to a problem that should be reported.

In this chapter, you will learn about each body system, including its structure (anatomy) and its functions (physiology). We will also discuss the changes that happen with aging. You will learn to recognize signs of abnormal changes in residents and also become familiar with common illnesses and problems that affect various body systems. The observations you report to the charge nurse can significantly improve the quality of a resident's care.

OBJECTIVES:

- List the body systems and name and describe the major structures and functions of each system.

- Provide examples of age-related changes in each body system.

- Differentiate between acute and chronic conditions.

- Explain the importance of early detection of cancer.

- Explain how the body responds to infection.

- Provide at least five examples of information and observations that should be reported to the charge nurse.

- Name and describe common diseases and conditions that affect each body system, along with their associated signs and symptoms.

- Describe the nurse assistant's role in observation and care of residents with these diseases and conditions.

Body Systems

A group of organs and structures that work together to perform certain vital functions are known as a **body system**. The body systems all work together to support life. Each individual organ and system must function properly, and the body systems must work together to ensure health. The systems of the human body are:

- Integumentary system (skin)
- Musculoskeletal system
- Respiratory system
- Circulatory system (heart, blood vessels, and lymphatic tissues and vessels)
- Digestive system
- Urinary system
- Nervous system (and special senses)
- Endocrine system (glands)
- Reproductive system

There is no one pattern of aging for everyone, and different body systems age in different ways. Aging causes general changes that happen gradually over time. These changes include reduced functioning of the body systems.

Residents and the Aging Process

Aging is the process of growing older. Aging begins at birth, and it is a natural process that we all experience. Many factors influence aging. Our family history and lifestyle choices affect how we will age.

Some people try not to think about aging because they are afraid of growing old. People have differing ideas and fears about aging. By asking questions of residents, you can better understand the psychological effects of aging on each person in your care. You can learn if certain health conditions make their daily life more difficult or make them more fearful of particular activities. An important part of your job is observing and reporting any abnormal signs and symptoms they may have.

In this chapter, you will learn about the signs and symptoms of common illnesses, diseases, and conditions. You must carefully observe all signs and symptoms and report any changes to the charge nurse.

Acute Versus Chronic Problems

Acute health problems are those that develop rapidly or suddenly. An acute problem usually lasts for a limited period of time. The common cold, for example, is an acute problem. It comes about quickly, and it takes seven to 10 days for the infection to resolve. It is important to identify an acute problem as soon as possible so that it can be treated effectively.

In contrast, **chronic** problems last a long time or recur often. Diabetes and cardiovascular disease are examples of chronic conditions. Residents with chronic problems may experience signs and symptoms on some days but not on others. Some residents live with constant pain from chronic illness or disease. Chronic back pain and arthritis are two problems that involve constant pain.

Many chronic conditions have both acute and chronic phases. A chronic condition can also affect an acute problem. At times, a chronic condition can worsen and need medical treatment. This is one reason you must monitor residents and identify and report any changes. When you report accurate information, treatment can be started before a problem gets worse. Cancer is an example of a chronic disease that can also involve acute episodes where symptoms require immediate medical attention.

Cancer

Cancer describes a group of diseases characterized by the uncontrolled growth of abnormal cells. **Malignant** (cancerous) cells can grow locally, within a specific organ or tissue, and can also spread throughout the body via the blood and lymph systems. *Primary site* refers to the first organ or body system affected by cancer, and *metastasis* refers to the spread of cancer cells to other parts of the body.

There are some warning signs for cancer, but these signs do not automatically mean that a resident has cancer. They are observations that need to be reported to the charge nurse. Cancer warning signs include:

- Fever
- Fatigue
- Pain
- Weight loss
- Skin changes, such as a sore that does not heal or changes in a wart or mole (Figure 11-1)
- Change in bowel or bladder habits
- Unusual bleeding or discharge from a body opening
- Lump or thickening in the breast or elsewhere on the body
- Difficulty swallowing
- Digestive problems
- Nagging cough or hoarseness

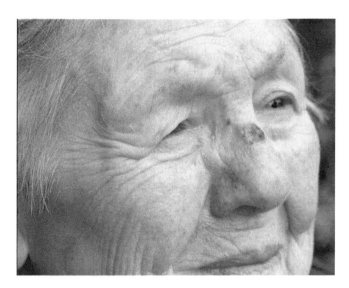

Figure 11-1 A sore that does not heal can be a warning sign of skin cancer.

Because cancer can spread rapidly, early detection is important so treatment can begin as soon as possible. Cancer treatments include surgery, radiation, chemotherapy, or a combination of these methods. Dietary changes and stress management techniques may also be part of the recommended treatment. Surgery may be performed to remove an organ, part of an organ, or tissues that are cancerous. Some surrounding tissue may also be removed. Radiation therapy uses high-energy radiation or radioactive material to destroy cancer cells. Chemotherapy involves the use of drugs to kill cancer cells or stop cell division.

Unfortunately, radiation therapy and chemotherapy kill not only cancer cells but some normal cells, as well. Residents receiving these treatments may experience nausea, vomiting, and hair loss, and they have a higher risk for bleeding and infection. A resident undergoing cancer treatment may tell you that they felt better before they started the treatment. Listen to their concerns and help them through the challenges of their treatment program. The charge nurse can provide you with special care measures for these patients based on their physician orders and type of treatment.

Infection

An infection can begin in one place in the body and spread to other areas or systemically. The body's immune system responds to an infection in multiple ways. The response depends on the type of microorganism causing the infection and its severity. The immune system weakens as we age, so the older adult may have a harder time fighting infections. The three general types of responses are localized, whole-body, and silent responses.

Inflammation

Inflammation is a localized response to injury or the destruction of tissue. Signs of inflammation are heat, redness, swelling, pain, and loss of function. Some of these signs may be observed by looking carefully at a resident's skin. Localized responses are limited to a specific site of infection, such as a wound or the site of damaged tissue. A localized response may also include drainage of fluid or pus.

Whole-Body Responses

Whole body (systemic) responses affect the entire body. Body temperature rises due to fever. In older people, fever is usually not as high as occurs in children and younger adults. A temperature slightly over 100°F in an 80-year-old resident may be as serious as a temperature of 102°F in a small child. A resident's change in temperature should be reported to the charge nurse as soon as it occurs.

Signs and Symptoms of Infection

In addition to inflammation and fever, other signs and symptoms include respiratory distress, pain, cough, sputum production, and sometimes a change in mental status. When a resident doesn't feel well, has a fever, and exhibits a change in behavior such as lethargy, unusual irritability or agitation, or increased confusion, these may be signs that they are developing an infection.

Signs of infection are not as clear in older adults as they are in younger people. Also, a resident with cognitive impairment may not be able to tell you when they experience symptoms. You should be alert when providing daily care and look for signs that indicate change. Signs may include drainage from a wound, dark urine or a strong urine odor, and thick, greenish sputum. Remember that even a small change, such as a change in skin coloration, mood, or activity level, can be an important clue that something may be wrong. You know when a resident looks, acts, or sounds different than usual. You must report your observations to the charge nurse so that action can be taken, if needed.

Latent Infections

A latent infection is one that is hidden or dormant in the body. In these cases, the infection is present but causes no symptoms. It may only be discovered through lab tests.

Some microorganisms, such as the varicella-zoster virus that causes chickenpox during childhood, can remain in the body silently for many years. As some people age and their immune system weakens, the varicella virus "wakes up" and causes a painful skin rash known as shingles.

Integumentary System

The integumentary system consists of the skin and accessory structures. The condition of the skin often reflects a person's overall health status. Maintaining intact, healthy skin is a major goal of care in all health care settings. The skin is the largest organ of the human body that protects internal organs and prevents loss of too much water. The skin is the first line of defense against infection. Bacteria normally live on the skin surface. Once this protective skin layer is broken, bacteria and other disease-causing pathogens can enter the body. A skin infection or other type of infection may result.

One of the biggest challenges and goals in providing care for residents is to prevent wounds and the formation of pressure injuries. Pressure injuries are a source of much pain and suffering for residents, and they take time to heal. Treatment for pressure injuries is complex. All members of the interdisciplinary team must do everything they can to help prevent pressure injuries.

Structures

As shown in Figure 11-2, the skin has two main layers. The epidermis is the top layer that you can see and feel. The dermis is the thicker layer beneath the epidermis. Beneath these two layers is a cushion of subcutaneous tissue called the hypodermis. This cushion of fatty tissue helps the skin look smooth.

Five structures within the skin and subcutaneous tissue have specific protective functions:

- Sebaceous glands (oil glands) help keep the skin moist.
- *Sweat glands* help the body get rid of heat and waste products.
- *Hair roots and hair on parts of the body* help protect the skin.
- *Melanocytes* are cells containing pigment (melanin) that provides color to the skin and protection from the ultraviolet rays of the sun.
- *Blood vessels* nourish the skin and help control body temperature.

The hair, fingernails, and toenails are outgrowths of the skin, and mucous membranes line the inside of the nose, mouth, and other body structures.

Functions

The skin protects the body in two very important ways. It prevents microorganisms (germs) in the environment from entering the body. This is the first line of defense against infection. The skin also helps control body temperature. We sweat when we are hot, and the blood vessels in the skin dilate (expand) to let heat out. When it is cold, blood vessels constrict (narrow) to keep heat in.

Age-Related Changes

The skin often shows signs of aging sooner than other body systems. This is especially true in people who have had long-term exposure to sun, wind, cold air, and drying soaps. Table 11-1 lists common changes that occur in the skin and hair as a person ages.

Table 11-1   Changes in the Integumentary System with Aging

Change	Result
Inability of skin to retain moisture	- Dryness of skin and hair
Thinning of the dermis layer of the skin	- Wrinkling of the skin
Decreased elasticity of the skin	- Sagging skin
Shrinkage of the hypodermis layer of skin, due to loss of fatty tissue	- Difficulty adjusting to heat loss, especially on the face and back of hands

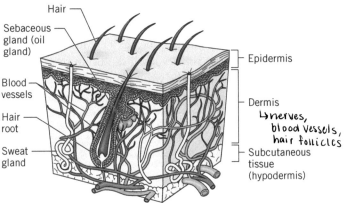

Figure 11-2 Layers and structures of the skin.

Change	Result
Decreased production of melanin in hair bulbs	▪ Graying hair
Decrease in rate of growth of hair follicles	▪ Thinning hair
Thinning of the epidermis	▪ Skin tears

Preventing Skin Problems

You should report immediately the slightest change in a resident's skin. Table 11-2 lists signs and symptoms you must look out for. Your role in caring for the resident's skin includes specific strategies to prevent skin breakdown. The keys to maintaining skin integrity involve promoting circulation and movement, keeping the resident clean, and ensuring that the resident has good nutrition and adequate fluid intake. Guidelines for preventing skin problems are shown in Table 11-3.

Table 11-2   Integumentary System Signs, Symptoms, and Observations

Signs and Symptoms	Related Observations to Report
Change in color or size of any skin growth such as a mole, freckle, wart, etc.	▪ What does the resident's skin normally look like? ▪ Is it different now? ▪ Is a growth new or has it always been there? ▪ Has a growth changed?
Bleeding or open sores	▪ What does the resident's skin normally look like? ▪ Is it different now?
Rash (red bumps on skin) or reddened areas	▪ Does the resident have a history of allergies or sensitivities? ▪ Has the resident made a change such as wearing new clothing or using new products? For example, trying a new lotion that may have caused a rash? ▪ Does the reddened area go away when you change the resident's position? ▪ Is the resident concerned about the appearance of their skin? ▪ Has the resident's personal hygiene habits changed?

Signs and Symptoms	Related Observations to Report
Flaking skin, rough skin, or other change in skin texture	▪ What has the weather been like? ▪ Is the resident's skin dry and flaky due to a change in weather? ▪ Is the resident concerned about the appearance of their skin? ▪ Has the resident's personal hygiene habits changed?
Cuts or bruises	▪ What does the resident's skin normally look like? ▪ Is it different now?
Swollen areas	▪ What does the resident's skin normally look like? ▪ Is it different now? ▪ Does the resident have a history of allergies or sensitivities?
Complaints of itching or pain	▪ Does the resident have a history of allergies or sensitivities?
Very hot skin or cold, damp skin	▪ Has the resident been ill recently? ▪ Does the resident have a fever?

Table 11-3   Strategies to Prevent Skin Problems

Preventive Strategies	Nurse Assistant's Role
Mobility	▪ Help the resident walk. Walking increases the circulation of blood to the skin, supplying nourishment the skin needs to be healthy. If a resident cannot walk, frequent changes in position are needed to relieve pressure and keep blood flowing to all areas of the body. ▪ Never slide the resident across the bed sheets. Always use available lifting devices.
Nutrition	▪ Ensure that the resident eats enough food. Adequate protein, vitamins, and minerals are needed for healthy skin. Report any change in the resident's weight or how much food they eat. Make sure the resident drinks enough fluid. Adequate fluid intake helps all body systems and keeps the skin moist.
Observation	▪ Inspect the resident's skin daily, especially if they cannot move or use the toilet independently. ▪ Check under all skin folds daily. Keep the area clean and dry.

Preventive Strategies	Nurse Assistant's Role
Range-of-motion (ROM) exercise	▪ Exercise is important for maintaining strength and muscle tone. It also increases the blood supply to an area.
Toileting	▪ Help the resident with toileting as needed. Monitor them frequently for incontinence. If the resident is incontinent, clean their skin after each episode. Make sure the resident is not left in wet clothes or a soiled incontinent product.
Bathing and moisturizing	▪ Keep the resident's skin clean and dry. Moisturize their skin daily. Use the resident's own products; if they do not usually use such products and you notice their skin is dry, ask the charge nurse what to use.
Reporting	▪ Immediately report any change in the condition of the resident's skin to the nurse.

redden skin that doesn't return to normal color

Common Chronic Diseases and Problems of the Integumentary System

Common problems involving the skin include pressure injuries, dry skin, and contact dermatitis.

Pressure Injuries

Pressure injuries are also called pressure sores, or bedsores. They are a breakdown of the skin caused by pressure, including pressure from rubbing, friction, or shearing. Pressure injuries form when a resident cannot or does not change positions often enough. Pressure over short periods of time decreases the flow of blood to an area of the body. This reduces the nourishment and oxygen the skin receives. Skin cells die, blood vessels break, and an open wound forms.

Pressure injuries occur most often where the skin is thin and you can easily feel bone underneath. Common locations are the elbows, shoulder blades, hips, base of the spine (coccyx or "tailbone"), and heels. Other problem areas are the ears, under the breasts, between the buttocks, and other areas experiencing frequent rubbing or friction. Friction and shearing forces occur when skin rubs against an object or another area of skin. Frequent rubbing can damage blood vessels and other tissue, along with skin breakdown. This can also happen when the resident is moved or pulled across the bed, such as during positioning.

Moisture is another factor that can contribute to skin breakdown. Moisture can build up in areas such as under the breasts, between the buttocks, or in the groin area if a resident is incontinent. Prolonged moisture can cause the skin to weaken. A resident who is incontinent is at greater risk for skin damage.

Your observations and prompt reporting of early pressure injuries signs and symptoms can prevent the development of a more serious ulcer. Signs and symptoms include:

▪ Any reddened area of the body that does not return to its original color after repositioning — the area may look bruised

▪ Blistering or breakdown of skin

▪ Increased sensitivity or pain

▪ Change in skin temperature

Preventing pressure injuries is one of the most important parts of your job. Your primary role in treatment is to report information to the nurse. Even when an ulcer first looks "healed," the skin area is still damaged and can become an ulcer again. Be sure to use the strategies outlined in Table 11-3 to prevent pressure injuries and other skin problems. These strategies are particularly important for residents at risk, but you should monitor the condition of all residents' skin on a daily basis. If the resident is at risk, inspect their skin at least every two hours and whenever providing personal care.

The following guidelines are important for prevention, treatment, and healing of pressure injuries.

To promote circulation:

▪ Change the resident's position and inspect bony skin areas at least every two hours.

▪ Perform passive ROM exercises as directed in the resident's care plan.

▪ Assist the resident with walking as appropriate.

To relieve pressure:

▪ Use a pressure-reducing device, such as an air mattress, circulating air mattress, or a mattress containing water or gel. These special mattresses help distribute the resident's weight evenly to reduce pressure on certain areas.

▪ For residents on bed rest, use devices that completely relieve pressure on their heels. This can be done by raising their heels off the bed.

▪ Inspect the heels when repositioning the resident and during bathing.

- Minimize skin-to-skin contact by using positioning devices like pillows between the resident's knees or under their elbows and forearms.
- Be sure that residents wear socks or stockings with shoes. Check the heels and toes to be sure that shoes fit properly and do not rub.

To prevent injury:
- Keep the resident's skin clean and dry.
- Prevent friction on the skin. For example, lift the resident in bed from underneath instead of pulling them up. Use padding on wheelchair arms and legs.
- Keep the bed clean and free of objects like crumbs, combs, and glasses, and keep the bedding free of wrinkles.
- Use cornstarch on the bedpan or commode seat to prevent the resident's skin from sticking.
- Keep skinfold areas clean and dry.
- Keep the head of the bed lower than 30 degrees, if possible. This prevents the resident from sliding down, which can cause friction.

To promote proper nutrition:
- Closely monitor the resident's fluid and food intake. Encourage good nutrition and drinking enough fluids.
- Offer snacks or nutritional supplements between meals as ordered. Notify the nurse if the resident has poor food or fluid intake.
- Weigh the resident often and report any change immediately.

Specific treatments are used to promote healing of pressure injuries. The health care team will use different treatments in each stage, but you must always continue the preventive strategies. Your primary role is to prevent and observe pressure injuries and report any skin changes right away.

An interdisciplinary team (led by a physician) may examine the pressure injury and assesses the need for any treatment change each week. The nurse usually performs treatments and assesses the area to help the physician decide if the treatment is working. You may be asked to help the nurse with positioning the resident or gathering supplies. Various treatments are used depending on the stage of the ulcer. Box 11-1 outlines treatment of pressure injuries during each stage.

Dry Skin

With aging and weather changes, skin dryness is a common problem. Dryness may also result from other factors such as irritating clothing fabrics or rough sheets or linens. Dry skin is annoying but can usually be handled easily.

Signs and Symptoms
- Flaky or reddened areas
- Complaints of itchiness
- Scratching

Nurse Assistant's Role in Observation and Intervention
- Pay attention to a resident's skin when giving care. You may find reddened areas, or the resident may tell you their skin feels itchy. The skin may itch more at night.
- Inspect the skin for flaking, redness, or scratch marks. These can be signs of a problem.
- Always report signs and symptoms to the charge nurse.
- Keep the resident's skin well lubricated (moisturized).

Goals of Care
- Eliminate dryness and itchiness of the skin.
- Help the resident feel more comfortable.
- Prevent problems such as skin damage caused by scratching.

Interventions or Skills for Care
- Limit the amount of soap used on the skin.
- Use a moisturizing cream on the affected area. Massage the cream gently into the skin to enhance absorption. Let residents choose the cream they want used. If the resident does not have a preference, any moisturizing cream will work.
- Add bath oil to the bath if the resident prefers and the charge nurse says you may.
- Use a therapeutic bath solution if ordered by the physician.
- Encourage the resident to drink more fluids, especially water (unless they are on fluid restrictions).
- Keep the resident's nails trimmed and clean.

Contact Dermatitis

Contact dermatitis is a skin inflammation and/or rash that results from contact with an object or substance that causes irritation or an allergic reaction.

Box 11-1

TREATMENT OF PRESSURE INJURIES

Stage I: Skin intact

- Notify the charge nurse immediately about any change. Ask them to inspect the area.
- Focus on preventing pressure on the area. Use all prevention methods.

Stage II: Partial-thickness skin loss

- May present as an intact or ruptured serum filled blister.
- The nurse cleans the area, and covers it with a dry sterile dressing or a protective dressing.

  Note: The key is prevention. All members of the team are responsible for preventing any skin breakdown.

Stage III: Full-thickness skin loss

- The nurse cleans the area and applies medications and dressings ordered by the physician. The wound may require packing or irrigation. Assist the nurse as asked. Observe and report if the dressing becomes saturated or dislodged.
- Closely watch the resident for infections. Watch for any foul smell, discharge, or redness around the area. Report these findings to the nurse.

Stage IV: Full-thickness skin and tissue loss

- May present with muscle or bone involvement
- The nurse cleans the area and applies medications and dressings as ordered by the physician. The wound may require packing or irrigation. In some instances a "wound vac" (which promotes healing by removing excess drainage from the wound) may be used. Assist the nurse as asked. Observe and report if the dressing becomes saturated or moves, or if the "wound vac" moves.
- Surgery may be needed to remove dead tissue or provide a new top skin layer (a "flap").

Unstageable

- Where there is full-thickness and/or tissue loss but the injury is unable to be staged because the wound bed cannot be clearly seen.
- The nurse cleans the area and applies medications as ordered by the physical. Assist the nurse as asked. Watch the resident for signs of infection and report if the dressing becomes dislodged.

Deep Tissue Pressure Injury

- Persistent non-bleachable discoloration. May present as a blood filled blister.
- Focus on keeping pressure off of the area.

Signs and Symptoms
- Rash (skin lesions that may be red and/or bumpy)
- Complaints of itchiness

Nurse Assistant's Role in Observation and Intervention
- Identify and report to the charge nurse any changes that occurred before the rash developed. For example, residents may react to new clothing or jewelry, a change in laundry detergent or personal care products, or a new food or medication.
- Report any rash to the charge nurse because it may indicate an infection or an allergic reaction.

Goals of Care
- Identify the source of the irritation or allergic reaction.
- Relieve the itchiness.

- Prevent problems such as skin damage caused by scratching.

Interventions or Skills for Care
- Help the charge nurse with the use of topical ointments if the physician recommends. (Most of these ointments contain hydrocortisone to relieve itching.)
- Assist the nurse in covering the area with a dry dressing if the physician orders.
- Use therapeutic bath solutions if the physician orders.

Wound Care

Remember that a wound is a break in the continuity of the skin. Wound healing involves restoring the skin to its intact state. Wounds can be classified by the type of injury to the skin:

- Incision — made by a sharp instrument, such as a surgical scalpel
- Contusion — made by blunt force, causing a break in small blood vessels (bruising) and swelling
- Laceration — made by an object, causing an irregular, jagged wound
- Puncture wound — made by a pointed object
- Lesion or skin breakdown — caused by a disease such as cancer, HIV, or poor circulation

The type of wound determines the type of care needed. Your role may include helping the nurse with dressing changes. You will of course monitor all wounds and report any changes such as signs of infection. If a wound becomes red or swollen, or has a foul smell and discharge, this means infection is likely. You must report this immediately.

To promote wound healing, be sure that the wound is protected from further injury and that the resident has good nutrition and gets enough rest. Different types of dressings are used on wounds (Box 11-2).

Dressings are not used on all wounds. For example, a day after surgery, the wound may be dry and skin edges intact, and a dressing may not be used. Leaving a wound uncovered has two benefits: It allows for easy observation of wound healing and helps prevent conditions that may cause infection, like warmth, darkness, and too much moisture.

Musculoskeletal System

The musculoskeletal system is made up of bones, muscles, tendons, ligaments, and joints. It provides support for the body and allows for movement (Figure 11-3).

Box 11-2

COMMON TYPES OF DRESSINGS

DRY DRESSING

This type of dressing is primarily used for surgical incisions. A dry dressing protects the wound and absorbs drainage.

WET-TO-DRY DRESSING

This type of dressing is rarely used because it pulls away good tissue as well as bad tissue. It is only used for infected wounds or wounds that contain dead or poor tissue. Gauze soaked with a sterile saline or antiseptic solution is first packed into the wound. This is covered by a dry dressing.

WET-TO-WET DRESSINGS

This type of dressing is used on clean open wounds. Sterile saline or antiseptic solution is put on the dressing. This wet dressing is placed on the wound. A moist wound generally heals more naturally.

PROTECTIVE AND ABSORPTIVE DRESSINGS

These dressings protect as well as absorb drainage from a shallow wound. They are changed every two or three days. These are called hydrocolloid dressings and include Duoderm® and Tegasorb® dressings. The dressing provides a moist environment for more natural wound healing.

PROTECTIVE OR 2ND SKIN® DRESSINGS

These dressings cover and protect a superficial wound. Because the dressing is transparent, the nurse can observe how the wound is healing.

The primary purposes of any dressing are to protect the wound and absorb excess drainage.

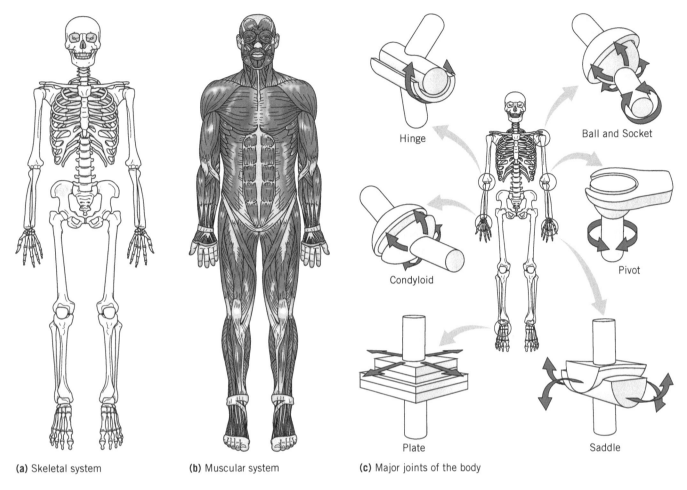

(a) Skeletal system　　　(b) Muscular system　　　(c) Major joints of the body

Figure 11-3　Overview of the musculoskeletal system: (A) bones in the body; (B) muscles in the body; (C) major joints of the body.

Structures and Functions

The musculoskeletal system provides the framework for the body and enables it to move.

- *Bones* are the supporting structure for the body.
- *Muscles* generate movement.
- *Tendons* attach muscles to bones.
- *Ligaments* attach bones to other bones.
- *Joints* are the point at which two or more bones come together and allow for movement.

Age-Related Changes and Important Observations

Table 11-4 lists the changes that occur in the musculo-skeletal system as a person ages, and Table 11-5 lists signs, symptoms and important observations related to musculoskeletal problems.

Table 11-4　Changes in the Musculoskeletal System with Aging

Change	Result
A shortening of the spinal column due to compression of vertebrae and changes in posture	Loss of height
Loss of minerals from bones	Greater risk of broken bones
Loss of muscle mass	Loss of strength
Loss of elasticity	Muscle stiffness

Calcium [handwritten annotation pointing to "Loss of minerals from bones"]

Table 11-5 Musculoskeletal System Signs, Symptoms, and Observations

Signs and Symptoms	Related Observations to Report
Swollen, reddened joints	- Is there a change in the appearance of joints? - Does the resident favor a certain position? - Is the resident's position changed often?
Bumps and/or bruises on arms or legs	- Is there a change in the appearance and/or function of the arms or legs? - Does the resident favor a certain position? - Is the resident's position changed often? - Has the resident bumped into any objects or fallen recently?
Complaints of stiffness or inability to move	- Does the resident favor a certain position? - Is the resident's position changed often? - Does the resident get up and move often enough? - Does the resident have problems moving in the morning or after sitting for a period of time? - Do they need assistance to move? - What can you do to support the resident's ability to move (offer your arm, move things out of the way)?
Complaints of pain	- Does the resident favor one arm or leg over the other? - Do the resident's shoes and assistive devices fit properly? - Has the resident bumped into any objects or fallen recently?

Common Chronic Diseases and Problems of the Musculoskeletal System

Common problems affecting residents include arthritis, osteoporosis, and bone fractures.

Arthritis

Arthritis is the inflammation of a joint that causes pain and often limits movement. The two most common types are osteoarthritis and rheumatoid arthritis. **Osteoarthritis** is more common. It is caused by age and long-term wear and tear on the joint. The cartilage in joints between bones thins and breaks down, resulting in less shock absorbency. Because of this, the body produces bony protuberances (swellings, bumps) at the sides of the joints (Figure 11-4). **Rheumatoid arthritis** is an autoimmune disease that causes inflammation, pain, and deformity of the joints.

Signs and Symptoms
- Stiffness
- Painful joints
- In rheumatoid arthritis, red, swollen joints that feel hot to the touch

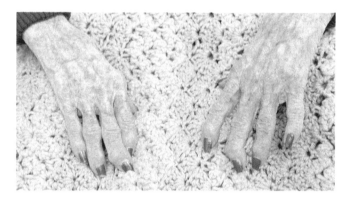

Figure 11-4 Arthritis can cause swollen, disfigured joints.

Nurse Assistant's Role in Observation and Intervention
- Promote the resident's capabilities and encourage them to do whatever they can.
- Plan care around scheduled pain management.
- Encourage independence. Recognize the resident may need more time to complete an activity.
- Help the resident maintain as much mobility as possible. Residents may resist movement due to pain, but it is important for the joints to move as much as possible to prevent problems. When a resident does not use a joint, muscle fibers may shorten (a contracture) and movement is inhibited.
- Encourage the resident to use adaptive equipment.

Goals of Care
- Minimize pain.
- Prevent injury.
- Promote mobility.
- Keep joints movable by providing range-of-motion (ROM) exercises.

Interventions or Skills for Care

When caring for a resident with joint pain, you should:

- Let the resident know you care, understand, and want to help. People in constant pain can feel hopeless and depressed.

- Plan your schedule for care and other activities such as ROM exercises so that residents can receive their pain medication first. Talk to the charge nurse about this.

- Help the resident with ROM exercises. Never move a joint that is very painful, red, or swollen.

- Properly position a resident in bed or a wheelchair. Encourage good posture.

- Help the resident put on splints or braces (if worn).

- Plan your schedule to help the resident back to bed for rest periods as needed. Don't push a person to be active when they are tired because this can damage joints.

- Report any joint problems to the charge nurse.

- Encourage residents to do as much as possible to help maintain their independence.

Osteoporosis

Osteoporosis, also called thinning of the bones, is a loss of bone tissue that most often occurs in older adults. Bones become weak and brittle, increasing the risk for fractures. Often this condition is not diagnosed until a resident is injured. Osteoporosis is most common in women after menopause. Many postmenopausal women have a bone density screening as part of their physical examination.

Calcium supplements and prescription drugs may be used as part of treatment.

Signs and Symptoms
- Loss of height
- Falling
- Bone fractures

Nurse Assistant's Role in Observation and Intervention
- Monitor residents who are frail and/or have a history of falling and previous fractures.

- Anticipate problems when residents move and use safety measures.

- Encourage weight-bearing exercise and activities, as appropriate for each resident.

Goals of Care
- Promote safety.

- Encourage good nutrition and exercise as tolerated.

Interventions or Skills for Care
- Always use assistive devices, such as a gait belt, when moving a resident from bed to chair or chair to bed and when assisting with walking.

- Encourage residents to use a cane or walker as needed for support and stability.

- Be sure the resident has a clear path from the bed or chair to prevent injury from bumping into things.

- If a resident starts to fall when you are with them, support them and guide them to the floor.

- If you find a resident on the floor, call the charge nurse immediately and follow their instructions.

- Encourage residents to eat healthy, balanced meals, especially foods that are rich in calcium, other minerals, and vitamin D (needed for calcium absorption).

Bone Fracture

A **fracture** is a break in a bone or other hard tissue, caused most often by a fall. The most common type of fracture in elderly residents is a fractured hip.

Signs and Symptoms
- Swollen, black and blue area at the break site
- Complaints of pain or altered sensation
- Inability to put weight on a leg or foot or to use an arm or a hand
- Abnormal shape of arm or leg, including possible shortening of the limb

Nurse Assistant's Role in Observation and Intervention
- Report any abnormality you see in a resident's arms, legs, hands, or feet.

- Report any pain.

- Provide a safe environment. Keep the call button within the resident's reach.

- Promote activities that enhance healing and mobility. Follow the recommendations of the nurse and physical therapist.

Goals of Care
- Prevent complications from the fracture, such as muscle weakness and joint abnormalities.

- Help the resident regain their former level of mobility (before the fracture).

Interventions or Skills for Care

- Support a resident going to physical or occupational therapy and assist with mobility according to their care plan (such as using a walker).

- Do ROM exercises (per the care plan) to keep joints and muscles moving.

- Use proper transfer techniques to avoid further injury at the fracture site.

- Encourage the resident's independence to the degree possible.

- Help with toileting, if necessary.

- Encourage and assist the resident in dressing in comfortable clothing.

- Recognize that a resident may fear falling again and may avoid certain activities. Be supportive and offer help until the person feels secure.

- Follow the instructions of the charge nurse and physical therapist in positioning the resident properly in bed and in a chair. Improper positioning can slow the healing of a fracture.

Respiratory System

The body needs a continuous supply of oxygen to survive. The respiratory system works to supply oxygen to the blood and remove waste products.

Structures

- The main structures of the respiratory system include the nasal cavity, oral cavity, the air passages, and the lungs (Figure 11-5):

- The pharynx (commonly called the throat) has several sections: the nasopharynx (nasal passage), oropharynx (mouth and oral passage), and the laryngopharynx, which opens into the larynx (voice box) and esophagus.

- The *trachea* (windpipe) descends from the larynx and connects to the bronchi.

- The right and left bronchi enter the lungs, and bronchioles branch from each bronchus.

- The two *lungs* are large, lobed organs.

- Alveoli are small air sacs within the lungs.

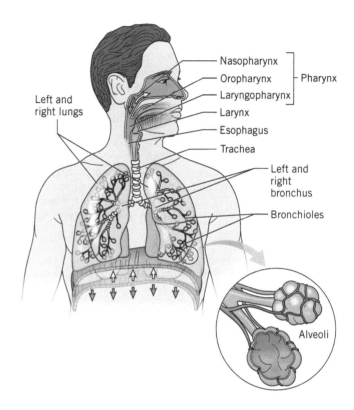

Figure 11-5 Structures of the respiratory system.

Functions

Respiration (breathing) is the process of gas exchange between the atmosphere and body cells. We inhale (breathe in) oxygen and exhale (breathe out) carbon dioxide. This is one of the most basic and important body functions.

The respiratory system takes in air containing oxygen through the nose or mouth. The oxygen passes through the bronchi and bronchioles, into the alveoli and then into small blood vessels. The heart and lungs work together to supply oxygenated blood to all body parts.

The process works in reverse to expel carbon dioxide from the body. The air we breathe out contains carbon dioxide that has been removed from the blood.

Age-Related Changes and Important Observations

Table 11-6 lists changes that occur in the respiratory system as a person ages, and Table 11-7 lists signs, symptoms and important observations related to respiratory problems.

Table 11-6 Changes in the Respiratory System with Aging

Change	Result
The chest wall and lung structures become more rigid. Respiratory muscle strength decreases.	There is not as much room for air in the lungs, and it is more difficult to take deep breaths.
A decreased amount of air is exchanged with each breath.	During exercise, illness, or stress, a person has to breathe faster to get enough oxygen in and carbon dioxide out.

Table 11-7 Respiratory System Signs, Symptoms, and Observations

Signs and Symptoms	Related Observations to Report
Cyanosis (bluish coloration of skin)	■ What do the resident's lips, nail beds, and skin usually look like? ■ Are they different now?
Gasping, shortness of breath, or labored breathing	■ Has the resident's breathing changed? ■ Does the resident take frequent rest periods?
Rattling or gurgling breathing sounds	■ Does the resident's breathing sound strange?
Abnormally fast or slow chest movements	■ Has the resident's breathing changed?
Needing to sit up to breathe	■ Is the resident sitting upright? Is it difficult for the resident to lie flat?
Pain with breathing	■ Does the resident complain of shortness of breath, difficulty breathing, or decreased ability to do normal tasks?
Very hot or very cold skin or excess sweating	■ What do the resident's lips, nail beds, and skin usually look like? ■ Are they different now?
Foul-smelling breath, unusual color sputum (respiratory tract secretions), or funny taste in the mouth	■ Does the resident have foul-smelling breath? ■ Has the resident coughed up unusual sputum?

Common Chronic Diseases and Problems of the Respiratory System

People who live in residential facilities are at risk for respiratory infections because of the close living quarters and contact with staff and other residents. Common infections include colds, influenza (flu), and pneumonia. Some residents may have chronic obstructive pulmonary disease (COPD).

Colds and Influenza

The common cold is an upper respiratory infection caused by a virus. Influenza (flu) is a highly contagious and more serious infection that causes more symptoms. A resident with the flu will typically have cold-like symptoms along with fever, body aches, and headache. An annual flu vaccine is available, and it may be given to most residents.

Cold Signs and Symptoms
- Runny nose
- Nasal congestion
- Facial pain or a sense of fullness or pressure
- Cough and/or sore throat
- Watery eyes

Flu Signs and Symptoms
In addition to the cold symptoms listed above, the flu may also result in:
- Aching muscles and joints
- Fever
- Headache
- Weakness and fatigue

Nurse Assistant's Role in Observation and Intervention
- Report symptoms early to prevent further illness.
- Provide care to relieve symptoms.
- Practice infection control procedures, especially proper handwashing, to keep the infection from spreading to other residents and yourself.

Goals of Care
- Help the resident to be comfortable and monitor their symptoms.
- Prevent the spread of infection with proper handwashing and other infection control measures.

Interventions or Skills for Care

- Wash your hands before and after contact with a resident.
- Observe symptoms and report even a small change to the charge nurse.
- Encourage the resident to drink plenty of fluids (unless they are on fluid restrictions) and to get plenty of rest.
- Encourage the resident to get out of bed for short periods. If they cannot get out of bed, be sure they change position often. Keep the head of the bed elevated to prevent or reduce respiratory distress (Figure 11-6).
- Remind the resident to breathe deeply and cough often to prevent mucous secretions from building up in the lungs.
- Keep tissues handy. Use gloves when handling tissues containing secretions, and dispose of tissues properly.
- Provide comfort by fluffing pillows, giving back rubs, etc.
- Measure the resident's vital signs as directed and report any changes.

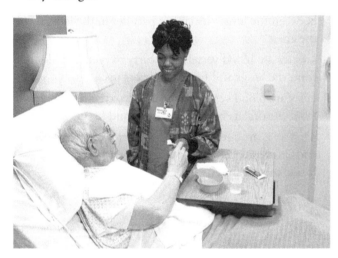

Figure 11-6 Keeping the head of the bed elevated can prevent or reduce a resident's respiratory distress.

Pneumonia

Pneumonia is a lung infection caused by a virus or bacteria. It may follow a cold or bronchitis (infection of the bronchial tubes).

Signs and Symptoms

- Difficulty breathing and/or shortness of breath
- Complaint of painful breathing
- Cough, sometimes with increased sputum
- Elevated temperature

- Lethargy or weakness

Nurse Assistant's Role in Observation and Intervention

- Report symptoms to the charge nurse.
- Give care to relieve symptoms and provide comfort.

Goals of Care

- Keep the resident comfortable and encourage rest.
- Relieve symptoms.

Interventions or Skills for Care

- Perform hand hygiene before and after contact with a resident.
- Observe symptoms and report even a small change to the charge nurse.
- Encourage the resident to drink plenty of fluids (unless they are on fluid restrictions) and to get plenty of rest.
- Encourage good nutrition to aid in the healing process.
- Encourage the resident to get out of bed for short periods. If they cannot get out of bed, be sure they change position often. Keep the head of the bed elevated to prevent or reduce respiratory distress.
- Remind the resident to breathe deeply and cough often. This helps prevent mucous secretions from building up in the lungs.
- Keep tissues handy. Use gloves when handling tissues containing secretions and dispose of tissues in proper receptacles.
- Provide comfort by fluffing pillows, giving back rubs, etc.
- Monitor the resident's vital signs as directed and report any changes.

Chronic Obstructive Pulmonary Disease

Chronic obstructive pulmonary disease (COPD) is the term used to describe a group of chronic inflammatory diseases that affect the bronchial passageways and lungs, obstructing air flow. Chronic bronchitis, emphysema, and some forms of asthma are types of COPD. These diseases cause a chronic inflammation that narrows the bronchioles and alveoli. This narrowing results in a loss of lung elasticity.

Signs and Symptoms

- Difficulty breathing and/or shortness of breath
- Wheezing
- Coughing
- Increased sputum production

- Cyanosis (bluish tone to the skin)
- Activity intolerance

Nurse Assistant's Role in Observation and Intervention

- Maintain adequate respiration.
- Monitor the resident for secondary conditions such as infection.
- Reduce the resident's anxiety.

Goals of Care

- Keep the resident breathing comfortably.

Interventions or Skills for Care

- If the resident is able, encourage them to take four or five deep breaths in and out several times during the day. Deep breathing helps fill the lungs with air and helps the chest wall stay flexible.
- Encourage the resident to rest between meals, bathing, exercise, and social activities.
- Encourage the resident to breathe slowly and deeply while walking, and to rest often for a minute during longer walks.
- When the resident is seated, ask them to lean forward and cross their arms in front to make breathing easier.
- Watch for any change in a resident's ability to perform the activities of daily living. Report even a small change to the charge nurse.
- Monitor the resident's vital signs. Even a small change in temperature, pulse, respiration, or blood pressure may indicate a complication of the disease.

Some residents may need oxygen occasionally or continuously. To care for residents on oxygen, you should:

- Elevate the head of the bed to help the resident breath more easily.
- Check the resident's nasal passages. Oxygen therapy can be very irritating to tissues in the nose. Report redness, bleeding, or discomfort to the charge nurse.
- Do not change the oxygen flow-rate setting. Only the nurse may do this. Too much oxygen can depress the respiratory centers of the brain and be life-threatening.
- Never allow smoking or flames near oxygen. Make sure that "No Smoking, Oxygen in Use" signs are posted.
- Check the tubing and connection to prevent twists.

Sputum Specimens

Sputum is a mixture of saliva and mucus coughed up from the respiratory tract. It may at times also contain purulent (infected) secretions or drainage. Usually, it is thicker than saliva. A sputum specimen is often used to diagnose diseases and conditions of the respiratory system. Procedure 11-1 describes how to collect a sputum specimen.

Circulatory System

The **circulatory system** circulates blood and lymph fluids throughout the body. It consists of the heart, blood vessels, lymphatic vessels and tissues, blood, and lymph. The heart, blood, and blood vessels are also known as the *cardiovascular system*. The lymphatic system plays a role in removing excess fluid and wastes from body tissues and supports the immune system in protecting the body from infection.

Structures

- The *heart* is a muscular organ with four chambers (Figure 11-7). It is located behind the ribs and between the lungs; its largest part lies in the left side of the chest.
- **Arteries** are blood vessels that carry oxygenated blood from the lungs and heart to the organs.
- **Veins** are blood vessels that carry deoxygenated blood from the organs back to the heart and lungs.
- **Capillaries** are tiny blood vessels that connect arteries and veins and exchange oxygen for carbon dioxide inside the organs.

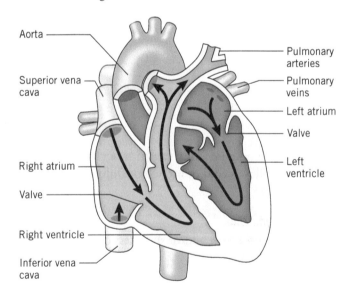

Figure 11-7 Structures of the heart.

11-1: Collecting a Sputum Specimen

PREPARATION STEPS

1. Check the care plan.
2. Knock, introduce yourself, and address resident by preferred name.
3. Perform hand hygiene.
4. Gather supplies and secure assistance if needed.
5. Explain procedure and ask about resident preferences. Respect privacy and rights at all times.

ITEMS NEEDED

- Specimen container and label
- Gloves
- Biohazardous bag or specimen bag

Make sure that a resident who chews tobacco has not done so before you collect the specimen. If the resident has just eaten, ask them to rinse out their mouth. Try to collect the specimen in the morning. Often, large amounts of sputum are coughed up first thing in the morning.

1. Put on gloves. Give the resident the sputum collection container or hold it yourself. Take care not to touch its inside surface.

2. Ask the resident to take several deep breaths and cough deeply from the chest. They may need to cough several times to get enough sputum for the sample. Ask them to try not to spit only saliva into the container.

3. Place the lid securely on the specimen container. Label it with the resident's name, room number, and the date and time of collection. Place the specimen in a biohazardous bag. Remove gloves and perform hand hygiene.

4. Report the color, amount, and consistency of the specimen to the charge nurse.

COMPLETION STEPS

1. Determine the resident's preferred position for comfort and ask them if they need anything else.
2. Examine the environment for safety and cleanliness.
3. Secure the call light and any other needed items within reach of the resident.
4. Perform hand hygiene.
5. Document the procedure and report any findings to the staff in charge.

Functions

The heart pumps blood through the blood vessels to every part of the body. Every time you count a resident's pulse, you are counting how fast the heart pumps blood through the body. The blood vessels carry oxygen from the lungs and other vital nourishment to all the cells of the body. Waste products are also transported to certain organs so the body can get rid of them.

Deoxygenated blood (oxygen has been used by the organs) flows to the right atrium of the heart. The blood passes through an opening (valve) into the right ventricle. The right ventricle pumps it through blood vessels to the lungs, where the blood is oxygenated. Then the blood returns to the left atrium. The blood passes through a valve into the left ventricle, which pumps it out of the heart into the largest blood vessel, the *aorta*. The aorta branches off to the upper and lower parts of the body and connects with smaller blood vessels that carry oxygenated blood to every organ and cell in the body.

Age-Related Changes and Important Observations

Table 11-8 lists changes that occur in the circulatory system as a person ages, and Table 11-9 lists signs, symptoms and important observations related to cardiovascular problems.

Table 11-8   Changes in the Circulatory System with Aging

Change	Result
The heart muscle wall thickens, becomes stiffer, and may increase in size.	The heart has to work harder to pump the same amount of blood.
	The heart can become overworked during strenuous activity, forcing an older person to take more frequent rest periods.

Change	Result
The blood vessels become more rigid and stiff.	The heart has to work harder to pump blood through rigid vessels; blood pressure is higher.
Sensors that regulate blood pressure with position changes are less sensitive.	Dizziness occurs when changing position.
The heart rate decreases.	May cause no symptoms. If the heart rate becomes too low, dizziness may result.

Table 11-9 Circulatory System Signs, Symptoms, and Observations

Signs and Symptoms	Related Observations to Report
Swollen extremities due to edema	■ Are the resident's feet or ankles puffy or swollen? ■ In a bedridden resident, is the area around the sacrum (bone at the base of the spine) swollen?
Shortness of breath, especially with exertion	■ Is the resident suddenly unable to do things they could do before (such as walk to the dining room or climb stairs)?
Fast, slow, or irregular pulse	■ Is the resident's heart rate normal or abnormal?
Increased or decreased blood pressure	■ Is the resident's blood pressure normal or abnormal? ■ Does the resident complain of dizziness?
Cold, damp skin	■ What does the resident's skin normally look and feel like? ■ Is it different now?
Feet have pale color	■ What does the resident's skin normally look like? ■ Is it different now?
Weight gain or loss	■ Has the resident suddenly gained or lost weight?
Complaints of chest pain, indigestion, fatigue, headache, dizziness, vision problems, difficulty swallowing, or weakness or paralysis of a limb or one side of the body	■ Does the resident have pain while not moving or while engaged in activity? ■ When did these symptoms occur? Are they ongoing?
Face drooping, slurred speech, or difficulty speaking	■ When did these symptoms occur? Are they ongoing?

Signs and Symptoms	Related Observations to Report
Loss of balance or coordination or difficulty walking	■ When did these symptoms occur? Are they ongoing?
Change in mental status such as confusion or inability to understand speech	■ When did these symptoms occur? Are they ongoing?

Common Chronic Diseases and Problems of the Circulatory System

Diseases of the cardiovascular system include congestive heart failure, peripheral vascular disease, and coronary artery disease. A cerebral vascular accident (stroke) is a serious and life-threatening condition that requires immediate medical assistance.

Congestive Heart Failure

Congestive heart failure (CHF) occurs when the heart muscle weakens and blood moves through the body less effectively. CHF is common in people who have had high blood pressure and coronary artery disease for years.

Signs and Symptoms
- Shortness of breath
- Edema (swelling of the legs and ankles due to excess fluid in body tissues)
- Cyanosis
- Noisy respiration
- Complaints of tiring easily

Nurse Assistant's Role in Observation and Intervention
- Identify any changes that suggest the condition is worsening, such as an inability to perform one or more activities of daily living.
- Monitor vital signs as directed by the charge nurse.
- Monitor the resident's weight.
- Follow the resident's dietary restrictions if any have been ordered.

Goals of Care
- Help maintain the resident's level of independence.
- Help maintain the resident's level of cardiac function.
- Help maintain the resident at an appropriate weight.

Interventions or Skills for Care

- Give the resident opportunities to perform their own personal care to the degree possible.
- Encourage the resident to rest frequently.
- Encourage the resident to take deep breaths.
- Weigh the resident as ordered, and report any weight change to the charge nurse.
- Maintain accurate intake and output records.
- Encourage the resident to exercise and walk regularly.
- Make sure the resident's shoes are not too tight.

- For a resident with edema in the lower legs: Have the resident sit with their legs elevated on a footstool or lie in bed with legs stretched out for one to two hours, three times a day. Legs should be elevated higher than the buttocks, and pressure should be off the resident's heels.

Elastic stocking may be used to help with blood flow in the legs, they may be used to help control swelling or to help prevent blood clots. If the doctor has ordered elastic stockings, follow the guidelines in Procedure 11-2 for applying these stockings. Elastic stockings should

PROCEDURE

11-2: Applying Elastic Stockings

PREPARATION STEPS

1. Check the care plan.
2. Knock, introduce yourself, and address resident by preferred name.
3. Perform hand hygiene.
4. Gather supplies and secure assistance if needed.
5. Explain procedure and ask about resident preferences. Respect privacy and rights at all times.

ITEMS NEEDED

- Elastic stockings of correct size and length
- Basin with warm water
- Soap
- Washcloth
- Towel

It is important to use the correct size of support stockings. Stockings should be snug enough to provide support but not too tight or too loose. Check with the charge nurse if you are unsure about the stocking size. **Apply the stockings in the morning before the resident moves their legs off the bed.** *This helps to prevent pooling of fluid in the feet.*

1. Make sure the stockings are clean and dry.

2. Help the resident lie on their back.

3. Expose only the person's legs.

4. Observe the person's legs for swelling, moles, cuts, bruising, or other changes in skin color or appearance.

5. Clean and dry the legs and feet before applying elastic stockings.

6. Apply one elastic stocking at a time. Begin by rolling the stocking with your hands so that only the toe section is exposed. Put the stocking on the person's leg, positioning the opening over the top of the toes. Make sure the heel is properly placed. Then roll the stocking up the leg as far as it will go.

7. Repeat the process on the other leg. The stockings should fit firmly and have no wrinkles.

8. Check for good circulation and movement by observing the person's toes for color and ability to move freely.

9. Make sure the resident knows not to roll the stockings down. Doing so can greatly reduce circulation in the legs.

10. Ask the resident to call you if they become uncomfortable.

COMPLETION STEPS

1. Determine the resident's preferred position for comfort and ask them if they need anything else.
2. Examine the environment for safety and cleanliness.
3. Secure the call light and any other needed items within reach of the resident.
4. Perform hand hygiene.
5. Document the procedure and report any findings to the staff in charge.

be applied before the resident gets out of bed in the morning.

Check the resident's toes every hour to ensure that they are warm and a normal color. Check the stockings to make sure there are no wrinkles. Remove elastic stockings at least twice a day for 30 minutes or according to the care plan and/or instructions from the charge nurse. Removing the stockings lets you observe the skin and allows the legs to rest (Figure 11-8).

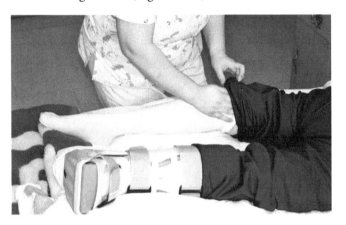

Figure 11-8 Elastic support stockings may be part of the care plan for residents with circulatory problems.

Peripheral Vascular Disease

Peripheral vascular disease (PVD) is a progressive circulatory disorder caused by narrowing or blockage of a blood vessel, resulting in diminished blood flow to the extremities. Tissues in the arms and legs then do not receive enough oxygen-containing blood. This condition most commonly affects the legs and feet. Residents with this condition should avoid:

- Crossing legs at the knees or dangling the feet for an extended time
- Restrictive clothing such as tight garter straps or panty girdles
- Smoking
- Spending time in cold environments, which narrow blood vessels
- Sitting too close to a heat source

Signs and Symptoms

- Paler than normal color in the feet and/or hands
- Complaints of feet and/or hands being cold
- Tingling sensation ("pins and needles") in hands, arms, legs, or feet
- Loss of feeling in hands, arms, legs, or feet

Nurse Assistant's Role in Observation and Intervention

- Identify any changes in a resident's skin.
- Monitor the environment to prevent injury.

Goals of Care

- Promote circulation.
- Prevent injury.
- Maintain skin integrity.

Interventions or Skills for Care

- Inspect the resident's feet.
- Feel the temperature of the resident's skin. If circulation is decreased, the skin feels cool.
- Observe the color of the skin. When circulation is decreased, skin looks bluish or pale in a light-skinned person or dusky gray in a dark-skinned person.
- Observe the color of the nail beds. Poor circulation can cause a bluish tinge to the nail beds. Watch for and report reddened areas, cracked skin between the toes, or skin breakdown.
- Report any changes you observe in any wounds.
- Feel for pulses in the lower extremities: the popliteal pulse behind the knee, the posterior tibial pulse at the ankle, and the pedal pulse on the upper part of the foot. Report the results of these pulse checks to the charge nurse.
- Keep the resident's skin clean, dry, and lubricated (moisturized).
- Keep the resident's room uncluttered.
- Make sure shoes fit properly.
- Maintain a clear path for the resident when walking.
- Check bath water temperature for the resident.
- Encourage the resident to change position every one to two hours while awake. If a resident reads or watches television sitting or lying down, encourage them to get up and walk around for a few minutes every hour or so.
- Encourage the resident to take daily walks and participate in exercise programs to the degree possible.
- Encourage the resident to keep their legs elevated when seated and to wiggle their toes and make circles with the feet to promote circulation.

Coronary Artery Disease

Coronary artery disease (CAD) results from decreased blood flow through the coronary arteries, which nourish the heart. The major blood vessels that supply the heart become damaged or diseased, often due to plaque build-up and/or inflammation. The exact cause of coronary artery disease is not known. A number of factors can contribute to its development, including family history, high blood pressure, high cholesterol, diabetes, a high-fat diet, obesity, smoking, stress, and lack of exercise.

Signs and Symptoms

- Complaints of chest pain
- Feeling light-headed
- Shortness of breath
- Abnormal pulse rate or rhythm (palpitations)
- Elevated blood pressure
- Elevated cholesterol level

Nurse Assistant's Role in Observation and Intervention

- Monitor and watch for changes in the resident's vital signs.
- Follow all treatment programs as prescribed.

Goals of Care

- Maintain the person's independence to the degree possible.

Interventions or Skills for Care

- Encourage the resident to exercise.
- Encourage an appropriate therapeutic diet.
- Limit stress: Talk with the resident about anything that is upsetting to them, and work with other staff to reduce the resident's stress.
- If pain occurs:
  - Have the resident immediately stop all activity.
  - Have the resident sit or lie down. When the resident is lying down, elevate the head of the bed.
  - Call the charge nurse. Follow his/her instructions.
  - Monitor the resident's vital signs.
  - Help with the delivery of oxygen.
  - Reassure the resident.
  - Communicate to other staff what factors seem to cause pain (precipitating factors).

Cerebral Vascular Accident

In chapter 6, you learned about emergency care for someone having a cerebral vascular accident (CVA). A CVA commonly called a stroke, can be caused by many things, including narrowing of a blood vessel due to plaque build-up, a blood vessel rupture, or a traveling blood clot that blocks the blood flow.

Signs and Symptoms

CVA signs and symptoms vary depending on the location in the brain affected, the extent of the interruption in blood supply, and the resulting tissue damage. It is important to tell the nurse immediately if a resident has any of the symptoms listed below. Prompt medical intervention can prevent or limit the effects of a stroke. The most common signs and symptoms are:

- Face drooping or numbness, especially on one side
- Weakness, numbness, or paralysis of a limb or of one side of the body
- Difficulty swallowing
- Slurred speech or difficulty speaking
- Change in mental status, such as sudden confusion or inability to understand speech
- Vision problems
- Loss of balance or coordination or difficulty walking
- Sudden, severe headache

Nurse Assistant's Role in Observation and Intervention

- Report signs and symptoms and get immediate medical help.
- Support the resident's rehabilitation.

Goals of Care

- Prevent complications such as paralysis, muscle atrophy (wasting), and contractures.
- Improve the resident's level of functioning and promote independence.

Interventions or Skills for Care

To help a resident with paralysis:
- Recognize that paralysis changes a person's life drastically. Residents with paralysis may feel angry, frustrated, and/or depressed.
- Per the physical therapist's plan, assist the resident with ROM exercises three or four times a day (or as prescribed) to prevent contractures and maintain muscle strength. Check the care plan or ask the charge nurse for specific guidelines for exercises.
- Position and turn the resident at least every 2 hours. Support affected limbs with pillows.
- Make sure that a footboard is used at the end of the bed and that the resident's affected foot or feet are against it to prevent foot drop.
- Keep items the resident uses where the resident can see and reach them.

- Check with the charge nurse about how to support the work of the physical therapist and occupational therapist to help the resident relearn skills such as eating, moving, and dressing.

To help a resident with difficulty swallowing:

- Always place the resident in an upright sitting position when eating.
- Encourage or give small bites of food.
- Encourage or give small sips of fluid to moisten food.
- Give verbal cues when the resident is eating.
- Be prepared to perform the Heimlich maneuver if the resident chokes (see Chapter 6).
- Offer small sips of fluid often throughout the day to ensure adequate fluid intake.
- Notify the charge nurse of the resident's food and fluid intake and if the ability to swallow declines further or if any signs of illness (such as fever or rapid pulse rate) occur.

To help a resident who has difficulty communicating and/or understanding:

- Make sure you are familiar with the care plan.
- Talk to the resident in a calm, reassuring manner.
- Speak slowly, using simple sentences.
- Recognize that a resident may understand written messages but not verbal communication.
- Point to objects and use gestures as much as possible to reinforce what you are saying.
- Be patient and gently touch the resident often if they are comfortable with that.

To help a resident who understands speech but cannot put their thoughts into words:

- Speak with the resident in a normal way. Explain everything you do with or to them.
- Remember that the resident can understand you and is not confused.
- Give the resident time to try to speak to you. They may be able to speak some words.
- See if they can write messages. Sometimes residents can still write when they cannot speak.

Digestive System

The **digestive system** consists of the gastrointestinal tract (alimentary canal) and accessory organs of digestion. Its function is to ingest food, convert food, into the nutrients needed to provide energy and sustain life, and to expel waste from the body.

Structures

The main structures of the digestive system are shown in Figure 11-9. They include:

- The *mouth* is the oral cavity that is the beginning of the digestive system.
- The *esophagus* is a muscular tube that connects the throat to the stomach.
- The *stomach* is a sac-like organ, and the small intestine is a long tube-like structure.
- The *liver, gallbladder,* and *pancreas* are accessory organs.
- The *large intestine* is a long tube-like structure that leads to the rectum and anus.

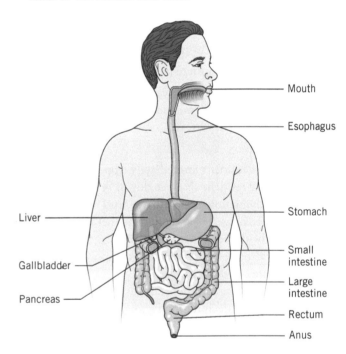

Figure 11-9 Structures of the digestive system.

Functions

Food enters the mouth and is chewed and mixed with saliva, beginning the digestive process. Chewed food travels to the stomach via the esophagus, where it mixes with digestive juices, which break down food to prepare it for absorption. Most nutrient absorption takes place in the small intestine. The liver produces bile, which helps digest fatty foods, and bile is stored in the gallbladder.

The pancreas produces digestive juices and insulin, which regulates the body's blood sugar level. The large intestine absorbs fluid and moves waste toward the rectum, where it is excreted through the anus as feces.

Age-Related Changes and Important Observations

Table 11-10 lists changes that occur in the digestive system as a person ages, and Table 11-11 lists signs, symptoms and important observations related to digestive system problems.

Table 11-10   Changes in the Digestive System with Aging

Change	Result
Food passes through the digestive system more slowly.	Constipation, decreased frequency of bowel movements
	Decreased ability to tolerate food or large meals
The amount and effectiveness of digestive juices are decreased.	Decrease in specific nutrients being absorbed

Table 11-11   Digestive System Signs, Symptoms, and Observations

Signs and Symptoms	Related Observations to Report
Loss of appetite and/or food left on tray	▪ Do I know the resident's normal eating habits? ▪ Are they different now? ▪ Does the resident enjoy meals?
Decreased frequency of bowel movements (as reported on record or communicated by resident)	▪ Do I know the resident's normal bowel patterns? ▪ Are they different now? ▪ Is the resident getting enough exercise, fluid, and fiber?
Increased frequency of bowel movements (as reported on record or communicated by resident)	▪ Do I know the resident's normal bowel patterns? ▪ Are they different now?
Excessive straining during bowel movements	▪ Is the resident getting enough exercise, fluid, and fiber?

Signs and Symptoms	Related Observations to Report
Loss of bowel control (incontinence)	▪ Do I know the resident's normal bowel patterns? ▪ Are they different now?
Change in consistency or texture of feces: loose, watery, sticky, slimy, or hard (rock-like)	▪ Do I know the resident's normal bowel patterns? ▪ Are they different now?
Change in color of feces: black, green, or red (containing blood)	▪ Do I know the resident's normal bowel patterns? ▪ Are they different now?
Foul odor of feces	▪ Do I know the resident's normal bowel patterns? ▪ Are they different now?
Nausea and/or vomiting	▪ When do these symptoms occur? ▪ How frequently do they occur?
Swollen abdomen or one that is abnormally firm or tender to the touch	▪ How long has the abdomen been abnormal?
Complaints of pain or feeling bloated	▪ When do these symptoms occur? ▪ How frequently do they occur?
Weight loss	▪ Is the resident gaining or losing weight?

Common Chronic Diseases and Problems of the Digestive System

Diseases and problems of the digestive system include constipation, diarrhea, and bowel incontinence.

Constipation

Constipation is a slowing of bowel processes resulting in difficulty in eliminating feces. It is common among residents but occurs more often in residents who do not get enough exercise or enough fluid or fiber in their diet.

Fecal impaction may occur if a resident's constipation is not treated. This is uncomfortable for residents and may lead to a serious bowel obstruction. You must monitor, record, and report any problems concerning a resident's bowel movements to the charge nurse. One sign of fecal impaction is that a resident may have small amounts of loose, watery stool that pass by the blockage. This loose, watery stool is sometimes mistaken for diarrhea.

Signs and Symptoms
▪ Decreased number of bowel movements from the resident's usual pattern

- Passing hard stool
- Swollen or enlarged abdomen
- Complaints of feeling bloated and/or having gas
- Loss of appetite

Nurse Assistant's Role in Observation and Intervention
- Identify change in bowel movement pattern.
- Help the resident maintain their regular pattern of bowel movements.
- Recognize complications such as fecal impaction.

Goals of Care
- Help the resident return to a normal pattern of bowel movements.
- Prevent future bowel problems.

Interventions or Skills for Care
- Encourage the resident to drink plenty of fluids (unless they are on fluid restrictions).
- Encourage the resident to eat fruits, vegetables, and other high-fiber foods, such as bran.
- Encourage exercise, especially walking.
- Follow any prescribed orders for enemas or rectal suppositories.

If an enema or suppository is ordered, make sure to check with the nurse to make sure that you are allowed to perform these procedures.

Procedure 11-3 provides directions on giving an enema that must be prepared onsite and is usually a larger volume. Many doctors will order a commercially prepared enema, these are single use. They come prepackaged and ready to use. To use a commercially prepared enema:

- Perform hand hygiene and put on gloves.
- Place a disposable pad under the resident's buttocks.
- Assist the resident to a left side-lying position with knees bent.
- Remove the cover of the enema tip.
- With gentle steady pressure insert the tip of the enema into the rectum, the tip should be pointing toward the navel. Stop and report to charge nurse if the tip is hard to insert.
- Squeeze the bottle until most of the fluid is expelled.
- Remove tip from rectum while still squeezing the bottle.
- Discard of disposable items.

- Remove gloves and perform hand hygiene.
- If leaving the room, make sure resident is in a comfortable position and call light in in reach.
- Assist the resident to the bathroom once they have the urge to have a bowel movement.
- Document and report results and observations to the charge nurse.

Diarrhea

Diarrhea is caused by many factors, including food to which a person has a sensitivity (such as lactose intolerance) or allergy. It can also be caused by influenza (flu) and other types of infections. Infectious diarrhea can be a major problem in a facility because the infection can spread rapidly among residents and cause other complications.

Signs and Symptoms
- Frequent watery stool
- Complaints of cramping
- Increased gas

Nurse Assistant's Role in Observation and Intervention
- Help the resident maintain a regular pattern of bowel movements.
- Identify a change in the resident's pattern of bowel movements.

Goals of Care
- Prevent the complications of dehydration and skin breakdown.
- Prevent the spread of infectious diarrhea.

Interventions or Skills for Care
- Offer the resident clear liquids to prevent dehydration.
- Keep the resident's skin clean and dry. Apply protective cream to reddened areas to protect the skin.
- Keep the charge nurse informed about the number, color, and consistency of the resident's stools.
- Practice all infection control procedures as instructed by the charge nurse.
- Collect specimens as directed.

Gastroesophageal Reflux Disease

Gastroesophageal Reflux Disease (GERD) is a digestive disorder that occurs when stomach contents leak back into the esophagus causing irritation.

PREPARATION STEPS

1. Check the care plan.
2. Knock, introduce yourself, and address resident by preferred name.
3. Perform hand hygiene.
4. Gather supplies and secure assistance if needed.
5. Explain procedure and ask about resident preferences. Respect privacy and rights at all times.

ITEMS NEEDED

- Three pairs of gloves
- Plastic trash bags
- Disposable enema kit with prescribed solution
- Lubricant
- Two disposable protective pads
- Bath blanket or sheets
- Bedpan
- Toilet paper

Enema kits may contain a prepared commercial product (already mixed and ready to administer) or may have to be mixed. Different types of enemas are used: tap water, oil retention, cleansing, and medicated. In the case of a medicated enema, the nurse adds the medication and supervises the enema. Make sure that your facility allows you to do this procedure. Check with the charge nurse to confirm the proper equipment and supplies and for specific instructions.

1. Put on gloves.

2. Place disposable protective pad under the resident's buttocks. Place a second protective pad at the end of the bed to place under and over bedpan when resident is finished.

3. Position the resident on their left side, helping them turn if necessary. Make sure their hips are near the edge of the bed on the side where you're working.

4. Hold the rectal tube over the bedpan. Open the clamp on the tubing and let the solution run through into the bedpan until it flows smoothly, so that no air is left in the tubing to cause discomfort for the resident. Close the clamp.

5. Turn back the bath blanket so that the resident's hips are exposed but the rest of the body is covered. Hold the lubricated rectal tube about five inches from the tip. Gently put it into the rectum to the red line on the tube.

6. Raise the container about 15 inches above the resident's hips. Never hold the container any higher.

7. Open the clamp and let the solution run in slowly. If the resident complains of cramps, tell them to breathe deeply through their mouth, as you clamp the tubing for a minute or so. You may also lower the irrigating bag.

8. When all the solution has run in, close the clamp.

9. Remove the rectal tube. Place the tubing in a plastic trash bag.

10. Turn the resident on their back and slip the bedpan under them. Ask the resident to try to hold the solution as long as possible. Raise the head of the bed. Ensure that the call button and toilet paper are within reach.

11. Give the resident privacy, but do not leave them for a long period of time. Check on the resident after five minutes.

12. When the resident feels they are done, put on gloves, and assist with perineal care if necessary. Remove the bedpan and place it on a protective pad. Remove your gloves, and help the resident into a comfortable position. Put on gloves and remove the covered bedpan.

COMPLETION STEPS

1. Determine the resident's preferred position for comfort and ask them if they need anything else.
2. Examine the environment for safety and cleanliness.
3. Secure the call light and any other needed items within reach of the resident.
4. Perform hand hygiene.
5. Document the procedure and report any findings to the staff in charge.

Signs and Symptoms

- Residents may complain of heartburn (a burning feeling in their chest), that may worsen when lying down or bending over
- A bitter taste in their mouth
- Difficulty swallowing
- Persistent nausea or vomiting
- The feeling of food caught in the throat
- Coughing
- Sore throat

Nurse Assistant's Role in Observation and Intervention

- Identify and report and signs and symptoms of GERD.

Goals of Care

- Prevent any complications of GERD.
- Decrease symptoms.

Interventions or Skills for Care

- Help the resident avoid foods and drinks that can trigger symptoms, such as: spicy foods, citrus juices, caffeinated, alcoholic, or carbonated beverages.
- Eat smaller, more frequent meals.
- Avoid eating at bedtime.
- Wear loose-fitting clothes.
- Avoid foods high in fat, such as fried foods.
- Encourage the resident to sleep with the head of the bed elevated.

Vomiting

Vomiting, also known as emesis, is when stomach contents exit through the mouth. Nausea often accompanies the urge to vomit. **Nausea** is an uneasy or sick feeling in the stomach.

Vomiting can be caused by many different things including:

- Foodborne illnesses
- Bacterial infections
- Motion sickness
- Medications
- Migraine headaches
- Chemotherapy
- Drinking too much alcohol
- A blockage in the bowel

- Problems with the gall bladder
- Brain injury

Some complications associated with vomiting, are aspiration, electrolyte imbalance (dehydration), or injury to the esophagus. Prolonged vomiting can lead to weight loss and nutritional concerns.

Nurse Assistant's Role in Observation

- Report any episodes of vomiting to the nurse.
- Note the characteristics of the vomit, such as, amount and what the appearance.

Goals of Care

- Prevent aspiration.
- Decrease or prevent episodes of possible.

Interventions or Skills for Care

- If vomiting occurs, follow standard precautions and don the appropriate PPE.
- If the resident is lying down, turn their head to the side and place an emesis (kidney) basin under their chin.
- Notify the nurse immediately.
- Note the amount, odor, and appearance of the emesis.
- Allow the nurse to see the emesis before discarding.
- Assist the resident with personal care as needed (brushing teeth or changing clothes).

Urinary System

The **urinary system** is one of the most important systems in the body. It helps the body maintain fluid balance (the amount of water in the body) and eliminate liquid waste. The major structures of the urinary system are shown in Figure 11-10).

Structures

- The right and left *kidneys* maintain the body's fluid balance by filtering out waste products and producing urine.
- The right and left *ureters* are tubes that carry urine from the kidneys to the bladder.
- The *bladder* is a sac-like muscle that stores urine until it is eliminated.
- The *urethra* is the tube that carries the urine from the bladder outside the body.
- The **urinary meatus** is the opening at the end of the urethra where the urine exits out of the body.

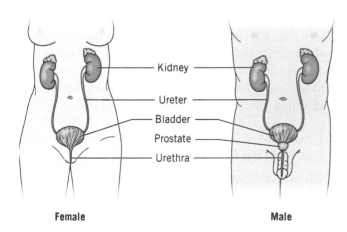

Female   Male

Figure 11-10 Structures of the urinary system.

Functions

The urinary system consists of organs involved in producing, collecting, and eliminating liquid waste from the blood stream in the form of urine. It functions to remove waste products from the blood, to regulate the balance of electrolytes (salts and minerals such as sodium, potassium, and calcium) and acids and bases in the body, and to help regulate blood volume and blood pressure.

Age-Related Changes and Important Observations

Table 11-12 lists changes that occur in the urinary system as a person ages, and Table 11-13 lists signs, symptoms and important observations related to urinary system problems.

Common Chronic Diseases and Problems of the Urinary System

Diseases and problems of the diseases system include urinary tract infections, kidney disease, and urinary incontinence (as discussed in chapter 9)

Urinary Tract Infections

An infection in the urinary system is called a *urinary tract infection (UTI)*. The bladder is most commonly affected. UTI's are one of the most common infections in long-term care facilities. Urinary tract infections occur more often in women, in people who are incontinent, and in those with poor fluid intake. A UTI can occur when bacteria enters the urethra and travels to the bladder. *Escherichia coli (E coli)*, is one of the most common causes of urinary tract infections. This bacteria is found in the intestine and can present in the stool.

Signs and Symptoms

- Increased urinary frequency
- Complaints of burning or stinging during urination
- Urine that is dark yellow, cloudy, or has a foul odor
- Blood in urine
- A change in cognitive status (confusion)
- Pain in lower back

Nurse Assistant's Role in Observation and Intervention

- Identify residents at risk for a urinary tract infection.
- Report any changes in a resident's urinary pattern to the charge nurse.

Goals of Care

- Prevent urinary tract infections.
- Help reduce discomfort experienced by the resident.

Interventions or Skills for Care

- Encourage residents to drink enough fluids every day, mainly water. Cranberry juice may be recommended for residents with a UTI.
- Encourage residents to urinate at least every three to four hours when awake.
- Encourage proper perineal hygiene, as discussed in chapter 5 (such as females wiping from front to back after urination) and daily washing of the perineal area.
- For residents who have incontinence, perineal care should be performed after each incontinent episode.
- Remind residents that are able to toilet themselves the proper procedures for perineal care.

Table 11-12 Changes in the Urinary System with Aging

Change	Result
Decreased size of kidneys	Slowing of kidneys' ability to filter the blood
	Less efficiency in concentrating urine
Decreased bladder capacity	More frequent urination
Decreased bladder muscle tone	Decreased ability to empty bladder: residual (leftover) urine present after urination
Decrease in hormones that regulate fluid volume	Increased risk of dehydration

fluids, toilet q2h, peri-care

Table 11-13　Urinary System Signs, Symptoms, and Observations

Signs and Symptoms	Related Observations to Report
Very dark yellow urine, bloody or orange urine, or cloudy urine	▪ Do I know the resident's normal urinary patterns? ▪ Are they different now? ▪ Is the resident getting adequate fluids? ▪ When did you first notice this change?
Urine with very strong odor	▪ Do I know the resident's normal urinary patterns? ▪ Are they different now? ▪ Is the resident getting adequate fluids? ▪ When did you first notice this change?
Passing very small amounts of urine	▪ Do I know the resident's normal urinary patterns? ▪ Are they different now? ▪ Is the resident getting adequate fluids? ▪ Is the resident's fluid intake and output about equal?
Sense of urinary urgency	▪ Do I know the resident's normal urinary patterns? ▪ Are they different now?
Complaints of burning or stinging during urination	▪ When did you first notice this change? ▪ Is the resident getting adequate fluids? ▪ Does the resident have good hygiene? ▪ Does a female resident wipe the urethral area correctly from front (near pubic bone) to back (toward anus)?
Frequent urination in small amounts (urinary frequency)	▪ Does the resident feel the need to urinate again just a short time after urinating?
Loss of urinary control (incontinence)	▪ When did you first notice this change? ▪ Do I respond fast enough when the resident needs assistance with elimination?

Kidney Disease

Kidney disease occurs when the kidneys are damaged and unable to filter blood the way they should. Kidney disease can be acute or chronic. Acute kidney disease occurs suddenly and is known as acute kidney injury or acute renal failure. Causes of acute kidney injury:

▪ Not enough blood flow to the kidneys
▪ Damage to the kidneys
▪ Urine backed up in the kidneys

Chronic kidney disease (CKD) involves a gradual loss of kidney function. In the early stages of the disease, signs and symptoms may not be present but gradually gets worse over time. According to the CDC, more than one in seven American adults are estimated to have CKD. Two of the main causes of chronic kidney disease are diabetes and high blood pressure.

Risk factor for chronic kidney disease includes:

▪ Diabetes
▪ High blood pressure
▪ Heart disease
▪ Smoking
▪ Obesity
▪ Older age
▪ Family history

Signs and Symptoms
▪ Nausea and vomiting
▪ Loss of appetite
▪ Urinating less or more
▪ Feeling tired
▪ High blood pressure
▪ Swelling in hands, ankles, or feet

Nurse Assistant's Role in Observation
▪ Monitor and report and signs and symptoms to the nurse.

Interventions or Skills for Care
▪ Monitor the resident's blood pressure as directed by your nurse.
▪ Encourage resident to adhere to dietary restrictions.
▪ Monitor intake and output.

If chronic kidney goes untreated it may lead to kidney failure, requiring dialysis.

Nervous System

The **nervous system** is made up of the brain, spinal cord, and nerves. Its components work together to control bodily functions and receive, interpret, and respond to stimuli. The system has two main divisions; the brain and spinal cord make up the *central nervous system,* and the nerves and other structures outside of the brain and spinal cord make up the *peripheral nervous system* (Figure 11-12).

Structures

- The *brain* is the body's communication and control center. It is located within the protective skull.

- The *spinal cord* is a thick cord of nerve tissue that extends down the back, protected within the spine (vertebral column).

- *Nerves* are fibers that extend from the spinal cord to all parts of the body. The nerves carry messages back and forth between the body and brain.

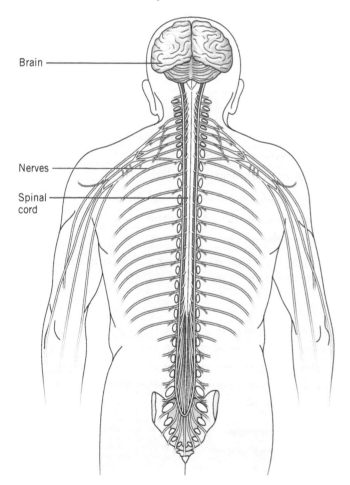

Brain

Nerves

Spinal cord

Figure 11-12 Structures of the nervous system.

Functions

The nervous system, along with the endocrine system, coordinates the body's response to internal and external stimuli and directs all other body systems. Information enters through sensory receptors and is carried to the brain, where it is interpreted, processed, and stored. The brain sends messages back to the body that control all body functions, including physical movement. Thinking, reasoning, learning, and emotions all originate in the brain.

Age-Related Changes and Important Observations

Table 11-14 lists changes that occur in the nervous system as a person ages, and Table 11-15 lists signs, symptoms and important observations related to nervous system problems.

Table 11-14   Changes in the Nervous System with Aging

Change	Result
Slowing of nerve impulses	Longer time for residents to learn new information
	Slower response time to situations, which may result in injury
Decreased blood flow to certain areas of the brain	Decrease in short-term memory

Table 11-15   Nervous System Signs, Symptoms, and Observations

Signs and Symptoms	Related Observations to Report
Loss of interest in learning	■ Do I reinforce the resident's recently learned behavior? ■ Do I take every opportunity to review new information with the resident?
Memory loss, confusion, or feeling isolated	■ Do I reinforce the resident's recently learned behavior? ■ Do I take every opportunity to review new information with the resident? ■ Do I encourage the resident to interact with others?
Impatience	■ When did you first notice this change?

Signs and Symptoms	Related Observations to Report
Reduced sensation or paralysis	■ Does the resident have any tremors or weakness? ■ Is the resident steady on their feet? ■ Can the resident move without help?
Involuntary motions or tremors	■ Does the resident have any tremors or weakness?
Unsteadiness while walking	■ Is the resident steady on their feet? ■ Can the resident move without help?
Speech problems	■ When did you first notice this change?
Complaints of not remembering where things are	■ Do I reinforce the resident's recently learned behavior? ■ Do I take every opportunity to review new information with the resident?
Complaints of not being able to react as quickly as in the past	■ When did you first notice this change? ■ Can the resident move without help?

Nurse Assistant's Role in Observation and Intervention

■ Provide care the resident needs because of the progression of the disease.

Goals of Care

■ Help the resident maintain their independence as long as possible.
■ Prevent complications.

Interventions or Skills for Care

■ Help with ROM exercises of the arms and/or legs that are affected by the disease.
■ Use proper positioning methods.
■ Maintain the resident's skin integrity.
■ Ensure proper nutrition.
■ Provide adequate fluids.
■ Identify the resident's bowel and urination patterns and ensure compliance with the resident's toileting routine.
■ Provide support by listening to the resident's concerns about changes occurring in their body.
■ Attend to the resident's requests regarding personal hygiene or social interactions with family and friends.

Parkinson's Disease

Parkinson's disease is a degenerative disease of the central nervous system that affects a person's motor skills (movement of muscles). Its exact cause is not known. The disease usually begins when adults are age 60 or older.

Parkinson's-like symptoms can occur following a stroke and as a side effect of certain drugs.

Signs and Symptoms

■ Musculoskeletal: muscle weakness and stiffness, tremors, slumped posture, shuffling walk, poor balance and coordination, and mask-like facial expression
■ Gastrointestinal: constipation, difficulty chewing and swallowing
■ Personality: confusion and/or mood changes

Nurse Assistant's Role in Observation and Intervention

■ Identify changes in a resident's status.

Goals of Care

■ Help the resident maintain their mobility.
■ Ensure adequate nutrition and fluid intake.
■ Maintain a safe environment to prevent falls.
■ Help the resident maintain their independence.

Interventions or Skills for Care

■ Keep the resident's room free of clutter.
■ Encourage the resident to use assistive walking devices as ordered.
■ Encourage frequent rest periods.
■ Offer small, frequent meals high in fiber.
■ Encourage adequate fluid intake.
■ Keep tasks simple.
■ Support residents by listening to their concerns about physical changes and loss of abilities.

Multiple Sclerosis

Multiple Sclerosis (MS) is a chronic disease affecting the central nervous system. This disease causes damage to the myelin sheath, the material that forms around the nerve. The damage slows down or blocks message between the brain and the body.

Signs and Symptoms

■ Visual disturbances
■ Muscle weakness
■ Unsteady gait
■ Problems with coordination

- Feeling of numbness or tingling
- Fatigue

Usually, the disease is mild, but a resident can lose the ability to speak, write, or walk. For some the losses may be temporary, but others it can be long lasting. Rehabilitation and physical therapy may be ordered for these residents.

Symptoms of MS usually appear when a person is between the ages of 20 and 50 but can occur in other age groups as well. Recent studies suggest that women are three times as likely as men to have MS.

Goals of Care
- Help the resident maintain their mobility.
- Ensure adequate nutrition and fluid intake.
- Maintain a safe environment to prevent falls.
- Help the resident maintain their independence.

Interventions or Skills for Care
- Keep the resident's room free of clutter.
- Encourage the resident to use assistive walking devices as ordered.
- Encourage frequent rest periods.
- Encourage adequate nutrition and fluid intake.
- Keep tasks simple.
- Support residents by listening to their concerns about physical changes and loss of abilities.

Special Senses

Vision, hearing, equilibrium (balance), smell, taste, and touch are referred to as the special senses. The associated *sense organs* are the eyes, ears, nose, tongue, and skin. We rely on the special senses to give us information from the outside world and send information to the brain. Aging influences the function of all the senses, but sight and hearing are the most commonly affected.

The Eye

The eye is the organ of vision. The eye is delicate. It sits in the eye socket, which provides protection for the eye. The major structures of the eye are shown in Figure 11-13.

Structures

- The *sclera* is the "white" of the eye.
- The *iris* is the colored part of the eye. It regulates the amount of light that enters the eye by controlling the size of the pupil.

- The *pupil* is the opening through which light passes to get to the retina.
- The *cornea* protects the iris.
- The iris and *lens* direct and focus light on the retina.
- The *retina* is the membrane lining the inner eyeball that is connected to the brain by the optic nerve.

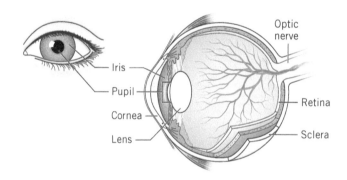

Figure 11-13 Structures of the eye.

Functions

Sight gives us knowledge about our surroundings. Visual stimuli enter the eye and are converted into nerve impulses transmitted to the brain. The brain interprets and processes the impulses into visual images.

Age-Related Changes and Important Observations

Table 11-16 lists changes that occur in the eye as a person ages, and Table 11-17 lists signs, symptoms and important observations related to eye and vision problems.

Table 11-16 Changes in the Eye Due to Aging

Change	Result
The cornea flattens.	Resident has decreased ability to focus at normal reading distances.
The lens becomes more yellow.	Greens and blues are difficult to see, and reds and oranges easier to see.
The lens becomes more rigid or less elastic.	Resident can see objects clearly only at a greater distance.
The pupil becomes smaller.	Because less light reaches the inner eye, it is more difficult to see in poorly lit conditions.
The retina becomes less efficient.	Resident's spatial discrimination decreases.
The iris becomes more rigid.	Eyes do not adjust well to changes in amount of light.

Table 11-17 Signs, Symptoms, and Observations of the Eye

Signs and Symptoms	Related Observations to Report
Discharge from one or both eyes	- When did you first notice this change?
Excessive watering of the eyes	- When did you first notice this change?
Inability to find things; bumping into things	- Do I leave things where the resident can find them? - Does the resident have enough light? - Is the resident wearing eyeglasses? - Are glasses clean and of the correct prescription?
Complaints of not being able to see well, not being able to focus clearly, or having double vision	- Does the resident have enough light? - Is the resident wearing eyeglasses? - Are glasses clean and of the correct prescription? - Is the resident concerned about loss of sight? - Is the resident having trouble distinguishing color? - Do I address the resident directly?
Complaints of eye pain or a burning sensation in one or both eyes	- When did you first notice this change?

Common Chronic Diseases and Problems of the Eye

Eye and vision problems include cataracts, glaucoma, and blindness.

Cataracts

A **cataract** can occur in one or both eyes. It is a partial or complete opacity (loss of transparency) of the lens of the eye, which impairs vision. Surgery can be performed to correct this condition and improve vision.

Signs and Symptoms

- Increase in nearsightedness
- Complaints of double vision or dim or blurry vision
- Problems with glare
- Inability to distinguish color

Nurse Assistant's Role in Observation and Intervention

- Identify the resident's capabilities.
- Ensure a safe environment.

Goals of Care

- Improve the resident's ability to perform the activities of daily living.
- Protect the resident from injury.
- If cataract surgery is performed, ensure that recovery proceeds smoothly.

Interventions or Skills for Care

- Be sure that the resident's things are kept in the same place and always returned there.
- Help the resident with personal belongings as needed. Open lids, put toothpaste on their toothbrush, help them pick out color-coordinated clothing, etc.
- Describe where foods are on the resident's plate, using clock-face directions (Figure 11-14). For example, "The potatoes are at three o'clock, the vegetables are at 11 o'clock, and the meat is at six o'clock."

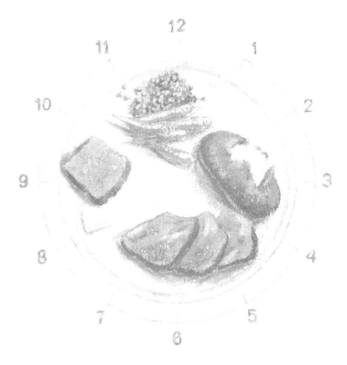

Figure 11-14 For residents with impaired vision, you can describe the location of food on the plate using the numbers on a clock face.

- Make sure the resident wears their glasses. Clean and store them properly.
- Read to the resident if necessary.

- Keep the room well-lit and uncluttered.
- Let the resident know when you enter the room and identify yourself.
- Stand where the resident can see you.
- Encourage the resident to touch and feel objects around them.
- Support the resident emotionally if they are having cataract surgery, and provide assistance during their recovery.

Glaucoma and Blindness

Glaucoma is a disease that is linked to increased fluid pressure in the eye. This pressure damages the optic nerve and causes vision loss. Glaucoma is treated with eye drops, and sometimes surgery is needed. If left untreated, it can lead to blindness. Some residents who are considered "legally blind" are visually impaired but still have some sight.

Signs and Symptoms
- Difficulty with activities of daily living
- Difficulty moving from place to place
- Pain, nausea, and vomiting (with sudden-onset glaucoma)
- Gradual blurred or tunnel vision
- Halos of light around objects

Nurse Assistant's Role in Observation and Intervention
- Identify the resident's capabilities.
- Ensure a safe environment.

Goals of Care
- Improve the resident's abilities to perform the activities of daily living.
- Protect the resident from injury.
- Help the resident to remain active and not become socially isolated.

Interventions or Skills for Care
- Be sure that the resident's things are kept in the same place and always returned there.
- Help the resident with personal belongings as needed. Open lids, put toothpaste on their toothbrush, help them pick out color-coordinated clothing, etc.
- Describe the location of foods on their plate, using clock-face directions.

- If the resident has partial vision and has glasses, encourage them to wear them. Clean and store them properly.
- Read to the resident if necessary.
- Keep the room well-lit and uncluttered.
- Let the resident know when you enter the room and identify yourself.
- Encourage the resident to touch and feel objects around them.
- Help the resident walk: Have them hold your elbow or use an assistive device as you guide them along.
- Position their furniture in a simple arrangement.
- Orient the resident to their surroundings.

Age-Related Macular Degeneration

Age-related macular degeneration (AMD) is an eye disease that affects the central vision. Central vision is what you see in the center of your visual field and allows you to see fine details. According to the CDC, AMD is the leading cause of vision loss and blindness in Americans 65 and older.

There are two types of AMD, wet and dry. Wet AMD is when abnormal blood vessels behind the retina grow under the macula, causing blood and fluid to leak. Wet AMD can lead to a rapid loss of vision. An early warning sign of wet AMD is that straight lines appear wavy.

Dry AMD is when the macula thins over time, gradually blurring the central vision. Dry AMD is more common than the wet form. A common warning sign of dry AMD are tiny yellow or white deposits under the retina.

The Ear

The ear is the organ of hearing. Structures of the inner ear are involved in maintaining equilibrium (balance).

Structures

- The ear has three primary regions: the inner, middle, and outer ear (Figure 11-15).
- Sound enters the *outer ear* and is transmitted through the *middle ear* to the *inner ear.*
- Nerve impulses travel from the inner ear to the brain for interpretation.

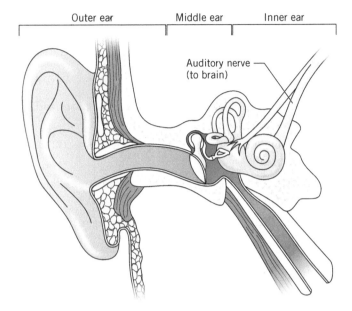

Outer ear   Middle ear   Inner ear

Auditory nerve
(to brain)

Figure 11-15 Major regions and structures of the ear.

Functions

The structures of the ear allow us to hear. Hearing, like vision, provides awareness of the world around us. Sounds provide clues to dangers as well as communication and pleasure. Structures of the inner ear are involved in maintaining balance. If these structures are not working properly, a resident may experience vertigo (a sensation of spinning or whirling motion) or dizziness (lightheadedness, unsteadiness, or imbalance).

Age-Related Changes and Important Observations

Table 11-18 lists changes that occur in the ear as a person ages, and Table 11-19 lists signs, symptoms and important observations related to ear and hearing problems.

Table 11-18   Changes in the Ear with Aging

Change	Result
Hearing structures in the ear become stiff.	Loss of hearing of high-frequency sounds
Structures in inner ear related to balance begin to degenerate.	Harder to maintain balance
Production of soft ear wax decreases.	Buildup of hard, dry wax in the ears, which can cause hearing loss

Table 11-19   Signs, Symptoms, and Observations of the Ear

Signs and Symptoms	Related Observations to Report
Discharge from the ear	▪ When did you first notice this change?
Repeated tugging or scratching of the ear	▪ Do I speak directly and clearly to the resident? ▪ Do I lower the tone of my voice? ▪ Does the nurse check the resident's ear frequently for wax? ▪ Does the resident wear a hearing aid and know how to use it? ▪ If so, is it clean and operating properly?
Speaking in an overly loud voice, yelling, and/or turning the television or radio volume to a high setting (very loud)	▪ Do I speak directly and clearly to the resident? ▪ Do I lower the tone of my voice? ▪ Does the nurse check the resident's ear frequently for wax? ▪ Does the resident wear a hearing aid and know how to use it? ▪ If so, is it clean and operating properly?
Feelings of anger or isolation	▪ Does the resident exhibit anger toward others? ▪ Does the resident avoid group activities? ▪ Does the resident seem withdrawn or fearful?
Complaints of ringing in the ear or feeling dizzy or unsteady	▪ When did you first notice this change?

Common Chronic Diseases and Problems of the Ear

The most common problem experienced by older adults is hearing loss.

Hearing Loss

Residents may experience hearing loss for a number of reasons, including injury, disease, and age-related changes.

Signs and Symptoms

- The resident may not respond to other people talking to them.
- The resident may not interact with other residents.
- The resident may not participate in activities.
- When listening, the resident may turn their head or cup their hand over their ear.
- The resident may look like they do not understand you when you speak.

Nurse Assistant's Role in Observation and Intervention

- Report any changes in how a resident who is hard of hearing communicates to the charge nurse to ensure that proper interventions are arranged.

Goals of Care

- Maintain and improve the resident's communication with others, including caregivers, other residents, friends, and family.

Interventions or Skills for Care

- When the resident is standing, position yourself in front of them when you are speaking. When the resident is seated, position yourself at their eye level when speaking.
- Speak slowly and clearly because the person may be reading your lips.
- Speak in your normal voice, not a louder or a high-pitched voice.
- Reduce background noise.
- For a resident who cannot hear you or read your lips, use writing to communicate.
- Point to objects you are talking about.
- If the resident uses a hearing aid, make sure that they wear it. Check the battery each day before they put it in. Become familiar with the type of hearing aid the resident uses. Hearing aids should be labeled with the resident's name. Always keep the hearing aid in a safe place when it is not being worn.

The Other Senses

As we age, changes occur in our sense of smell, taste, and touch. Table 11-20 lists changes that occur in these senses as a person ages, and Table 11-21 lists signs, symptoms and important observations.

Table 11-20 Changes in the Other Senses with Aging

Change	Result
Smell The ability to identify or detect odors decreases with age, more commonly in men than in women.	Resident may not be able to detect odors that signal a danger, like chemicals or smoke from a fire.
Taste The ability to taste salty and sweet tastes may decrease because of changes in the tongue.	Resident may request more seasoned foods.
Touch Decreased sensitivity of touch receptors Decreased response to painful stimuli	Resident may not be able to tell how hot an object is, leading to a burn.

Table 11-21 Signs, Symptoms, and Observations of the Other Senses

Signs and Symptoms	Related Observations to Report
Inability to taste or smell food	- Does the resident like the type of food served? - Does the resident enjoy meals? - Is the resident getting adequate nutrition?
Loss of appetite or complaints that the food is bland	- Does the resident like the type of food served? - Does the resident enjoy meals? - Is the resident getting adequate nutrition?
Burns on the skin	- Is the water temperature adjusted correctly for the resident's personal care? - Does the resident check water temperature using the inner part of the wrist?

Endocrine System

The **endocrine system** includes many different glands (Figure 11-16). Glands are organs that make and release hormones, which are substances that regulate the activity of various cells, tissues, and organs throughout the body.

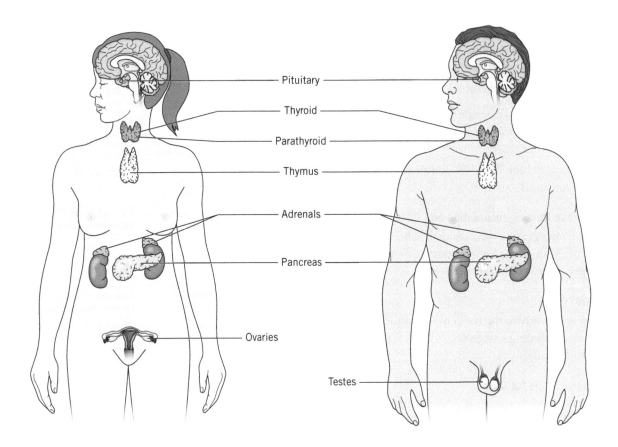

Figure 11-16   Structures of the endocrine system.

Structures

The following are the major structures of the endocrine system:

- The *pituitary gland,* located in the brain, secretes hormones and regulates other glands. It is often called the "master gland."
- The *adrenal glands,* located on top of the kidneys, secrete hormones that regulate metabolism (the process of producing energy). They also help regulate sodium, water, and potassium levels in the body. Adrenal glands release hormones that increase blood sugar, control blood vessel constriction, and help us to react in emergency situations.
- Cells called the *islets of Langerhans,* located in the pancreas, secrete insulin, which controls the breakdown of carbohydrates (sugars) in the body.
- The *thyroid* and *parathyroid glands,* located in the neck, secrete hormones that regulate metabolism.

- The female ovaries, located in the pelvic area, secrete hormones that control sexual function and are involved in pregnancy.
- The male testes (testicles), located in a sac behind the penis, secrete a hormone controlling sexual function and sperm production.

Functions

The endocrine system makes hormones that control many important body functions. Hormones play a role in regulating many activities, including growth, metabolic processes, and sexual function.

Age-Related Changes and Important Observations

Table 11-22 lists changes that occur in the endocrine system as a person ages, and Table 11-23 lists signs, symptoms and important observations related to endocrine/hormonal problems.

Table 11-22   Changes in the Endocrine System with Aging

Change	Result
Glands have a slower rate of releasing hormones.	This change affects the resident's blood studies but should not affect the overall health of the resident.
Decreased insulin production	The body takes longer to process sugar; resident may have less energy.
Dramatically decreased amount of hormones produced by the ovaries	Menstruation stops, along with the ability to have children; this is known as menopause.
Male hormone production decreases but does not stop.	May have decreased sexual response.

Table 11-23   Endocrine System Signs, Symptoms, and Observations

Signs and Symptoms	Related Observations to Report
Excessive thirst (drinking large amounts of fluids)	Have the resident's requests for water or other beverages dramatically increased?
Dramatic increase in urine output	Does the resident go to the bathroom more often than normal?
Increased food intake	Is the resident eating a lot more food than normal?
Complaints of feeling tired or cold	Is the resident lethargic?

Common Chronic Diseases and Problems of the Endocrine System

The most common disease of the endocrine system is diabetes mellitus (often referred to simply as diabetes).

Diabetes

According to the Centers for Disease Control and Prevention, 37.3 million children and adults in the United States have diabetes. In addition, 96 million Americans aged 18 and over have *prediabetes,* a serious condition that increases a person's risk of developing diabetes and other chronic diseases. Prediabetes is indicated when a person's blood sugar is higher than normal but not high enough to be diagnosed as diabetic.

In diabetes, either the pancreas does not produce enough insulin, or the body does not use insulin effectively. Insulin controls the body's use and distribution of carbohydrates. When an insulin problem occurs, a person's blood sugar level becomes too high or too low.

There are three types of diabetes:

- *Type 1 diabetes* is an autoimmune disease that accounts for about 5% of cases. For unknown reasons, the immune system destroys insulin-producing cells in the pancreas, so it cannot produce enough insulin. A person with type 1 diabetes must have insulin injections or use an insulin pump.

- *Type 2 diabetes* is the most common type. In this case, the pancreas produces insulin, but for unknown reasons, the body does not use it effectively. Type 2 diabetes usually occurs later in life, but due to poor diet and lack of exercise, many children and young adults have developed this disease. Type 2 can usually be controlled with diet, exercise, oral medication, and/or insulin injections.

- *Gestational diabetes* develops during pregnancy.

People with diabetes are at risk of developing complications, generally caused by damage to nerves and/or blood vessels. Diabetics are at increased risk for heart disease, stroke, and kidney disease. The blood vessels narrow, causing reduced blood flow. Poor circulation to the legs can cause reduced sensation, changed skin color, and leg cramps. A decrease in blood flow to the eyes can cause pain, vision problems, and blindness. Nerve damage can occur in any part of the body. A nerve problem in the legs can cause symptoms such as numbness, tingling, or a shooting or stabbing pain. Serious damage to blood vessels and nerves can lead to limb amputations. Nerve damage to internal organs can affect many body functions, such as digestion and elimination.

Diabetes also decreases the body's ability to fight off infection. High blood sugar levels may lead to bacterial overgrowth or infection. Common infection sites for diabetics include the feet, kidneys, bladder, and skin. It is important to observe and report any changes in diabetic residents. With early detection, it may be possible to reduce or prevent complications. To prevent or slow the progression of diabetic complications, the health care team works to control the resident's blood sugar level, blood pressure, and cholesterol levels.

Signs and Symptoms

- Change in behavior, such as irritability
- Excessive thirst
- Excessive hunger
- Excessive urination

- Blurred vision
- Itching of the skin
- In females, itching of the vagina and vulva
- Tingling and/or numbness of hands and feet
- Slow healing of a wound or sore
- Fatigue
- Weight loss

Nurse Assistant's Role in Observation and Intervention

- Identify and report any physical changes and any changes in the resident's behavior.
- Closely monitor the resident's nutrition. Residents with diabetes typically are on special diets.
- Monitor and encourage the resident's daily exercise program.
- Provide a safe environment to prevent injury.

Goals of Care

- Prevent complications by observing and reporting changes in the resident.
- Help maintain a proper diet.
- Encourage exercise.

Interventions or Skills for Care

- Promptly provide meals and snacks specially prepared for residents with diabetes. All residents with diabetes must eat on time and must eat the correct amount of the foods prepared for them. Carefully observe the food intake. Record and report it if the resident does not eat all their meals and snacks or if they eat foods not on their diet.
- When helping a diabetic resident with personal care, inspect their skin daily and report any changes immediately. Wash, rinse, dry, and inspect the resident's skin thoroughly, especially their feet. Observe the skin for any reddened areas or skin breakdown. Report any skin changes to the charge nurse. Tell the nurse if the resident's fingernails or toenails need to be cut. A nurse or physician must cut a diabetic resident's toenails because of the high risk of injury.
- Observe the resident for any skin discolorations or sores that are not healing. This may indicate decreased circulation to the area. Report any complaints of numbness or tingling in the hands or feet immediately.
- Some residents must have their blood sugar (glucose) levels checked daily with a blood glucose device or monitor. Many different glucose monitoring devices are available. If blood glucose testing is part of your

responsibilities, make sure you are familiar with the device used in your facility and that testing is done according to the resident's care plan. Procedure 11-4 describes the steps involved in checking a resident's blood sugar level.

- Although urine testing is no longer recommended for controlling blood sugar, it still gives the health care team valuable information. Urine tests may show the presence of ketones or protein in the urine. Ketones are byproducts created when the body burns fat instead of glucose for fuel. Ketones in the urine can signal a serious problem (see Chapter 10, Proce-dure 10-11, Testing Urine for Ketones). The physician may order a diabetic resident's urine to be tested for protein. Protein in the urine is an early sign of kidney disease. Make sure to check with the charge nurse for your facility policy before you provide any type of testing.
- Pay close attention to a diabetic resident's behavior. *[handwritten: SUDDEN CONFUSION]* Note and report any changes. Changes may be import-ant because they may indicate a problem in blood sugar level. Aggressiveness, irritability, or difficulty concentrating may indicate high blood sugar. Weak-ness or shakiness may indicate low blood sugar. Very low blood sugar is a medical emergency that requires immediate treatment; it can lead to coma and death.
- Monitor the resident's physical activity. All residents with diabetes need exercise, but each resident's pro-gram must be designed for their individual needs.

Male Reproductive System

The **reproductive system** in males is the body system responsible for sexual function and human reproduction. It consists of external and internal *genitalia*. In males, this system includes glands and a duct system.

Structures

The main structures of the male reproductive system are shown in Figure 11-17:

- The *penis* is used for sexual intercourse and urination.
- The *testes* are two oval-shaped glands, sometimes called the sex glands or gonads.
- The *scrotum* is the sac that holds the testes outside the body.
- The *prostate gland* secretes one of the fluids that make up semen.
- Semen is produced by the *seminal vesicle*.

PREPARATION STEPS

1. Check the care plan.
2. Knock, introduce yourself, and address resident by preferred name.
3. Perform hand hygiene.
4. Gather supplies and secure assistance if needed.
5. Explain procedure and ask about resident preferences. Respect privacy and rights at all times.

ITEMS NEEDED

- Gloves
- Soap and warm water or alcohol wipe
- Testing device (glucometer)
- Lancets and test strips
- Gauze pads
- Adhesive bandage
- Sharps container
- Disposable trash bag
- Resident's chart or record

Before you proceed, check with the charge nurse to confirm that your facility allows you to do glucose testing. Make sure that you have all necessary supplies on hand. If you have not previously used the glucometer, read the manufacturer's directions before beginning.

1. Explain the procedure if the resident is not familiar with routine glucose testing.

2. Have the resident wash their hands using warm water and soap or use an alcohol wipe to cleanse the fingertip. Dry thoroughly.

3. Perform hand hygiene, and put on gloves.

4. Turn on the meter and insert a test strip. Some devices activate when the test strip is inserted. The goal is to keep the process as painless as possible for the resident while obtaining an adequate blood sample.

5. Place the blood on the test strip in the correct area. Follow the guidelines for your specific device to obtain the glucose reading.

6. Read and record the results.

7. Cover/clean the prick site with an alcohol wipe, gauze, or tissue until the bleeding stops. If needed, apply an adhesive bandage.

8. Dispose of supplies in the appropriate containers and return the meter to the proper storage location

COMPLETION STEPS

1. Determine the resident's preferred position for comfort and ask them if they need anything else.
2. Examine the environment for safety and cleanliness.
3. Secure the call light and any other needed items within reach of the resident.
4. Perform hand hygiene.
5. Document the procedure and report any findings to the staff in charge.

Functions

The reproductive system is involved in sexual function and human reproduction. The testes produce sperm cells and the male sex hormone testosterone. Sperm cells leave the body in semen.

Age-Related Changes and Important Observations

Table 11-24 lists changes that occur in the reproductive system as a male ages, and Table 11-25 lists signs, symptoms and important observations related to reproductive system problems.

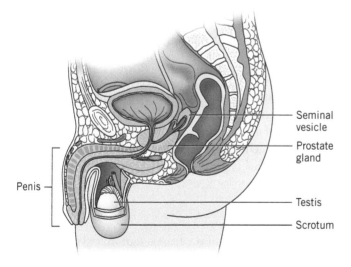

Figure 11-17   Structures of the male reproductive system.

Penis — | — Seminal vesicle
— Prostate gland
— Testis
— Scrotum

Table 11-24 Changes in the Male Reproductive System with Aging

Change	Result
Male hormone production decreases but does not stop.	Possibly decreased sexual response
Prostate gland enlarges.	Mild urinary retention
Testicular tissue mass decreases.	Decreased rate of sperm cell production

Table 11-25 Male Reproductive System Signs, Symptoms, and Observations

Signs and Symptoms	Related Observations to Report
Foul-smelling discharge from penis	▪ When did you first notice this change?
Bleeding or open sores on genitals	▪ When did you first notice this change?
Difficulty starting to urinate	▪ Do I know the resident's normal urinary patterns? ▪ Are they different now? ▪ When did you first notice this change?
Difficulty with sexual intercourse	▪ Do I consider the resident's need for physical intimacy? ▪ Do I consider the resident's need for privacy? ▪ Has the resident been sexually active? ▪ When was this change first experienced?

Common Chronic Diseases and Problems of the Male Reproductive System

Two conditions affecting older males are benign prostatic hyperplasia and prostate cancer.

BPH and Prostate Cancer

Benign prostatic hyperplasia (BPH), also known as benign prostatic hypertrophy, is the enlargement of the prostate gland. This condition is common in men over 50.

According to the Urology Care Foundation, about half of men between the ages of 51 and 60 have BPH, and the condition affects up to 90% of those over 80. Prostate enlargement causes narrowing of the urethra and a weakened bladder, leading to difficulty with urination. BPH can be treated with medication or surgery.

As men age, they are at a greater risk of prostate cancer, the most common non-skin cancer among men in the United States. Most men with this type of cancer are over age 65 and die of causes not related to the cancer because it usually grows slowly and may cause no symptoms. In cases involving fast-growing tumors, treatment options include surgery, radiation, chemotherapy, hormone therapy, and radioactive seed implants.

Signs and Symptoms

- Problems with urination, such as frequent or urgent need to urinate or increased frequency of urination at night
- Weak urine stream, stream that stops and starts, or dribbling at the end of urination
- Difficulty starting urination or straining while urinating
- Inability to completely empty the bladder
- Blood in the urine (less common)
- In physical examination, prostate feels enlarged and has an abnormal shape.

Nurse Assistant's Role in Observation and Intervention

- Identify and report any changes in the male resident's urinary pattern.

Goals of Care

- Help restore the resident to optimal health.
- Support the resident emotionally during treatment.

Interventions or Skills for Care

- Help the resident to the bathroom, especially at night.
- Record the resident's urine pattern and note changes.
- Be available to talk to the resident about any fears or concerns during treatment.

Female Reproductive System

The reproductive system in females is the body system responsible for sexual function and human reproduction. It consists of external and internal *genitalia*. In females, this system includes glands, organs, and structures designed to enable pregnancy and support the growth of a fetus.

Structures

The main structures of the female reproductive system are shown in Figure 11-18:

- The *ovaries* are two almond-shaped glands located in the pelvis. The *fallopian tubes* are two tubular structures connected to the uterus.
- The *uterus* is a muscular organ. During pregnancy, it holds the fetus. The *vagina* is the muscular passage leading from the uterus to the vulva. The *vulva* consists of the external female sex organs. It includes the mons pubis, the labia majora and labia minora, and the clitoris.

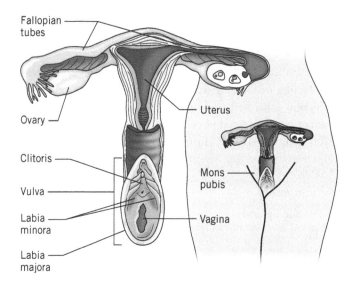

Figure 11-18 Structures of the female reproductive system.

Functions

The reproductive system is involved in sexual function and human reproduction. The ovaries hold the eggs and produce the hormones estrogen and progesterone. Eggs travel from the ovaries to the uterus via the fallopian tubes. The uterus holds the fetus during pregnancy and when a woman is not pregnant, the uterine lining is shed during menstruation.

Age-Related Changes and Important Observations

Table 11-26 lists changes that occur in the reproductive system as a female ages, and Table 11-27 lists signs, symptoms and important observations related to reproductive system problems.

Table 11-26 Changes in the Female Reproductive System with Aging

Change	Result
Dramatic decrease in the amount of hormones produced by the ovaries	Monthly menstrual cycles stop, along with the ability to have children.
Decreased vaginal lubrication	Dryness in vaginal walls

Table 11-27 Female Reproductive System Signs, Symptoms, and Observations

Signs and Symptoms	Related Observations to Report
Foul-smelling discharge from vagina	▪ When did you first notice this change?
Vaginal itching	▪ When did you first notice this change?
Bleeding or open sores on genitals	▪ When did you first notice this change?
Pain or burning with urination	▪ Do I know the resident's normal urinary patterns? ▪ Are they different now? ▪ When did you first notice this change?
Mood changes	▪ Do mood changes affect the resident's interactions with others or her sleep patterns? ▪ When did you first notice this change?
Difficulty with sexual intercourse	▪ Do I consider the resident's need for physical intimacy? ▪ Do I consider the resident's need for privacy? ▪ Has the resident been sexually active? ▪ When was this change first experienced?

Common Chronic Diseases and Problems of the Female Reproductive System

Vaginal infections are a common problem affecting women of all ages.

Vaginal Infections

Bacterial vaginosis (sometimes called vaginal bacteriosis; caused by bacteria) and vaginal yeast infections (caused by yeast overgrowth) are the most common types of vaginal infections.

Signs and Symptoms
- Vaginal discharge and/or odor
- Vaginal itching
- Red, irritated skin around vaginal opening and labia
- Pain when urinating

Nurse Assistant's Role in Observation and Intervention
- Identify any changes such as odor, redness, or irritation.
- Report any signs or symptoms to the charge nurse.

Goals of Care
- Assist with treatment.
- Help relieve the resident's signs and symptoms.

Interventions or Skills for Care
- Give perineal care often to decrease odor.
- Help the nurse administer medication in the vagina.
- Pour warm water over the vaginal area while resident is on the bedpan or toilet. This soothes the irritated, swollen perineal area.

Sexually Transmitted Diseases

Sexually transmitted diseases (STDs) are acquired through sexual activity with an infected partner. This group of diseases includes human papillomavirus (HPV), genital herpes, gonorrhea, chlamydia, and HIV/AIDS. STDs affect both men and women. Sometimes symptoms are present, and sometimes people can be infected and not experience any symptoms.

Common Chronic Diseases and Problems of the Reproductive System

One of the most devastating diseases related to the reproductive system is the human immunodeficiency virus (HIV), which can lead to acquired immune deficiency syndrome (AIDS). While HIV can be transmitted in other ways, the most common way is through sexual contact.

HIV/AIDS

AIDS is a collection of symptoms caused by the human immunodeficiency virus. HIV lives in blood, vaginal fluid, breast milk, and semen. The virus can be transmitted by sharing needles or syringes or through unprotected oral, vaginal, or anal sex. An infected mother may also transmit the virus to her baby before or during birth or after birth through her breast milk. HIV cannot be eliminated from the body, and there is no cure for AIDS. But many drugs are available today that allow HIV-infected people to stay healthier and live longer.

Signs and Symptoms
A person can be infected with HIV for many years without feeling or looking sick. A definitive diagnosis of HIV infection must be based on a blood test. The virus slowly damages the infected person's immune system, leading eventually to AIDS. Common signs and symptoms are:

- Night sweats
- Skin rashes
- Swollen glands
- Fever
- Weight loss
- Diarrhea
- Fatigue

Nurse Assistant's Role in Observation and Intervention
You may care for residents who have HIV and/or AIDS. Because you cannot always know if a resident is HIV-positive (infected with the virus and able to transmit it to others), you must use standard precautions and blood-borne pathogen precautions with every resident.

Goals of Care
- Help relieve the resident's discomfort and alleviate symptoms.
- Provide emotional support.

Interventions or Skills for Care
- Follow standard precautions at all times.
- Teach the resident to follow standard precautions.
- Elevate the head of the bed for a resident with pneumonia.
- Treat all skin conditions as directed by the care plan.
- Always treat the resident with respect and dignity.

- A group of organs and structures that work together to perform certain vital functions are known as a body system.

- The systems of the human body are: integumentary (skin), musculoskeletal, respiratory, circulatory (heart, blood vessels, and lymphatic tissues and vessels), digestive, urinary, nervous (and special senses), endocrine (glands), and reproductive.

- Acute health problems develop rapidly or suddenly and usually last for a limited period of time. Chronic health problems last a long time or recur often.

- Cancer describes a group of diseases characterized by the uncontrolled growth of abnormal cells. Many types of cancer can be treated, so early detection is important.

- The body's immune system responds to an infection with localized, whole-body, and/or silent responses.

- Changes occur in the body's structures with aging, which may lead to changes in function.

- One of your most important responsibilities is to understand, recognize, and report changes that occur in residents under your care. Therefore, you need to know how to recognize signs and symptoms that indicate abnormalities in the body systems.

- Nurse assistants play an important role using interventions and skills to help achieve the resident's goals of care.

- In this chapter you learned about changes that occur to the different body systems as we age. As a nurse assistant it is important to recognize abnormal changes in body functioning and the importance of reporting such changes to a supervisor:

  - Shortness of breath
  - Rapid respiration

- Fever
- Coughs
- Chills
- Pains in chest
- Blue color to lips
- Pain abdomen
- Nausea
- Vomiting
- Drowsiness
- Excessive thirst
- Sweating
- Pus
- Blood or sediment in urine
- Difficulty urinating
- Frequent urination in small amounts
- Pain or burning on urination
- Urine has dark color or strong odor
- Behavioral change
- Talks or communicates less
- Physical appearance/mental health changes
- Participates less in activities or refuses to attend
- Eating less
- Drinking less
- Weight change
- Appears more agitated/nervous
- Appears tired, weak confused or drowsy
- Change in skin color or condition
- Requires more assistance with dressing, toileting, transfers
- Observation for pressure injuries and skin tears

acquired immune deficiency syndrome (AIDS) — group of symptoms caused by the human immunodeficiency virus (HIV)

acute — problem that begins rapidly and lasts for a limited period of time

alveoli — air sacs in the lungs

arteries — blood vessels that carry oxygenated blood to all parts of the body

arthritis — joint inflammation that causes pain and limits movement

benign prostatic hyperplasia (BPH) — enlargement of the prostate gland

body system — group of organs and structures that work together to perform vital functions

bronchi — two main air passageways (right and left) into the lungs; singular form is *bronchus*

bronchioles — branches of each bronchus

cancer — group of diseases characterized by the uncontrolled growth of abnormal cells

capillaries — tiny blood vessels that connect the smallest arteries and veins; the site of gas exchange

cataract — clouding of the lens of the eye that reduces vision

cerebral vascular accident (CVA) — condition that occurs when blood flow to the brain is interrupted; also called a *stroke*

chemotherapy — type of drug therapy used as a treatment for disease, especially cancer

chronic — problem that usually begins gradually and lasts for an extended period of time

chronic obstructive pulmonary disease (COPD) — chronic inflammatory disease of bronchial passages and lungs; three most common types are bronchitis, emphysema, and asthma

circulatory system — body system that includes the heart, blood vessels, and lymphatic tissues and vessels

congestive heart failure (CHF) — condition that occurs when the heart muscle weakens and becomes ineffective in moving blood throughout the body

coronary artery disease (CAD) — condition in which the major blood vessels that supply the heart become damaged or diseased, often due to plaque build-up and/or inflammation

dermatitis — inflammation of the skin

dermis — inner layer of the skin beneath the epidermis

diabetes — disease in which the body either doesn't produce enough insulin or doesn't use insulin properly, resulting in high blood glucose

digestive system — body system involved in processing food, providing nutrients to the body, and expelling waste

edema — swelling of the legs and ankles due to excess fluid in body tissues

endocrine system — body system made up of glands that secrete hormones

epidermis — surface (outer) layer of the skin

fever — elevated body temperature

fracture — break in a bone or other hard tissue

gastroesophageal reflux disease (GERD) — a digestive disorder that occurs when stomach contents leak back into the esophagus

human immunodeficiency virus (HIV) — virus that attacks the body's immune system

hypodermis — layer of fatty tissue beneath the epidermis

inflammation — cellular and tissue response to injury and infection

influenza — viral respiratory infection; also called the *flu*

integumentary system — body system made up of the skin, nails, and hair

latent — in a resting or dormant state

malignant — cancerous tumor or cells that grow uncontrollably and spread to other parts of the body

multiple sclerosis — progressive disease that affects nerve fibers

musculoskeletal system — body system made up of bones, muscles, tendons, ligaments, and joints

nausea — an uneasy or sick feeling in the stomach

nervous system — body system made up of the brain, spinal cord, and nerves

osteoarthritis — degenerative joint disease caused by wear and tear of the joint

osteoporosis — bone disease that involves loss of tissue; bones become weak and brittle and prone to fractures

ovaries — female reproductive glands that secrete sex hormones and produce eggs

Parkinson's disease — neurological disease that affects motor skills

peripheral vascular disease (PVD) — condition that causes diminished blood flow to the extremities

pharynx — tube extending from the back of the nasal passages and mouth to the esophagus

pneumonia — serious bacterial or viral lung infection

prostate cancer — cancer of the prostate gland in males

pus — thick yellowish-white fluid formed in infected tissue

radiation therapy — treatment for cancer or other disease using x-rays or other forms of radiation

reproductive system — body system made up of reproductive organs and glands

respiration — process of breathing in which oxygen is inhaled and carbon dioxide is exhaled

respiratory system — body system that allows for the exchange of oxygen and carbon dioxide in the body

rheumatoid arthritis — autoimmune disease that causes inflammation of the joints

sebaceous glands — microscopic glands in the skin that secrete an oily substance called sebum

sexually transmitted disease (STD) — infectious disease transmitted through sexual contact

special senses — vision, hearing, equilibrium (balance), smell, taste, and touch

sputum — material coughed up from the lungs and expelled through the mouth; contains mucus, cellular debris, microorganisms, and may also contain blood or pus

stroke — condition that occurs when blood flow to the brain is interrupted; also called a *cerebral vascular accident (CVA)*

subcutaneous — under the skin

testes — two oval glands that produce sperm cells and secrete male sex hormones; also called *testicles*

urinary system — body system that helps maintain fluid balance and eliminates liquid waste

veins — blood vessels that carry deoxygenated blood from the body back to the heart and lungs

vomiting — also known as emesis, is when stomach contents exit through the mouth

1. **A condition that begins rapidly and typically lasts 7-10 days until the patient recovers is call a/an:**

   a. Chronic problem
   b. Epidemic
   c. Pandemic
   d. Acute problem

2. **The resident has pneumonia and has fever, difficulty breathing, aches and pains in her chest. This is an example of a/an:**

   a. Whole body response
   b. Absent response
   c. Silent response
   d. Localized response

3. **General characteristics of aging include that it reduces the functioning of the body systems and it happens:**

   a. Gradually
   b. Naturally
   c. To everyone
   d. All of these

4. **A body characteristic that can be observed objectively, like a rash or bruising, is called a:**

   a. Sign
   b. Symptom
   c. Diagnosis
   d. Pre-diagnosis

5. **Which of the following is a cancer warning sign?**

   a. Nagging cough or hoarseness
   b. Gradual weight gain
   c. Irritability in the morning
   d. A good appetite

6. **Early detection of cancer is important because:**

   a. Insurance may not pay for treatment of advanced cancer
   b. The resident needs time to adjust to having cancer
   c. Hair loss is greater later on
   d. The cancer may spread to other parts of the body and be more difficult to treat

7. **The function of the endocrine system is to:**

   a. Prevent germs in the environment from entering the body
   b. Produce hormones that help the body work properly
   c. Eliminate waste materials from the body
   d. Carry vital nourishment to all cells of the body

8. **Which of the following happens because of nervous system changes as we age?**

   a. Decreased short-term memory
   b. Slowing of respirations
   c. Slowing of heartbeat
   d. Decreased insulin production

9. **A tumor or condition that tends to spread abnormal cells throughout the body is called:**

   a. Benign
   b. Inconsequential
   c. Malignant
   d. Acute

10. **Swelling due to fluid gain, most commonly observed in the legs and ankles is called:**

    a. Blockage
    b. Constipation
    c. Thrombosis
    d. Edema

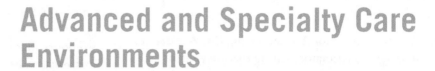

12

Advanced and Specialty Care Environments

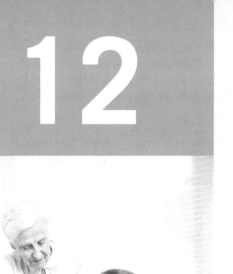

Nurse assistants care for residents in a variety of settings, and each environment requires specific approaches to care. Regardless of the setting, your primary goal is always to provide excellent care while maintaining the resident's quality of life. This chapter introduces you to providing care in environments such as assisted living facilities and post-acute care units. You will also learn about caring for residents with Alzheimer's disease and those who are intellectually or developmentally disabled. Special needs require special skills, and this chapter is devoted to the unique needs of these populations.

OBJECTIVES:

- Explain your role in caring for diabetic residents.

- Describe various methods used for oxygen delivery and your role in oxygen administration.

- List the signs and symptoms to observe and report when a resident is receiving dialysis.

- List types of hot and cold applications and the purposes of each.

- Explain your role in preoperative and postoperative care of residents undergoing surgery.

- Define developmental and intellectual disabilities.

- Describe your role in caring for residents who are developmentally disabled.

- Name five symptoms associated with each stage of Alzheimer's disease.

- State six principles that should guide your care of residents with

Alzheimer's disease and related disorders.

- List techniques used to responding to residents' behavioral symptoms.

- Explain your role in helping residents with Alzheimer's and related disorders with activities of daily living.

- Define mental health disorders and provide examples.

- List symptoms of substance abuse disorder.

Assisted Living

The National Center for Assisted Living (NCAL) defines *assisted living* as a residential setting that provides or coordinates personal care services, 24-hour supervision, scheduled and unscheduled assistance, activities, and health-related services. Assisted living facilities are designed to enable residents to live in a more home-like environment while accommodating individuals' changing needs. The goal is to provide assistance while maximizing residents' dignity, autonomy, privacy, independence, choice, and safety.

Many assisted living facilities employ nurse assistants. In this role, you may be called a personal care attendant or direct care staff member. You may work directly for the assisted living facility or for an agency that provides services to the facility.

Post-Acute Care

As health care has evolved, it became clear that there was a need for a new kind of service to provide care to patients after they left the hospital but before they could go home or to a long term care facility. This service is called post-acute, short-stay, or rehab care. As you learned in Chapter 1, a post-acute care unit or facility provides a higher level of care than is typically given in a long term care facility but a lower level of care than a hospital. The resident usually needs this care only for a short period of time, generally less than 30 days.

As a nurse assistant, you may work on a post-acute floor or unit that provides care for people with serious complications from diabetes, kidney disease, or respiratory or gastrointestinal problems. It is important for you to understand the impact these conditions have on the resident physically, psychologically, and socially.

Care of Residents with Diabetes

In chapter 11, you learned how the endocrine system breaks down carbohydrates (sugars) in the body. With diabetes, either the pancreas does not produce enough insulin or the body does not use insulin properly. Insulin controls how the body uses carbohydrates, which include sugar and starches. When insulin cannot do its job correctly, a person's blood sugar level may become either too low, a condition known as hypoglycemia, or too high, which is hyperglycemia.

The most common way to test a person's blood sugar level is to do a finger-prick test using a glucose meter (see Procedure 11-4). A fasting blood sugar (FBS) blood sample is taken after a person has not eaten for at least eight hours. A blood glucose test may also be performed two hours after eating a meal or at a random time. You may assist in these ways:

- Make sure the resident does not eat during the time prescribed before the test. Sips of water are allowed.
- Encourage the resident not to smoke. Smoking may affect the test results.
- For a random blood glucose test, note the time and content of the last meal.
- Listen to and talk with the resident about any concerns they have.

A person with diabetes is at risk for problems with their feet. Problems may include pressure injuries due to poor circulation, an inability to feel pain due to peripheral neuropathy (nerve endings are damaged), and susceptibility to infection. When giving foot care (Procedure 12-1), be sure to inspect, wash, and dry the feet thoroughly. Apply moisturizing lotion but not between the toes.

Care of Residents Needing Oxygen Therapy

Recall that the major function of the respiratory system is to deliver oxygen to the body's cells and remove carbon dioxide. Many residents need oxygen therapy, which involves giving them higher concentrations of oxygen than exist in the air. You may be asked to assist with the setup and to provide support to a resident receiving oxygen therapy. Oxygen is used to treat or prevent symptoms of respiratory distress. These symptoms can be caused by:

- Inability to inhale enough oxygen into the body
- Inability of the lungs or circulatory system to use oxygen
- Inability of the lungs to exhale or remove enough carbon dioxide

If the lungs or circulatory system cannot provide enough oxygen to cells, this condition is called hypoxia. A person experiencing hypoxia may have any of these signs and symptoms:

- Rapid breathing
- Fatigue
- Anxiety or restlessness
- Dizziness or confusion

12-1: Diabetic Foot Care

PREPARATION STEPS

1. Check the care plan.
2. Knock, introduce yourself, and address resident by preferred name.
3. Perform hand hygiene.
4. Gather supplies and secure assistance if needed.
5. Explain procedure and ask about resident preferences.
6. Respect privacy and rights at all times.

ITEMS NEEDED

- Basin of warm water
- Washcloth
- Nondrying soap
- Towel

1. Inspect the feet daily. Report to the nurse any calluses, corns, blisters, abrasions, redness, or nail abnormalities.

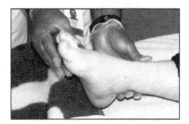

2. Wash the feet in warm water, using nondrying soap.

3. Dry thoroughly between the toes to prevent skin breakdown. Lotion the tops and bottoms of the feet, do not put lotion between toes.

4. Be sure the person wears well-fitting shoes and socks to prevent pressure on the feet.

5. Inspect the inside of shoes for foreign objects or areas of roughness.

6. Report any injury to the nurse immediately.

COMPLETION STEPS

1. Determine the resident's preferred position for comfort and ask them if they need anything else.
2. Examine the environment for safety and cleanliness.
3. Secure the call light and any other needed items within reach of the resident.
4. Perform hand hygiene.
5. Document the procedure and report any findings to the staff in charge.

- Cyanosis (bluish tint of lips, nailbeds, tongue, or other parts of the body)
- Unconsciousness

Unless treated, continuing severe hypoxia will lead to death. A person may have a temporary or chronic condition that causes respiratory distress and/or hypoxia. Temporary conditions include a broken rib, heart attack, severe anemia, unconsciousness, pneumonia or other respiratory condition, and recent surgery to nose, mouth, neck, chest, back, or abdominal area.

Chronic conditions include asthma, chronic obstructive pulmonary disease (COPD), and congestive heart failure.

Administering Oxygen Therapy

Oxygen therapy may be given using a piped-in system or oxygen concentrator. In emergency situations, oxygen may also be given from a cylinder (tank). In home care or transport situations, oxygen may be supplied from liquid oxygen in a cylinder. Oxygen can be administered via a nasal cannula, face mask, or an airway (Figure 12-1). Table 12-1 describes various oxygen delivery methods. A patient on a mechanical ventilator may also receive oxygen directly. The method of oxygen administration depends on the physician's orders. Procedure 12-2 outlines the steps involved in administering oxygen by nasal cannula, and Procedure 12-3 shows how to administer it using a face mask.

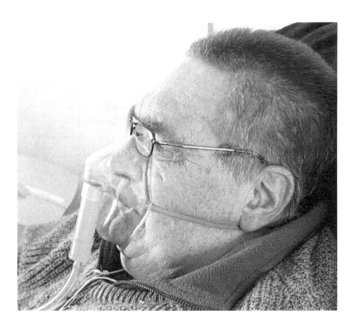

Figure 12-1 The face mask is one of several oxygen delivery devices.

Table 12-1 Oxygen Delivery Devices

Device	Description
Nasal cannula	A two-pronged tube. The prongs are carefully inserted into the person's nostrils and secured in place by wrapping the tubing around the ears and adjusting the tubing under the chin. This method can be used only if the person is able to, and does, breathe through his/her nose. It cannot be used if the person is a "mouth breather." It delivers a low oxygen concentration.
	Note: observe the nostrils and ears often and carefully for signs of pressure. Remove and reapply or reposition the cannula and ear tubing every two hours.
Face mask	This mask covers the person's entire nose and mouth. Holes in the mask allow exhaled carbon dioxide to escape. It can deliver a higher oxygen concentration.
Venturi mask (or venti-mask)	This mask allows an exact amount of oxygen to be delivered, using color-coded adaptors.
Partial rebreather mask	This face mask traps part of the exhaled carbon dioxide in a bag attached to the mask. It has valves that allow a mix of exhaled carbon dioxide and oxygen to be inhaled to stimulate normal breathing.
	Note: always be sure that the bag is inflated.

Device	Description
Non rebreather mask	This face mask allows only administered oxygen to be inhaled. Valves in the mask prevent room air from mixing with the oxygen. This mask also has a bag.
	Note: Always be sure that the mask fits securely to the person's face. Always be sure that the bag is inflated.

Positioning for Easier Breathing

Positioning the resident with the head elevated can help them breathe more easily and get more oxygen. Many people who are having difficulty breathing are more comfortable in a semi-Fowler's or Fowler's position (see Chapter 8). Some residents may also feel better sitting up with their head resting over the bed table (Figure 12-2). Place a pillow under the head for comfort. Encourage the person to change position frequently to prevent secretions from pooling in any one area of the lungs. Pooled secretions can cause an infection. Some residents may breathe easier if positioned on their side. The care plan should indicate the correct positioning for easier and more effective breathing.

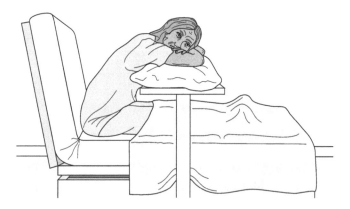

Figure 12-2 For some residents with respiratory difficulties, sitting with the head bent forward over the table allows for easier breathing.

Other measures used to help residents with respiratory problems include deep-breathing exercises (Procedure 12-4), assisting with deep breathing and coughing (Procedure 12-5), and deep-breathing exercises using an incentive spirometer (Procedure 12-6).

Artificial Airway and Mechanical Ventilation

You may at some time care for a resident with an artificial airway or one who is on a mechanical ventilator.

PREPARATION STEPS

1. Check the care plan.
2. Knock, introduce yourself, and address resident by preferred name.
3. Perform hand hygiene.
4. Gather supplies and secure assistance if needed.
5. Explain procedure and ask about resident preferences.
6. Respect privacy and rights at all times.

ITEMS NEEDED

- No-smoking signs
- Humidification container
- Distilled water
- Nasal cannula tubing
- Flow meter (if not already present)

1 Post no-smoking signs.

2 If ordered, fill the humidifier to the appropriate level.

3 Attach the connecting tube from the nasal cannula to the humidifier.

4 The nurse will set the flow rate at the prescribed liters per minute.

5 Assist the nurse in placing the tips of the cannula in the person's nose, and adjust the straps around ears for a snug, comfortable fit.

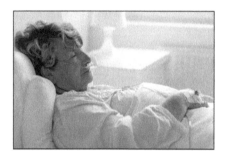

COMPLETION STEPS

1. Determine the resident's preferred position for comfort and ask them if they need anything else.
2. Examine the environment for safety and cleanliness.
3. Secure the call light and any other needed items within reach of the resident.
4. Perform hand hygiene.
5. Document the procedure and report any findings to the staff in charge.

An artificial airway is a tube that enters the person's respiratory system. Some patients may have an artificial airway but not require a mechanical ventilator or oxygen therapy. In other situations, the artificial airway allows the mechanical ventilator to deliver oxygen directly to the respiratory system. A person may need mechanical ventilation assistance because of a temporary or permanent condition such as:

- Acute respiratory failure
- Central nervous system depression with lack of consciousness or an inability for the body to trigger normal respiration
- Neuromuscular disease
- Pulmonary disease
- Upper airway obstruction caused by a tumor, inflammation, or foreign body
- Trauma to the respiratory system

The most common types of artificial airways are an oropharyngeal tube (placed through the mouth into the pharynx), endotracheal tube (placed through the mouth or nose into the trachea), and the tracheostomy tube (placed directly into the trachea through a surgical opening in the person's neck). You will not be responsible for the direct care of an artificial airway, but you must report to the nurse any abnormal or unusual situations, such as:

- The tube falls out, is pulled out, or is disconnected, or an alarm sounds.
- You hear gurgling sounds, indicating the need for suctioning.
- Any redness or discharge is present around the tube.
- The person seems restless or acts or moves differently (thrashing of limbs, attempts to pull out the tube, rapid eye movements, or other actions).

12-3: Administering Oxygen by Simple Face Mask

PREPARATION STEPS

1. Check the care plan.
2. Knock, introduce yourself, and address resident by preferred name.
3. Perform hand hygiene.
4. Gather supplies and secure assistance if needed.
5. Explain procedure and ask about resident preferences.
6. Respect privacy and rights at all times.

ITEMS NEEDED

- No-smoking signs
- Humidification container
- Distilled water
- Face mask and tubing (per orders)
- Flow meter for the wall if not already available

1 Post no-smoking signs.

2 If ordered, fill the humidifier to the appropriate level.

3 The nurse will adjust the flow meter.

4 Assist the nurse in placing the mask on the person's face and adjusting the straps so the mask fits securely.

5 If the tubing fills with water, drain the tubing by emptying the water. Do not drain it back into the humidifier.

6 If a heating element is used, check the temperature. The humidifier bottle should be warm, not hot, to the touch.

COMPLETION STEPS

1. Determine the resident's preferred position for comfort and ask them if they need anything else.
2. Examine the environment for safety and cleanliness.
3. Secure the call light and any other needed items within reach of the resident.
4. Perform hand hygiene.
5. Document the procedure and report any findings to the staff in charge.

The presence of a tracheostomy or the need for mechanical ventilator assistance does not necessarily mean that the resident cannot understand others or does not have a need to communicate. Always do your job as if the person understands everything, helping the person communicate with you. Offer pen and paper, a communication board, flashcards, chalk, or dry eraser board — anything to help the person communicate their needs, problems, and concerns.

Although a person with an artificial airway cannot talk normally, many people with tracheostomies have learned how to "plug" the tracheostomy and speak. Others learn to use ancillary muscles to speak with an amplifying device.

Care of Residents Receiving Dialysis

If a person develops chronic kidney disease or acute renal failure, the kidneys are not working properly or are not

functioning at all. When this occurs, the kidneys cannot filter and remove extra fluid and waste from the body. **Dialysis** is a form of artificial filtration of the blood. It is a temporary solution while the person waits for kidney function to return, if this is possible, or for a kidney transplant. The two methods used are peritoneal dialysis and hemodialysis. The physician decides which method is best for an individual.

Peritoneal Dialysis

There are three types of **peritoneal dialysis:**

- Continuous ambulatory peritoneal dialysis (CAPD) — the most common type.
- Continuous cycling peritoneal dialysis (CCPD)
- Intermittent peritoneal dialysis (IPD)

The most common problems or complications that occur with peritoneal dialysis are infection around the

PREPARATION STEPS

1. Check the care plan.
2. Knock, introduce yourself, and address resident by preferred name.
3. Perform hand hygiene.
4. Gather supplies and secure assistance if needed.
5. Explain procedure and ask about resident preferences.
6. Respect privacy and rights at all times.

ITEMS NEEDED

- Pillow for splinting (support for a painful site) if needed

It may take several sessions for a person to successfully perform diaphragmatic breathing. A resident with cognitive impairment may require slow and repetitive instruction or may not be able to perform this type of breathing.

1 Have the person place one hand on the abdomen and the other hand on the middle of the chest. If the person is not able, ask if you can place your hand on their abdomen.

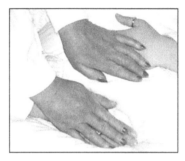

2 Have the person inhale (breathe in) slowly and deeply through the nose for a count of two while extending the abdomen as far as they can. You can help by counting out loud: one, two. You should be able to see, and the person should be able to feel, the abdomen push the hand outward.

3 Then have the person exhale (breathe out) through pursed or partially closed lips for a count of four while tightening their abdominal muscles. You can help by counting out loud: one, two, three, four. You should be able to see, and the person should be able to feel, the abdomen move inward.

4 With this type of breathing, you should be able to see and the person should be able to feel only movement of the abdomen (no chest movement).

COMPLETION STEPS

1. Determine the resident's preferred position for comfort and ask them if they need anything else.
2. Examine the environment for safety and cleanliness.
3. Secure the call light and any other needed items within reach of the resident.
4. Perform hand hygiene.
5. Document the procedure and report any findings to the staff in charge.

---

catheter site or inside the peritoneal cavity (peritonitis). It is important for you to watch for signs of infection and report them immediately. Your responsibilities will include measuring the person's weight before and after dialysis and taking and recording vital signs as ordered by the physician. You must notify the nurse immediately if there are any changes. Other important signs and symptoms to observe and report are:

- Redness, bleeding, or drainage around the catheter site
- Leaking fluid around the catheter site
- Catheter tubing that is twisted, kinked, or disconnected
- Catheter site pain or complaints of abdominal pain
- Blood in the drainage fluid
- Fluid not draining properly
- Complaints of feeling dizzy or lightheaded
- Abnormal abdominal distention
- Shortness of breath and/or chest pain
- Behavior changes such as becoming withdrawn, depressed, and/or refusing to talk

PROCEDURE

12-5: Assisting with Deep Breathing and Coughing

PREPARATION STEPS

1. Check the care plan.
2. Knock, introduce yourself, and address resident by preferred name.
3. Perform hand hygiene.
4. Gather supplies and secure assistance if needed.
5. Explain procedure and ask about resident preferences.
6. Respect privacy and rights at all times.

ITEMS NEEDED

- Pillow or splint
- Tissue
- Emesis basin
- Gloves

1 Explain that after surgery a person needs to take deep breaths and cough. This helps to remove anesthesia and prevent the accumulation of lung secretions. Coughing and deep breathing are also important for someone who has been on bed rest for a period of time.

2 When ready, ask them to take at least four diaphragmatic breaths as described in Procedure 12-4.

3 Put on gloves.

4 Elevate the head of the bed as much as the resident can tolerate.

5 Tell (or show) them how to hold a pillow or splint over the surgical site.

6 While holding the pillow, ask them to take a deep breath, hold it for three seconds, and then exhale. Repeat this at least five times, if the person is able. With the last two deep breaths, encourage them to take a deep breath and cough as hard as possible while you hold the emesis basin to catch any sputum.

7 Clean up any secretions using tissues and the emesis basin. Note the color and consistency of secretions. Report your findings to the nurse.

8 Instruct the person to continue the deep breathing and coughing exercises once each hour.

COMPLETION STEPS

1. Determine the resident's preferred position for comfort and ask them if they need anything else.
2. Examine the environment for safety and cleanliness.
3. Secure the call light and any other needed items within reach of the resident.
4. Perform hand hygiene.
5. Document the procedure and report any findings to the staff in charge.

Hemodialysis

Three access methods are used for hemodialysis:

- A venous catheter is a tube placed in the neck, chest, or groin. This type of catheter is usually used until a permanent access is placed.
- A fistula is the most common and most durable access site. The fistula is created by making a surgical connection of an artery to a vein in the lower forearm. It can take six to 12 weeks for the fistula to form.
- A graft is a tube implanted under the skin of the arm. The tube becomes an artificial vein that can be accessed within a week for hemodialysis.

Your role may include assisting a resident to and from a dialysis center and caring for them between sessions. The most common problems that occur with hemodialysis are:

- Low blood pressure
- Muscle cramps
- Nausea and vomiting
- Infection at the surgical site
- Blood clots

A person on hemodialysis may have food and fluid restrictions related to amounts of protein, sodium,

PREPARATION STEPS

1. Check the care plan.
2. Knock, introduce yourself, and address resident by preferred name.
3. Perform hand hygiene.
4. Gather supplies and secure assistance if needed.
5. Explain procedure and ask about resident preferences.
6. Respect privacy and rights at all times.

ITEMS NEEDED

- Pillow for splinting (if needed)
- Incentive spirometer
- Alcohol wipe

If the resident has had surgery, this procedure should be done approximately 30 minutes after the administration of pain medication. You should communicate with the nurse to ensure that medication times are coordinated with this procedure.

1. Clean the spirometer mouthpiece using disposable alcohol wipe.

2. Place the patient in a comfortable sitting or semi-Fowler's position. Place the pillow on top of the incision to splint it, if necessary.

3. Set the spirometer according to instructions provided by the nurse or as noted in the orders or care plan.

4. Instruct the person to exhale fully, place the mouthpiece into the mouth, and keep the lips sealed tightly around the mouthpiece.

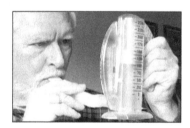

5. Direct the resident to inhale (breathe in) slowly and deeply, trying to reach the goal by watching the ball move up in the spirometer tube.

6. When the goal is reached, or if the ball will move upward no further, the person should hold the breath for three seconds, remove the mouthpiece, relax, and exhale (breathe out).

7. Encourage the person to cough, and praise their results.

8. Notify the nurse if the resident was not able to reach their spirometer goals.

COMPLETION STEPS

1. Determine the resident's preferred position for comfort and ask them if they need anything else.
2. Examine the environment for safety and cleanliness.
3. Secure the call light and any other needed items within reach of the resident.
4. Perform hand hygiene.
5. Document the procedure and report any findings to the staff in charge.

potassium, calcium, and phosphorus. The physician will determine how much fluid can be taken in a 24-hour period. You will take vital signs and weight measurements before and after treatments and monitor for changes. Blood pressure must never be taken in the arm used for dialysis. You must also monitor, measure, and record the person's fluid and food intake and output. Important signs and symptoms to observe and report are:

- Redness, bleeding, or drainage (pus) around the surgical site
- Complaints of pain at the fistula or graft site
- Changes in fluid and food intake and output
- Complaints of feeling dizzy, lightheaded, or unsteady when walking
- Swelling in the feet, legs, or other areas of the body
- Complaints of nausea, vomiting, and/or muscle cramps
- Shortness of breath or chest pain
- Behavior changes such as becoming withdrawn, depressed, and/or refusing to talk

Hot and Cold Applications

Hot and cold applications are used for treating specific conditions when ordered by the resident's physician. Heat or cold may be applied to the entire body for a general effect. More often, the application is ordered for a specific body area. Heat and cold may be applied either in either dry or moist form, depending on the physician's orders.

Heat

Moist heat applications involve placing warm moisture in direct contact with the skin. Moist heat works faster than dry heat. Sitz baths provide moist heat to the genitals or anal area. Tub baths provide moist heat to the whole body, and soaks provide moist heat to a specific area.

Hot, moist compresses using a cloth or disposable pack provide moist heat to a specific limb or body area. *Dry heat* can be applied using a hot water bottle or electric heat pad to a specific body area.

Before using a heat application, check with the nurse, make sure you understand all instructions, and follow these guidelines:

- Make sure that you know how to properly use the heat device or equipment.
- Never place an electric heating device over a wet dressing or compress. This could cause a burn because the moist heat may become too hot and intense. Using an electric device around moisture also increases the risk of electrical shock.
- Heat application should remain at the correct temperature the whole time. If the application becomes too cool, it won't have the desired effect.

Cold

Like hot applications, cold applications can be used body-wide (generalized) or on a specific area. Note that when a generalized cold application is used, there is a risk of shock caused by a sudden drop in blood flow in the body due to vasoconstriction (narrowing of blood vessels). Cold applications are used to:

- Reduce pain and swelling in an area.
- Help control bleeding. Bleeding is reduced or stopped because the cold constricts the blood vessels.
- Reduce sensitivity to pain by numbing the area.
- Help lower body temperature (as in the case of a fever).

Moist cold applications include cold compresses and disposable packs containing cooling solutions or alcohol sponge baths. *Dry cold* applications include ice packs and ice cubes inside bags or collars (special rubber collars that can be filled with ice). Before using a cold application, follow the care plan and consult the nurse for any special instructions and if you have questions.

Care of Residents Having Surgery

It is natural for a resident to experience some apprehension or fear about an upcoming surgical procedure. Report any signs of fear or anxiety to the health care team. An appropriate team member can help the person talk about and understand their fears and anxiety. Residents need to feel that they have adequate information and understand what will happen. If a resident asks you specific questions about the actual procedure, refer these questions to the nurse or surgeon.

Preoperative Care

The time period before the surgery is called the preoperative (pre-op) phase. Knowing the resident's baseline mental status before surgery is important. The trauma of surgery, medications, and anesthesia can have side effects that may alter a person's mental status. Knowing the patient's baseline status helps the health care team understand if abnormal changes occur after surgery.

Preoperative teaching involves providing the resident (and often the family) with information about what will happen before, during, and after the surgery. The nurse will explain the purpose of pre-op blood tests and other tests such as an EKG. Usually, the patient cannot have anything to eat or drink after midnight before surgery. This is called NPO, a medical order taken from the Latin phrase *nil per os,* which means "nothing by mouth." The nurse also explains what happens after the surgery.

Your role in the preoperative phase includes reinforcing the pre-op teaching and listening to the resident's concerns. Direct any questions about the surgery to the nurse. The resident will have a lot to remember and will look to you for added support.

The nurse assistant role may also include:

- Assisting with specimen collection for pre-op testing.
- Making sure that the person does not eat any food or drink anything after the specified time.
- Assisting with personal care, such as removing jewelry, nail polish, or makeup, bathing, and/or removing and taking care of dentures, hearing aids, eyeglasses, hair care items, or a prosthesis.
- Assisting in pre-op preparations, such as giving an enema before bowel surgery, cleansing the body area

with a special soap to help remove bacteria, and/or shaving the surgical area.

- Offering to call a clergy member to provide spiritual support.
- Helping the resident feel safe and comfortable.
- Assisting the nurse with checking that all the tasks on the preoperative checklist have been completed.
- Assisting the nurse with checking that all information is present in the resident's chart before surgery.
- Documenting and reporting the person's mental status prior to the surgery.

Following your facility's policy to safeguard the resident's personal belongings while they are in surgery.

Shaving the Surgical Site

The surgical site will need to be shaved for certain surgeries (Procedure 12-7). Shaving is usually done right before surgery. Before shaving the site, make sure you understand what type of surgery will be performed and the exact area to shave. Note any skin redness, moles, cuts, or any other skin issues at the prep site.

Postoperative Care

The time after the surgery is called the **postoperative** (post-op) phase. Immediately after surgery, the patient is transported to the recovery room, also known as the post-anesthesia care unit (PACU). The patient is brought to the PACU by operating room staff, and nursing care is provided here until the person is stable and awake. The

---

PROCEDURE

12-7: Shaving the Surgical Site

PREPARATION STEPS

1. Check the care plan.
2. Knock, introduce yourself, and address resident by preferred name.
3. Perform hand hygiene.
4. Gather supplies and secure assistance if needed.
5. Explain procedure and ask about resident preferences.
6. Respect privacy and rights at all times.

ITEMS NEEDED

- Gloves
- Washcloth
- Towel
- Basin filled with warm water
- Soap
- Plastic-covered pad
- Prep kit or disposable razor
- Bath blanket

Ask for help before beginning if you are unsure how to shave a surgical site.

1. Raise the bed to a good working height.

2. Assist the resident to a comfortable position.

3. Cover the person with the bath blanket. Fold the bed linens to the bottom of the bed.

4. Place the plastic-covered pad under the person. Remove clothing to expose only the surgical prep area.

5. Put on gloves.

6. Wash and lather the surgical prep site with warm water and soap, or use the surgical prep cleansing solution to clean the skin.

7. Hold the skin taut with one hand. With the other hand hold the razor at a 45-degree angle to shave the hair in the area of the surgical site. Shave in the direction of hair growth using short strokes. Be careful not to cut the skin or remove moles on the skin. If using an electric razor, gently move it over the area.

8. Wipe the skin with the washcloth to remove any remaining soap or lather. Dry the skin thoroughly.

COMPLETION STEPS

1. Determine the resident's preferred position for comfort and ask them if they need anything else.
2. Examine the environment for safety and cleanliness.
3. Secure the call light and any other needed items within reach of the resident.
4. Perform hand hygiene.
5. Document the procedure and report any findings to the staff in charge.

information provided by the PACU nurse is important and guides the resident's postoperative care.

A full report is given to the health care team, including:

- What surgery was done
- How the patient is doing
- Vital signs and urine output
- Any complications or anything unusual that happened during surgery
- Medications used for anesthesia
- Placement of any tubes or drains during surgery
- Administration of intravenous fluids
- Dressings present
- Any need for oxygen
- Other pertinent information

Your role is to assist the nurse with post-op care. Your tasks include:

- Taking vital signs as ordered and reporting any changes immediately to the nurse.
- Helping the person to a comfortable position and to change positions often (if allowed).
- Observing for mental status changes.
- Being alert to common conditions that occur after surgery, such as nausea, vomiting, gas pains, constipation, dry mouth, and postoperative pain.
- Helping to prevent nausea and vomiting by eliminating odors from the person's room, offering small sips of fluid if ordered, and encouraging deep breathing to help rid the effects of anesthesia. If vomiting occurs, offer an emesis basin, provide mouth care, change the sheets quickly to get the odor out of the room, and report the vomiting to the nurse.
- Helping to decrease gas and constipation by encouraging the person to move in bed and walk as soon as ordered by the surgeon. Often, assisting with walking a few steps is ordered just hours after surgery. Early ambulation helps gas move out, prevents constipation, and increases circulation.
- Offering sips of water or ice chips if ordered and providing mouth care to reduce dry mouth. When ordered by the surgeon, encourage the person to drink fluids to prevent dry mouth, to stay well hydrated, and to prevent constipation.
- Reporting any signs of pain immediately.

- Helping the resident with their ordered rehabilitation program.
- Helping the resident with personal care as needed. After surgery, the person often needs help with bathing and grooming. Since many surgical patients did not need this help previously, respect their feelings and provide privacy.
- Encouraging good nutrition, following the surgeon's orders.
- Always using standard precautions when handling any dressing or providing care.
- Observing for any signs of infection like redness, swelling, drainage, and odor at the wound site.
- Reporting observations to the nurse.
- Assisting with the use of elastic stockings (see Procedure 9-2) or other compression device, if ordered.

Sequential Compression Devices

Like elastic stockings, sequential compression devices are used postoperatively to increase blood flow and decrease the risk of blood clot formation. These devices can be used alone or with elastic stockings. There are many different types, so it is important to always read the directions before using them. The sleeves come in various sizes. The sleeve is attached to a pump that inflates and deflates the sleeve in a sequential motion. It is important that the sleeve is not too tight on the person's leg. You should be able to put two fingers between the sleeve and the leg. When the device is running, frequently check the toes for color, sensation, mobility, and warmth.

Deep Breathing and Coughing

Encourage deep breathing and coughing often to prevent post-op complications (see Procedure 12-5). The nurse will teach the resident to splint the wound with a pillow when coughing or moving. The surgeon may have the respiratory therapy department teach the use of a respiratory breathing exercise device such as, an incentive spirometer, to prevent postoperative breathing complications. Once the respiratory therapist has taught the resident how to use the device, you may assist (see Procedure 12-6) and remind them to perform the exercises. Make sure that you know how to properly use the device before providing assistance.

Care of Residents Who Are Developmentally Disabled

A **developmental disability** is a condition caused by a physical or mental impairment that affects language, learning, mobility, and the ability to perform activities of daily living. These disabilities are generally permanent conditions. You may work in a facility that provides care for residents who are developmentally disabled. These residents vary in age from the very young to the elderly.

Many people with developmental disabilities live in the community. Some people with developmental disabilities need very little assistance even though others need many services. They may live in their own home or apartment or in a shared living arrangement such as a group home, congregate housing, or an apartment with a roommate. A group home is a house where usually six or fewer individuals live together, usually with 24-hour support. Congregate housing is a managed home environment with some support services. Residents have their own space within the building for sleeping and eating. Congregate housing includes common rooms where residents can meet to watch television, eat, or socialize. Some individuals live and work in the community and need only limited services. Others live in long term care facilities.

The *habilitation model* of caregiving is used with residents with developmental disabilities. This is based on a principle known as *normalization*. Normalization involves creating an environment for individuals that is as close as possible to a normal environment. Caregiving emphasizes the resident's positive qualities and strengths rather focusing on weaknesses.

The goal of care is based on a philosophy of "person-centered" planning. An individualized habilitation plan, also called an individual service plan, is developed for each resident. This plan provides for special accommodations and sets the priorities of care for the resident. This approach encourages the resident to participate as fully as possible in all aspects of their life. This includes their family, community, and social life. Many people with developmental disabilities successfully meet their individual goals with the help of caring people, organizations, and facilities.

As a caregiver for a resident with a developmental disability, your main responsibility is to give guidance and support and help the resident function as independently as possible. You become a coach who helps them maximize their potential. Your role is to give them whatever help they need while allowing them do as much for themselves as they can.

Some conditions that cause developmental disability are Down syndrome, autism spectrum disorder (ASD), and cerebral palsy (CP). These are described in the following sections.

Intellectual Disability

According to the American Association on Intellectual and Developmental Disabilities (AAIDD), *intellectual disability* is a disability characterized by significant limitations in both **intellectual functioning** and in **adaptive behavior,** which covers many everyday social and practical skills. This disability originates **before the age of 22**. Adaptive behaviors include communication skills, skills used in the activities of daily living, social skills, and other skills used for leisure activities, health and safety, self-direction, basic literacy (reading, writing, and math), and involvement in the community and work.

Intellectual disability can be caused by hundreds of things. Any condition that damages the brain before birth, during birth, or during childhood can result in intellectual disability. Some common causes are listed in Box 12-1.

BOX 12-1

COMMON CAUSES OF INTELLECTUAL DISABILITY

- Down syndrome
- Fetal alcohol syndrome, caused by the mother's alcohol intake during pregnancy
- Fragile X syndrome: a genetic disorder and the most common hereditary cause of intellectual disability
- Problems or maternal habits during pregnancy, such as drug use, smoking, malnutrition, and certain infections such as rubella or syphilis
- Problems after birth, such as certain childhood diseases (whooping cough, measles, or chicken pox, for example), injuries (such as a blow to the head or a near drowning), or lead or mercury poisoning
- Problems resulting from malnutrition, inadequate medical care, or environmental hazards
- Cultural deprivation such as under-stimulation, which can result in irreversible damage

New methods are continually being developed to help prevent some of the causes, such as giving newborn screening tests, prescribing vitamins during pregnancy, using vaccines to prevent childhood illness, removing lead from the environment, using child safety seats and bicycle helmets, participating in early intervention programs for children, and administering other treatments to women before and during pregnancy.

Down Syndrome

Down syndrome, also known as trisomy 21, is a genetic disorder caused by the presence of all or part of a third copy of chromosome 21. It is usually associated with physical growth delays and mild to moderate intellectual disability. According to the CDC, Down syndrome is the most common chromosomal condition in the United States, occurring in about one in 700 births. The cause is not known, but women 35 years of age and older have a higher chance of having a baby with Down syndrome.

Common physical characteristics:

- A flattened face, especially the bridge of the nose
- Almond-shaped eyes that slant up
- A short neck
- Small ears
- A protruding tongue
- Poor muscle tone
- Small hands and feet

Individuals with Down syndrome need the same kinds of preventive health care and medical care as everyone else. In addition, they generally have problems requiring special attention. These problems include the following:

- hearing problems
- gastrointestinal problems
- eye problems
- heart problems

Autism Spectrum Disorder

Autism Spectrum Disorder (ASD) is a disorder that affects a person's ability to communicate and interact with others. ASD can vary greatly in severity from person to person: Some cases are relatively mild; others can be severe.

Some characteristics of ASD may include:

- repetitive actions or behaviors
- avoiding eye contact
- doesn't point at objects
- difficulty understanding what others are saying

- appears unaware when people are talking with to them
- unable to have a back-and-forth communication

The causes of ASD are still not known. There is no cure, but according to the CDC, research has shown that early treatment can improve a child's development.

Cerebral Palsy

Cerebral palsy (CP) is a disorder that affects movement and posture. It is caused by abnormal development or damage to the brain that occurs before, during, or after birth. The symptoms can vary greatly from person to person, ranging from mild to severe, where the person is unable to walk.

Additional common problems include the following:

- seizures
- speech, vision, and hearing problems
- intellectual disabilities
- language problems
- joint problems

There is no cure for cerebral palsy, but treatment can help children and adults reach their full potential. The treatment of cerebral palsy can include therapy and the use of braces, splints, and special appliances to help those affected perform activities as independently as possible. Range-of-motion exercises are used to minimize contractures.

Care of Residents with Alzheimer's Disease and Related Disorders

Dementia is the term used to describe a group of symptoms associated with cognitive impairment and memory loss that are severe enough to interfere with a person's daily activities. Dementia is characterized by memory disorders, impaired reasoning, and personality changes. **Alzheimer's disease** is a progressive disorder that involves damage to the brain's nerve cells (neurons); it results in memory loss, impaired cognition and language skills, and behavioral changes. It is the most common cause of dementia.

According to the Alzheimer's Association's 2021 report, more than 6 million Americans are living with Alzheimer's. This means that the disease affects more than one in nine people age 65 and older (11.3%) and over one-third of those age 85 and older (36.4%). By 2050, without a medical breakthrough to prevent or cure the disease, it is estimated that the number of Americans age 65 and older with Alzheimer's will rise to 12.7million.

Alzheimer's is the sixth-leading cause of death in the United States and the fifth-leading cause of death in those age 65 and older.

Since about half of LTC residents have a diagnosis of Alzheimer's disease, you can see that knowing how to care for residents with Alzheimer's and related disorders is important. To successfully care for these residents, you will need to adapt certain procedures to meet their needs. In most cases, residents you work with will recognize you and will remember events that happened yesterday or a few minutes ago. This is not the case with residents with Alzheimer's. When you greet these residents, you may have to introduce yourself each time as if it is your first time meeting them.

Think about your first day at a new job or in a new school. Wasn't it exhausting? You encountered many new things and met many new people. You tried to remember as much as possible, but you felt overwhelmed and wondered how you would make it through the day. Can you imagine feeling like that every day — feeling that everything you do is unfamiliar and you don't know the people around you? Would you be angry, frustrated, or frightened? Imagine what it would be like to not remember how to do even the simplest task. For many residents with Alzheimer's, each moment is a new experience. What we consider the "normal world" can be very frightening and overwhelming for them.

Cognitive Impairment and Dementia

Cognitive impairment means that a person's thinking skills and memory do not function normally. It can involve more than just memory loss. The person may also have impaired language comprehension (understanding language) and expression (speaking to others). They may also have a loss or reduction of attention span, impaired reasoning and judgment, and an inability to recognize and use common objects.

Cognitive impairment has many causes. Temporary causes include stress, medications, depression, vitamin deficiency, thyroid disease, alcohol, or head trauma. Permanent causes include severe head trauma, illness, brain disease, or brain damage at birth. In LTC facilities, most cognitive impairment in residents is caused by brain disease. Diseases that can cause cognitive impairment or dementia include:

- Degenerative diseases of the nervous system, such as Alzheimer's, Lewy body, Parkinson's, or Huntington's

- Diseases that affect blood vessels such as stroke or multi-infarct dementia (caused by a series of strokes that damage or destroy brain tissue)

- Toxic reactions, such as from excessive alcohol or drug use

- Nutritional deficiencies, such as vitamin B12 or folic acid deficiency

- Infections that affect the central nervous system, such as AIDS dementia complex or Creutzfeldt-Jakob disease

- Certain types of hydrocephalus (buildup of fluid in the brain), infections, injuries, or brain tumors

- Head injury — either a single severe injury or smaller injuries over time, as may happen with boxers and football players

- Other illnesses such as kidney, liver, or lung diseases

Alzheimer's disease is the most common incurable illness that causes dementia. No one knows exactly what causes the brain deterioration associated with this disease. We do know that nerve cells in the brain die, causing the symptoms of dementia.

Nurse assistants play an important role in compassionately caring for people with Alzheimer's or other forms of dementia (Figure 12-3). Your role is to help a resident with a cognitive impairment get through each new day. The term **behavioral symptoms** describes personality changes or behavior changes associated with the disease process. These symptoms may also be called behavioral and psychological symptoms of dementia (BPSD).

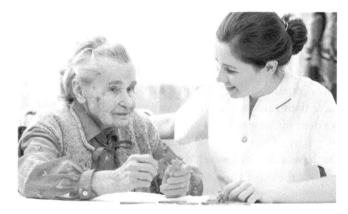

Figure 12-3 You must be patient and kind when assisting residents with Alzheimer's disease and related conditions.

Stages of Alzheimer's Disease

A resident with Alzheimer's disease may have both cognitive and behavioral symptoms. Cognitive symptoms include memory loss, disorientation, confusion, and problems with reasoning and thinking. Behavioral symptoms include agitation, anxiety, delusions, depression, hallucinations, insomnia, and wandering. Alzheimer's disease usually progresses in stages, and the earlier stages can last for many years. Understanding the different stages helps you know how to support residents and how to adapt your care to meet their changing needs (Box 12-2).

Your Role in Providing Care

Your role in caring for residents with Alzheimer's disease differs from your role with other residents. Instead of focusing on helping the resident regain lost function (rehabilitation), you focus on maintaining an ability to meet changing basic needs (habilitation). The problems caused by this type of damage to the brain cannot be reversed, and the disease cannot be cured. Your role is to support the resident and help them to be as productive and happy as possible. This involves doing all you can to reduce their anxiety, agitation, and fear. You can help meet many of their needs and work closely with their family to give support.

Current approaches to working with residents with Alzheimer's disease focus on maximizing their functional independence and maintaining morale. You must value what the resident can do instead of focusing only on what they cannot do. Work to help them have positive emotions and experiences. The following six principles apply to caring for residents with Alzheimer's disease or related disorders.

Anticipate Basic Needs

Anticipate the resident's basic needs so that you can meet them. In every situation, ask yourself, "Have this resident's basic needs been met?" Keep in mind Maslow's hierarchy of human needs. When did the resident last eat, have a drink of water, or go to the bathroom? Always address the most basic needs first when giving care.

Provide Guidance and Direction

Your first role is to gently guide and direct residents through the day. The amount of guidance and direction needed depends on the stage of the disease. Help the resident focus on the task they are trying to do. By late afternoon or early evening, they may be less able to cope. They may become irritable, combative, tearful, or withdrawn. This behavior is called sundowning or sundown syndrome. It is a state of increased agitation or confusion that occurs in the late afternoon and evening.

Discover and Use Residents' Abilities

As residents move through the stages of cognitive decline, they lose many abilities. You must continue your efforts to discover what they can still do. Try to involve these abilities in your caregiving. Whenever possible, do things with the resident, not for or to them. Involve residents in their care as much as possible, helping only as needed. Break directions into short statements. Think about helpful changes you can make in the environment, such as improving the lighting, eliminating clutter, and offering more limited choices of items such as clothing. Remember that these residents have difficulty making decisions.

As you notice a resident's abilities declining, talk with the charge nurse. Do not assume that the resident has lost a capability. Try to avoid situations that may cause the resident to fail because of their lost ability.

Promote Each Resident's Dignity

Another important role is to promote the resident's dignity in everything that you do. Be gentle as you offer assistance and be careful to not offend them. Do not simply assume that a resident doesn't understand what is happening or what you are saying. Residents sometimes experience moments of clarity or lucidity, and at these times they understand what is happening around them. Always treat residents with respect and dignity.

Provide Comfort and Reassurance

Your role also involves providing comfort and reassuring these residents (Figure 12-4). They are losing their abilities and often feel distress. Help them find physical, emotional, and spiritual support throughout the day.

Anticipate their needs, provide gentle touches, sit with them, read from familiar books, and ask clergy to visit (if the resident wishes). Be positive, polite, and enthusiastic as you interact with them. Compliment their clothing or how their hair looks. Mention positive things you know about their past. For example, while you serve a meal, you can mention that you know they were a great cook. Try to bring out positive emotions throughout the day.

BOX 12-2

STAGES OF ALZHEIMER'S DISEASE

Ealy Stage (mild)

Common difficulties include:

- Coming up with the right word or name.
- Remembering names when introduced to new people.
- Having difficulty performing tasks in social or work settings.
- Forgetting material that was just read.
- Losing or misplacing a valuable object.
- Experiencing increased trouble with planning or organizing.

Middle-stage (moderate)

Symptoms, which vary from person to person, may include:

- Being forgetful of events or personal history.
- Feeling moody or withdrawn, especially in socially or mentally challenging situations.
- Being unable to recall information about themselves like their address or telephone number, and the high school or college they attended.
- Experiencing confusion about where they are or what day it is.
- Requiring help choosing proper clothing for the season or the occasion.

- Having trouble controlling their bladder and bowels.
- Experiencing changes in sleep patterns, such as sleeping during the day and becoming restless at night.
- Showing an increased tendency to wander and become lost.
- Demonstrating personality and behavioral changes, including suspiciousness and delusions or compulsive, repetitive behavior like hand-wringing or tissue shredding.

Late-stage (severe)

At this stage, individuals may:

- Require around-the-clock assistance with daily personal care.
- Lose awareness of recent experiences as well as of their surroundings.
- Experience changes in physical abilities, including walking, sitting and, eventually, swallowing
- Have difficulty communicating.
- Become vulnerable to infections, especially pneumonia.

(Source: Alzheimer's Association, www.alz.org)

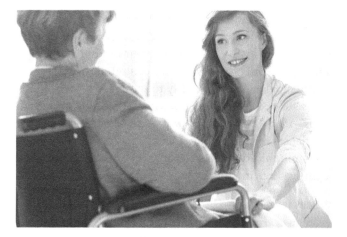

Figure 12-4 Providing comfort and a sense of security is essential in caring for residents with cognitive impairments.

Help Residents Enjoy Life

An important part of your job is enjoying the residents and helping them enjoy life moment to moment. Residents are happier when they feel successful and secure. You help them feel this way by implementing the principles just described. They need to feel that you are looking out for them and that they don't have to worry about their care. Your job will also go more smoothly when you fully appreciate and enjoy your residents. Residents with cognitive problems still respond to emotions. Smiles, laughter, and a caring touch often produce a positive response.

Techniques for Responding to Behavioral Symptoms

Residents with Alzheimer's disease and other cognitive impairments often misinterpret things around them. They may not understand what you are asking them to do or why, and they may resist your care. Always remember that behavioral symptoms such as outbursts and tearfulness show that the resident is in distress. Finding the cause of this distress is key to providing good care. Pay close attention and see if you can identify a time of day when they get upset or which tasks are frustrating or difficult. Share this information with other staff.

Enter a Resident's Reality

Reality orientation, a technique often used in long term care to help residents understand their surroundings and situation, does not work with residents with dementia because they no longer have the capacity to understand reality. If you try to convince them of something they cannot understand, they will become frustrated, agitated, and resistant to care.

Instead, use the practice known as validation therapy. With this approach, you first try to understand the resident's feelings (enter their world). Then you support their feelings (validate their perception of the world).

By doing this, you are reassuring and comforting the resident. For example, if a resident says that she saw her mother, but you tell her that her mother is dead, she will begin grieving. Minutes later she may forget that you said her mother died but still feel sad even if she doesn't know why. A better strategy is a positive approach: "I heard your mother was a wonderful lady. Tell me all about her." This approach can bring about positive emotions for the resident.

The world can be viewed in many different ways, so you must find out how the resident sees the world. You may feel that a resident's behavior is abnormal, but for that person, it is normal. Certain behaviors are normal at each stage of cognitive decline. When you understand how the resident views the world, you will see their behaviors in a whole new light and better understand how to care for them.

Know Your Resident

To care for residents, you need to know them well. Gather as much information as you can to help understand them. Ask questions of the resident (if they are capable of answering), other staff members, family members, and friends. Consider these questions:

- What did the resident do for a living?
- What is their religion?
- Did they have any hobbies or favorite social activities?
- What were they proud of?
- What made them feel sad or afraid?
- Did they experience major losses?
- How did they handle stress?
- What was a typical day like before their illness?

Agenda behavior is the tendency to want to follow a certain agenda during the day. Often a resident tries to follow a past routine, and disrupting this routine causes stress. Knowing their agenda and honoring it when you can helps the resident feel supported and secure.

Know Your Resources

In addition to knowing your residents, you must know what resources are available to help you provide care. Consider equipment in the facility and department resources. Have you read the resident's latest care plan? Can the nursing or dietary department suggest procedures that will make your job easier? Can the activities department provide items or activities the resident will enjoy? Be aware of all your resources. They will make your job easier.

Communicate Effectively

The most important skill you can learn is how to communicate with residents. This includes learning how the resident communicates. As their disease progresses, they may not be able to communicate their needs directly, and you will need to change how you communicate, as well. Eventually they lose the ability to speak and understand you (see Box 12-2). Watch for signals that show their needs. Adapt your communication to create positive experiences for the resident.

Communication techniques to use with residents with cognitive impairments include:

- **Body language** — Understanding residents' body language helps you anticipate their needs. Be mindful of your own body language, as well, to ensure that you are sending positive messages.
- **Facial expressions** — As their illness progresses, residents may "mirror" or copy your facial expressions, tone of voice, or body language. Residents take their

cues from you about how to respond. A smiling face is much more appealing than a frown.

- **Tone of voice** — Tone of voice often communicates more than words. Speaking with a gentle, patient tone tells residents they can feel safe and trust you. The resident's tone helps you understand their needs even when their words do not make sense. Is their tone angry or anxious? Is it lighthearted or sad?

- **Speaking** — Speak slowly and clearly, using simple statements and instructions. Give residents time to respond. For residents who can make choices, limit the options to two things. State each choice simply, and give them time to respond to the first choice before offering the second. With late-stage residents, use only the simplest words and communicate through pleasant tones of voice, facial expressions, and a gentle touch.

- **Listening** — Listen for a resident's verbal cues (simple statements such as "Do me" or "My mouth is dry").

- **Validation** — Validate a resident's perception of reality whenever possible. Try to distract them from any troubling thoughts. Do not try to force a resident to do something that upsets them.

- **Asking questions** — Do not test a resident, which may set them up for failure. For example, do not ask questions that require nouns or names, such as "Who came to visit today?" or "What is my name?" or "What is this called?" Ask simple questions they can answer with a "yes" or "no."

- **Giving directions** — When giving directions, use only one or two words. Include nonverbal cues whenever you can.

- **Nonverbal cues** — As a resident's communication skills decline, you will need to send nonverbal cues that will use their other senses. Watch for the resident's nonverbal cues that indicate signs of physical discomfort or needs.

Motivate the Resident

Learning what motivates residents helps you avoid unpleasant behavior and difficult caregiving.

Residents want to do things that feel physically and emotionally good. A warm washcloth is more inviting than a cold one. Unfamiliar people, places, and equipment can make residents feel threatened. Insisting that a resident do more than they can handle is emotionally distressing. Even residents with Alzheimer's disease like to feel successful.

Residents with Alzheimer's may be motivated by something funny such as a silly hat or a clown nose (Figure 12-5) or anything new, interesting, or unexpected. Curiosity is a big motivator. These techniques are also distractions that let you give care.

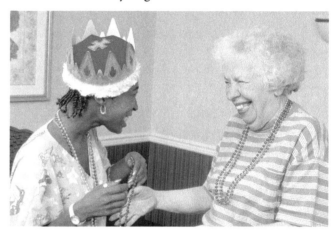

Figure 12-5   Humor and laughter often help motivate a resident.

Motivation also involves catching someone at the right time. Is the person ready to do something? Does it meet their needs at this time? For example, residents who are hungry or thirsty focus only on those needs until they are met. If you are trying to change their clothes at this time, they will not be very motivated to do this. Remember that you must meet their basic needs first before expecting motivation for other tasks.

Residents, like all of us, are motivated by pleasant things and people. Is the environment inviting and pleasant? Be pleasant in all your interactions, smell good, and be clean and neat. This encourages the resident to like you and feel safe and secure with you. Finally, almost no one is motivated by something that seems like work. So don't make it work — make it fun!

Stop When a Resident Resists Your Care

As you communicate with the resident and offer motivators, constantly check to see how well your approach is working. If you accomplish your task and the resident is happy, your technique is successful. Look for verbal and nonverbal signs that the resident is enjoying the activity or is becoming tired or agitated. When a resident resists your care, this signals that they are becoming distressed.

When a resident resists care, this tells you that the resident is stressed or feeling threatened. When this occurs, stop caregiving immediately! Consider the person and the situation to understand the cause of resistance. Make adjustments as needed. If you avoid confrontation, you will be successful. Sometimes you must give routine care to a resident who resists. In this case, validate the person's distress and try to provide comfort during and after the care. Offering a drink of water or juice when you complete the care may help.

Specific Behavioral Symptoms

Table 12-2 lists common behavioral symptoms along with strategies you can use to help residents. Common symptoms exhibited by residents with Alzheimer's disease are agitation, anxiety, depression, insomnia, wandering, delusions, and hallucinations. Remember that any change in a resident's behavior may mean that something is physically wrong—it may not be just a symptom of the disease. Report all changes to the charge nurse.

Table 12-2   Behavioral Symptoms, Observations, and Interventions

Symptom	Observations	Ways to Assist the Resident
Agitation	▪ Appears to be restless, uncomfortable, or distressed ▪ Sensitivity to noise ▪ Awake at night and sleeps during the day ▪ Repeats words, names, phrases, or questions ▪ Paces ▪ Swings an arm or leg back and forth ▪ Repeated finger-tapping on a surface ▪ Repeated rubbing or picking at the skin ▪ Bites, spits, or hits others ▪ Resists care	▪ Reduce the noise level around the person and speak in a soft tone of voice. ▪ Make sure that there is no physical problem, such as pain or needing to go to the bathroom, causing the behavior. ▪ Ask questions to determine what the resident needs. ▪ Try to divert the resident's attention from repeated behaviors by playing soft music, taking them for a walk, or sitting quietly with them. ▪ Provide an activity such as knitting, folding towels, or sweeping. ▪ Offer a nutritious snack, such as a piece of fruit. ▪ Make sure the resident is eating enough nutritious food. ▪ Limit caffeine by not offering chocolate or caffeinated tea or coffee. ▪ Allow the person to sleep as needed.
Anxiety	▪ Fearfulness or tension ▪ Increased pulse and/or blood pressure ▪ Sweating	▪ Be supportive, kind, and gentle. ▪ Assure the resident that they are safe. ▪ Provide simple choices. ▪ Provide quiet rest periods throughout the day. ▪ Watch for any anxiety triggers, and replace these triggers with a pleasant, quiet activity. ▪ Report any changes in nutritional intake to the nurse.
Depression	▪ Ongoing sadness or fatigue ▪ Difficulty concentrating ▪ Withdraws from others ▪ Trouble sleeping ▪ Reduced activity level ▪ Reduced appetite	▪ Let the resident talk about how they feel. ▪ Encourage participation in pleasant activities. ▪ Provide limited choices. ▪ Provide quiet rest periods throughout the day. ▪ Offer frequent, nutritious snacks.
Insomnia	▪ Restless and awake at night	▪ Help the resident get regular exercise. ▪ Offer frequent rest periods throughout the day. ▪ Play soft music. ▪ Give back rubs. ▪ Make sure the resident is eating enough nutritious food.

Symptom	Observations	Ways to Assist the Resident
Wandering	<ul><li>Walking with a purpose (may believe they are going to work or to visit someone)</li><li>Walking as if frightened or lost</li><li>Walking up and down hallways</li><li>Opening and closing doors</li><li>Looking for someone or something</li></ul>	<ul><li>Place signs on doors, wall, and hallways to help orient the resident to where they are.</li><li>Keep the room and hallways free of clutter.</li><li>Make sure the resident is wearing identification.</li><li>Be kind; do not argue with the resident.</li><li>Divert their attention by offering a pleasant activity.</li><li>Ask the resident to walk with you.</li><li>Help the resident get regular exercise.</li><li>Provide quiet rest periods throughout the day.</li><li>Make sure the resident is eating enough nutritious food.</li></ul>
Delusions	<ul><li>Fearfulness</li><li>Hiding</li><li>Suspicion of others</li><li>Accusatory remarks to staff or other residents</li></ul>	<ul><li>Be kind and supportive.</li><li>Reassure the person constantly.</li><li>Do not argue with the resident. Their thoughts and beliefs are real to them.</li><li>Participate in the resident's reality.</li><li>Make sure the resident is eating enough nutritious food.</li></ul>
Hallucinations	<ul><li>Fearfulness or distress</li><li>Acting as if they see or hear things that are not there</li><li>Speaking as if talking to a person who is not present</li></ul>	<ul><li>Be kind and supportive.</li><li>Listen to the resident.</li><li>Do not argue with the resident.</li><li>Participate in the resident's reality.</li><li>Make sure the resident is eating enough nutritious food.</li></ul>

Techniques for Activities of Daily Living

Residents with Alzheimer's and related disorders have unique needs. You must meet these needs as part of giving routine care and helping them with the activities of daily living. You will be challenged to give care in ways that do not cause distress.

Remember the stage of the resident's disease as you plan care. Tailor your methods to the individual resident to help them do daily activities more easily and with dignity. The goal is to help the resident have a positive experience with all activities. Whenever you give care, the resident should feel as though they are participating as fully as their ability allows.

Toileting

Residents with Alzheimer's eventually lose control of their bladder and bowels. Because of their cognitive impairment, they cannot identify the feeling of needing to go to the bathroom. They lose the ability to find the bathroom, to undress, to use the toilet, and to clean themselves.

They may reach this stage sooner if they have difficulty locating restrooms or communicating their need to go. Residents' verbal and nonverbal cues may show you when they need to go to the bathroom. You can prevent them from becoming incontinent at an early stage and maintain their dignity and independence longer if you recognize their cues.

As the disease progresses, you will see changes in their independence in toileting. Some residents can control their bowels and bladder if you help them find bathrooms and remind them to toilet. They will need your help with the mechanics of toileting, such as wiping, flushing, and pulling their underwear down and up.

Eventually they become completely incontinent. They may not hear or understand reminders to use the toilet and may resist your help and your offer of incontinence products.

Follow these guidelines to help a resident remain continent as long as possible:

- Always be ready to help residents find bathrooms and help as needed with toileting.
- Know residents' toileting schedules to predict when they may need your help. This also helps you recognize cues that a resident needs to use the bathroom.

- Help a resident with incontinence products when needed. You can ease the transition into using these products by placing underwear over them.

- Communicate slowly and gently with residents while toileting. Give them extra time to respond.

- Providing a distraction may be useful when a resident resists your help. A pleasant distraction may be to provide a favorite snack.

- Remember that toileting is personal. Wearing incontinence products can be embarrassing and upsetting. Keep in mind how you would like to be treated and maintain residents' dignity at all times.

Hydration

The body has a basic need for fluids (hydration). Water is the primary source of hydration. You may not understand how a resident can be thirsty when a water pitcher or water fountain is within easy reach. These objects become unfamiliar to them, and they do not notice or recognize them. The resident may go thirsty without your help in locating or providing water. Because these residents have difficulty telling you what they need, watch for verbal and nonverbal cues that show you their needs. As the disease progresses, residents may not be able to find water fountains or a water pitcher. They may not ask for something to drink when they are thirsty. Eventually they may not give you any cue at all.

Follow these guidelines to meet residents' hydration needs:

- Offer fluids according to their individual needs.

- Offer fluids more often and in smaller amounts, especially for residents who have difficulty swallowing. If a resident has trouble swallowing, tell the nurse immediately.

- Offer fluids in response to verbal cues such as "My mouth is so dry."

- Offer fluids when a resident shows nonverbal signs of thirst (dry mouth, agitation, tongue hanging out, or rummaging or searching behavior).

- Don't ask if the resident is thirsty; just bring water and let them drink.

Eating

Residents with Alzheimer's disease and other cognitive disorders need help finding the dining area and then eating. Tell the nurse about any changes in their abilities so that dietary trays are set up and the food choices are appropriate for each resident's abilities.

In the early stage of illness residents can eat by themselves but watch that they can still use their knife properly. They eventually lose eating skills and the ability to use utensils and straws. They may have problems with positioning and swallowing.

Follow these guidelines to help residents with eating:

- Ensure proper body positioning.

- Prompt them and give cues to keep eating, chewing, and swallowing as needed.

- Give them time to eat.

- Cut, season, and de-bone their food. Peel fruit if necessary. Their food should be ready to eat when the tray is put before them.

- Watch for any trouble using utensils. Give a fork and spoon to residents who cannot use a knife properly. Then give only a spoon when the fork is no longer manageable. When a spoon is no longer manageable, give the resident only finger foods. (It is okay for residents to use their fingers when they eat.)

- Watch for problems like the person ignoring one side of their plate (which may result from a visual problem), not being able to handle food and drinks served together, not eating other food if dessert is served with the meal or having trouble swallowing.

- Watch for a resident pouring their drink in their plate. If a resident does this, do not give food and drink at the same time.

- Add a sweetener to give food more appeal, if needed.

- If a resident will not sit long enough to eat, offer nutritious finger foods such as a sandwich or wrap, fruit, raw vegetables, nutrition or protein bar, etc.

Dressing

A resident's ability to dress and undress will change as the disease progresses. At first these residents can get dressed by themselves with limited supervision. You may only have to choose clothing appropriate for the season or occasion. Some residents may need coaxing to change their clothes or take off their clothes at night. Others may try to change their clothes repeatedly throughout the day.

Some residents need help putting their clothes on properly, like putting shoes on the right feet and tying their shoelaces. They may have problems wearing their glasses, dentures, and hearing aids all day. They may resist your help in dressing or undressing.

Eventually they need total assistance with dressing and cannot wear supportive appliances. They may remove their shoes and socks or clothes that fasten in front. They may fiddle constantly with buttons, zippers, or hems. They may resist changing their clothes and wearing underclothes.

Try to make dressing simpler and more enjoyable. Be ready to help whenever you see your help is needed. Simplify the process according to the person's individual needs.

Follow these guidelines for dressing residents as the disease progresses:

- Offer only two outfits and ask the person to choose one.

- Select clothing for the person to wear if they cannot choose for themselves.

- Simplify dressing by laying out clothes in the order they are put on.

- Dress residents in clothing that is easy to put on and take off. Avoid using belts and ties. You may have to help them place their arms, legs, and head in openings and fasten buttons, snaps, and zippers (Figure 12-6).

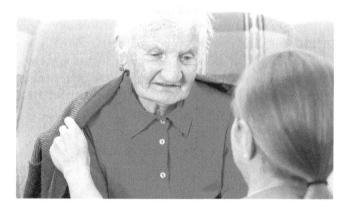

Figure 12-6 When helping residents to dress, choose clothing that is easy to put on and take off.

- If a resident resists your efforts to dress or undress them, they may need friendly coaxing. If they resist in the morning, wait until after breakfast. If they resist at night, encourage the family to bring in clothing they can wear day or night, like jogging suits, sweats, yoga pants, t-shirts, loose cotton dresses, etc. Then you can change their clothing only once a day, in the morning.

- If a resident resists wearing nonessential clothing like bras, slips, or stockings, do not force them to wear them.

- Make sure that the resident's shoes are on the correct feet. Residents who begin wearing only one shoe may need to be assessed for a foot problem, or their shoes should be checked for fit and condition. If no problem is found, they might wear slipper socks with non-slip soles instead of shoes. Talk to the nurse about this.

- Always be gentle and patient. Use words and gestures to communicate, move slowly, and give the resident time to understand what is happening. If the resident resists, leave and come back later. Try again with a big smile and a slow, patient manner.

Bathing

Bathing is often a traumatic experience for these residents, but it need not be. With your help, bathing can be done smoothly, without upsetting the resident. Consider each resident's needs and past routine.

Residents may rely on you to tell them when to bathe. They may need help finding the bathroom and supplies like soap, washcloth, towel, and shampoo. They may need help getting into and out of the shower or bath, adjusting the water, and washing and drying themselves. As a resident experiences more physical and cognitive decline, their ability to bathe may become limited to washing and drying their hands and face. Encourage any action a resident can do independently, even if it seems very small. Residents may develop a fear of water in a shower or tub and resist your efforts to help.

Follow these guidelines to help with bathing:

- Experiment to see what time of the day works best — not everyone needs to be bathed in the morning.

- Help them find the bathroom and get ready to bathe or shower. You should be ready to help if the resident is struggling.

- Make bathing more comfortable by warming the bathroom ahead of time.

- Help the resident undress, get into and out of the shower or bath, and wash and dry.

- Give directions to make sure that the resident cleans and dries themselves thoroughly. Talk the resident through it and/or demonstrate what to do.

- Encourage residents to wash easily reached areas like their face, chest, and thighs.

- Help with shampooing if assistance is needed. Instead of washing hair in the shower, you can wash hair at the sink and try to keep water off the person's face.

- Use simple one-step commands ("Rinse your arm ... now rinse your shoulder."). Place your hand over the resident's hand to guide them.

- Avoid actions that may make residents afraid of bathing. Use a hand-held shower nozzle, but do not wet a resident's face or hair directly with the spray. You can wet their feet first in the tub or shower before immersing them in the water. Give a sponge bath as needed instead of putting a resident completely in the water.

- Move slowly and give the person time to understand what you are communicating or doing.

- When a resident resists, you can distract them with a favorite snack or offer a drink after bathing.

Grooming

Good grooming helps preserve a resident's dignity. Grooming includes combing and brushing the hair, washing the face, brushing the teeth, removing and reinserting dentures, shaving, and applying makeup, lotion, and/or cologne. Some residents can groom themselves with your encouragement and supervision. As their skills decline, they need more help from you.

Residents may resist having their hair combed or brushed. They may stop using their glasses, hearing aids, or dentures. They may resist shaving and stop using supportive appliances. Eventually they depend on you completely for their grooming.

Follow these guidelines to make grooming easier and more pleasant:

- Be ready to help with any part of grooming.

- Simplify tasks as needed to encourage self-grooming. Help the resident get started with each task.

- Encourage residents to attend the facility's morning grooming program (if offered) and apply any finishing touches such as cologne and makeup. This promotes a positive self-image and good self-esteem.

- Gently communicate with residents during grooming. Use sensory cues to encourage grooming, like putting a warm washcloth on their face or applying warm shaving cream with a shaving brush. Move slowly to give them more time to understand what you are doing.

- When a resident stops using supportive appliances all day, give them to the resident only at beneficial times. For example, dentures are needed at meals but are not necessary at other times. Make sure you retrieve the resident's dentures after each meal.

- If a male resident resists shaving, check for pain, such as a razor burn, dry skin, oral problem, earache, or other discomfort. If they keep resisting, do not force shaving at this time. Try later using more sensory cues. If they still resist, try every day but do not force care on them. Let family members know that this is a normal behavior and that you will resume shaving the resident when they are more receptive to the activity.

Mental Health and Substance Use Disorders

Mental health and substance use disorders can affect anyone, regardless of race, sex, or socioeconomic status.

Mental health includes our emotionally, psychological, and social well-being. It affects a person's mood, thinking and behavior. Mental health is as important as our physical health and can have an effect on our physical health. A person's mental health can change over time. According to the CDC, mental illness (mental health disorders) are among the most common health conditions in the United States. More than 50% will be diagnosed with a mental illness or disorder at some point in their lifetime.

Some common types of mental health disorders are:

- **Anxiety** is a feeling of uneasiness, worry, fear or dread. Anxiety is a natural reaction to stress and usually dissipates once the stressor is removed. Anxiety disorders are conditions where the feelings of anxiety are not temporary and can become worse over time. Symptoms of anxiety disorders can interfere with daily activities such as work or school. Refer to Table 12-2 for additional information about anxiety.

- Obsessive-Compulsive Disorder (OCD) is a condition that is characterized by unwanted, repetitive thoughts (obsessions) or behaviors (compulsions) that the person feels they need to repeat over and over. A person with OCD usually have both symptoms of obsessions and compulsions but some may only have symptoms of one or the other. These behaviors can interfere with daily activities depending on the symptoms.

- Depression is a common mood disorder that causes a persistent feeling of sadness and loss of interest. Depending on the severity of symptoms, this can interfere with normal, everyday functioning. According to the CDC, one out of every 6 adults will have depression at some time in their life. There are many treatment options for depression, including therapy and medications. Some people with depression may have thoughts of harming themselves or committing suicide. Suicide is death caused by self-harm with the intent to die. The CDC reports that suicide is the tenth leading cause of death in the United States and was responsible for more than 47,500 deaths in 2019. It is the second leading cause of death for people between the ages of 10-34. If you, someone you know, or someone you are caring for has thoughts of harming themselves or having suicidal thoughts, reach out to someone immediately. If it is a resident you are caring for, report it to the charge nurse immediately. There are numerous outreach programs available, including the National Suicide Prevention Hotline, 800-273-8255.

- Bipolar disorder is a condition that causes severe fluctuations in mood, energy levels, concentration and affects their ability to carry out function of daily living. These fluctuations vary but can range from manic (feeling very high) to depressive (feeling very sad). Bipolar disorder is a lifelong condition and requires long-term treatment.

- Schizophrenia is a severe mental disorder that affects how a person acts, thinks, and behaves. Symptoms can include delusions, hallucinations, trouble thinking, decreased motivation or disorganized speech. These symptoms can greatly impact how a person is able to function and perform daily activities. There is no cure for schizophrenia but with proper treatment symptoms can improve.

According to the Substance Abuse and Mental Health Services Administration (SAMHSA), substance use disorders occur when the recurrent use of alcohol and/or drugs causes clinically significant impairment, including health problems, disability, and failure to meet major responsibilities at work, school, or home. The person with substance abuse disorder has the inability to control the use of the substance and is not confined to illegal drugs. SAMHSA's 2020 National Survey on Drug Use and Health reports that approximately 19.3 million people aged 18 or older had a substance use disorder in the previous year. Opioid overdose, in particular is considered an epidemic, with the CDC reporting that an average of 128 Americans die every day from an opioid overdose.

Depending on the substance consumed, the symptoms can vary, but may include:

- a change in behavior
- a sudden change in their weight
- tremors
- slurred speech
- impaired gait
- an increase in accidents or falls

Over time, people with a substance abuse disorder may need larger doses or more of the substance to achieve the desired effect. Withdrawal symptoms may occur when someone with a substance abuse disorder stops taking the substance.

As a nurse assistant it is important to know what symptoms to monitor for when it comes to mental health and substance abuse disorders, who to report symptoms to, and the community resources that are available.

Points to Remember

- Nurse assistants have many opportunities to work with residents in various types of care settings, including assisted living facilities, units or facilities that serve residents with Alzheimer's disease and related disorders, and units or facilities that provide post-acute care.

- In settings that serve residents with specialized needs, nurse assistants must learn how to adapt and modify the care provided to meet the resident's individual needs.

- Nurse assistants must develop the skills that allow them to care for residents with diabetes, those who require oxygen therapy or dialysis, those undergoing surgical procedures, residents who are developmentally disabled, those with Alzheimer's disease or other types of cognitive impairment, and those with mental health disorders or substance abuse disorders.

- It is very important to observe changes in residents and report information to the health care team.

- Special techniques are used to effectively respond to residents exhibiting behavioral symptoms.

- Nurse assistants learn how to adapt their care to help residents with cognitive impairments with activities of daily living.

agenda behavior — actions that follow a certain agenda, often a past routine

Alzheimer's disease — progressive brain disease that causes memory loss, other cognitive impairments, and behavioral changes

anxiety — a feeling of uneasiness, worry, fear or dread

artificial airway — tubular device placed into the respiratory tract to facilitate breathing or the removal of secretions

Autism Spectrum Disorder (ASP) — a disorder that affects a person's ability to communicate and interact with others

behavioral symptoms — actions caused by a disease or condition

Bipolar disorder — a condition that causes severe fluctuations in mood, energy levels, concentration and affects their ability to carry out function of daily living

Cerebral palsy (CP) — a disorder that affects movement and posture

cognitive impairment — measurable decline in memory and thinking skills

delusion — false thought that a person believes to be real

dementia — mental disorder characterized by memory loss, impaired reasoning, and personality changes

depression — a common mood disorder that causes a persistent feeling of sadness and loss of interest

developmental disability — chronic condition caused by physical and/or mental impairment that affects language, learning, mobility, and the activities of daily living; may prevent a person from living independently

dialysis — process of filtering and removing waste products from the blood used when the kidneys are not functioning properly

Down syndrome — also known as trisomy 21, is a genetic disorder caused by the presence of all or part of a third copy of chromosome 21

hallucination — false sensory experiences (visual images, sounds, smells, etc.) that appear to be real

hemodialysis — type of dialysis in which blood is removed from the body and filtered through a machine that removes waste products and excess fluid and returns the blood to the body

hyperglycemia — abnormally high blood sugar

hypoglycemia — abnormally low blood sugar

hypoxia — state in which not enough oxygen is reaching body tissues

obsessive-compulsive disorder (OCD) — a condition that is characterized by unwanted, repetitive thoughts (obsessions) or behaviors (compulsions) that they feel needs to be repeated over and over

peritoneal dialysis — type of dialysis in which waste and fluid are removed from the blood using a surgically placed catheter in the abdominal (peritoneal) cavity

postoperative — period of time after surgery

preoperative — period of time before surgery

preoperative orders — physician orders prior to surgery

schizophrenia — a severe mental disorder that affects how a person acts, thinks and behaves

sitz bath — bath in a tub or special basin in which only the perineum and buttocks are immersed

substance use disorder — occurs when the recurrent use of alcohol and/or drugs causes clinically significant impairment, including health problems, disability, and failure to meet major responsibilities at work, school, or home

suicide — when death is caused by self-harm with the intent to die

sundowning — worsening of symptoms of Alzheimer's disease and other types of dementia that occurs in the late afternoon or evening; also known as *sundown syndrome*

tracheostomy — creation of an opening into the trachea to facilitate breathing; also known as a *tracheotomy*

validation therapy — approach that validates and supports a person's perception of the world; used in treatment of Alzheimer's disease and related conditions

1. **Which of these statements about Alzheimer's disease is true?**

   a. Brain cells multiply uncontrollably
   b. Alzheimer's is incurable
   c. It leads to death within a few days
   d. It requires strict isolation procedures

2. **An important role for the nurse aide in caring for the patient on dialysis is:**

   a. Caring for the access site
   b. Taking an accurate weight before and after
   c. Getting the resident's favorite dessert for dinner
   d. Taking them to the bathroom to void

3. **Elastic stockings may be applied by the nurse aide when ordered by the physician after surgery to prevent:**

   a. Decrease the risk of blood clot formation
   b. Pneumonia
   c. Wound infection
   d. Bowel paralysis

4. **A form of temporarily or permanently altered thinking is called:**

   a. Schizophrenia
   b. Bipolar disorder
   c. Cognitive impairment
   d. Obsessive compulsive disorder

5. **A resident who is no longer able to communicate or care for oneself, loses control of the bladder and bowel, and experiences shutdown of the mind and body would be in which stage of Alzheimer's disease?**

   a. Early-stage (mild)
   b. Mid-stage (moderate)
   c. Late-stage (severe)
   d. Early cognitive loss

6. **The nurse may perform blood glucose monitoring by finger prick for the resident with diabetes to detect:**

   a. Hyperglycemia
   b. Hypoglycemia
   c. Both of these
   d. Neither of these

7. **The habilitation model of caregiving is used with residents with developmental disabilities and is based on a principle known as:**

   a. Normalization
   b. Agenda behavior
   c. Group therapy
   d. Self-help

8. **Cold applications are used for the following except to:**

   a. Help raise the body temperature
   b. Reduce pain or swelling to an area
   c. Help control bleeding
   d. Reduce sensitivity to pain by numbing the area

9. **Validation therapy is sometimes used in treatment of Alzheimer's disease and related conditions, this approach:**

   a. Supports a residents' perception of the world
   b. Reorients the resident to the real world
   c. Allows the resident to have time alone to think about their thoughts
   d. Supports reality orientation

10. **A persistent feeling of sadness and loss of interest is a symptom of:**

   a. Substance use disorder
   b. Autism spectrum disorder
   c. Cerebral Palsy
   d. Depression

13

Comfort Care and End of Life

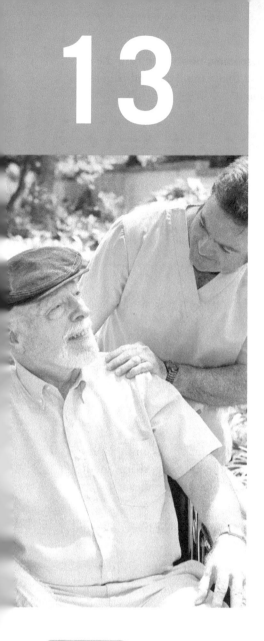

Pain and dying are two things that most people would like to avoid discussing or thinking about. Unfortunately, they are part of everyone's life. As a nurse assistant, a major aspect of your job is to help relieve pain and to assist in easing the dying process by providing comfort care. If a resident is in pain, their sleep and activities are disrupted, which affects their quality of life. In many health care facilities, pain is thought of as the fifth vital sign, along with temperature, pulse, respiration, and blood pressure. This perspective reminds staff to ask residents often about their pain. Some long term care residents are admitted for end-of-life comfort care. Others are admitted with a chronic illness that later becomes terminal, resulting in the need for end-of-life care. And others simply reach the natural end of life. In all of these situations, you provide care to keep the resident as comfortable and free of pain as possible.

OBJECTIVES:

- Explain the methods used to assess a resident's level of pain and your responsibility for reporting pain.

- Describe signs you may see that indicate a resident is in pain.

- List the possible side effects of pain medications.

- Describe complementary or alternative therapies commonly used to manage pain.

- List ways to promote comfort and sleep.

- Explain the purpose of advance directives such as a living will.

- Name and describe common feelings people have about death.

- Define the Kübler-Ross five stages of grief.

- Explain the goals of end-of-life care and your role in providing this care.

- Describe the care of the body after death.

Pain Management

In the past, pain was usually viewed as a symptom of a condition or disease affecting the body. Health care professionals often ignored the pain and focused only on treating the underlying cause. Today, we know that pain should never be ignored. Research is being done to find new ways to help manage pain and bring relief.

Pain affects socialization, ambulation, and overall well-being. Pain can create problems with the immune system and affect how the body fights infection. This can cause further deterioration in the resident's health.

Pain cannot be measured like temperature or pulse. Pain is what the resident feels. You must accept what a resident says about the pain they feel and its severity. Believe what the resident says and report their pain as they describe it. You cannot interpret another person's level of pain.

Pain management is a key part of caring for residents. What you report can determine whether residents are treated properly. Sometimes residents need pain medications around the clock. That means they must receive the medication on schedule. Your role in pain management is to report information about the resident accurately and in a timely manner and to perform other strategies as directed.

Understanding Pain

In health care, pain used to be defined as one of three types: acute pain (as caused by a sprain, strain, infection, inflammation, or surgical procedure), chronic pain (as caused by arthritis), and malignant pain (as in cancer). More recent research defines pain in relation to various forms of nervous system damage. This approach helps the interdisciplinary team more effectively treat residents' pain. Certain medications or alternative therapies work better with one kind of pain than with another. The goal is always to use the best pain management strategies for the resident's specific kind of pain.

Level of Pain

Most facilities have pain assessment tools that are used to rate the level of a person's pain. A numerical scale is often used for adults. You ask, "If zero is no pain and 10 is the worst pain possible, what is your pain right now?"

It may be easier for some residents, especially those who speak little or no English, to use a visual pain scale (Figure 13-1). Other scales may be used for residents with impaired cognitive ability. A resident's pain should be assessed regularly and whenever their condition changes.

Let the charge nurse know how much pain the resident is experiencing so that a more detailed pain assessment can be performed.

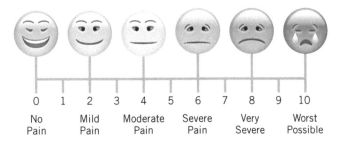

Used with permission, University of Colorado Health Sciences Center, Denver, Colorado.

Figure 13-1 Example of a visual pain scale used to help residents rate their level of pain.

The charge nurse, along with other members of the interdisciplinary team, may assess the resident's pain in more detail. Residents are asked about the following pain qualities:

- The location of the pain
- What the pain feels like, such as discomfort, pressure, achy, throbbing, sore, burning, sharp, shooting, crampy, or feeling like "pins and needles"
- When the pain started
- Whether the pain is always there or if it comes and goes
- What makes the pain worse or better
- How the pain affects their walking, eating, sleeping, and mood

The interdisciplinary team uses all this information to create a plan to help relieve the resident's pain. The charge nurse may ask you to report when the resident complains of pain or to observe how the resident responds after being given a pain medication. The physician may prescribe complementary or alternative therapies for pain relief. These may include the application of heat or cold. The charge nurse will explain your responsibilities with these therapies.

You play a key role helping the team assess a resident's pain. Listen carefully to how the resident describes their pain. You should also report any other signs or nonverbal cues to pain that you observe. Encourage residents to talk openly about their pain. They need to understand that pain is not a normal part of aging. Residents should never be made to feel that they should hide their pain. Pain can be managed, and they have the right to pain treatment.

In some situations, a resident may try to hide their pain due to cultural or religious beliefs that discourage showing pain. Always respect the resident's views while you work with the team to address the pain. Remember that it is crucial to report their pain so it can be treated appropriately.

Reporting Pain Accurately

Pain is very subjective. Remember that *subjective information* is what the resident tells you. You must report this subjective information exactly as the resident stated it. Each resident feels pain differently and responds in his or her own way. Researchers believe that cultural influences, the brain's release of endorphins, and previous experiences with pain may play a role in pain sensation, along with other individual factors.

It is important that you observe residents carefully and report both the person's description of the pain and your own observations. Table 13-1 lists common signs of pain that can be observed in the resident's movements, facial expressions, sounds, and speech.

Table 13-1 Signs of Pain

Observation	Signs of Pain
The resident's facial expression	■ Frown, wrinkled forehead ■ Furrowed brow ■ Grimace ■ Expression of fear ■ Expression of sadness ■ Tense muscles around the mouth and eyes
The resident's physical movements	■ Restlessness, fidgeting, agitation ■ Absence of movement, slow movements ■ Cautious movements, guarding, or bracing ■ Rigidity, generalized tension ■ Rubbing a body part
What you might hear	■ Groaning, moaning ■ Crying ■ Noisy breathing ■ Saying things like "Ouch!" or "Don't touch me"

Regardless of individual differences, unrelieved pain can lead to additional problems, such as a compromised immune system. Pain also affects other body systems.

Because of the constant effect of pain on the nervous system, even the lightest touch can cause a resident more pain.

It is difficult for a resident to feel happy when they are in pain. They cannot get comfortable and relax. They do not sleep well. They may feel that the quality of their life is poor. If a resident's pain is not managed, the resident may experience some or all of the following:

- Fear
- Depression
- Anxiety
- Distress
- Helplessness
- Hopelessness
- Decreased will to live

Resident Concerns and Beliefs about Pain

Some residents have certain beliefs about pain and its treatment. These beliefs may interfere with reporting their pain and good pain management. Table 13-2 lists common misconceptions or beliefs about pain along with the facts. Be aware of these misconceptions and beliefs.

When appropriate, talk about them with your residents.

Table 13-2 Misconceptions About Pain and Its Treatment

Misconceptions About Pain	Facts About Pain
"If I take too much pain medicine, I will get addicted."	The risk of addiction is rare (less than one in 10,000 people) when pain medications are taken for pain.
"Pain is inevitable as you get older — I just have to live with it."	As you age, conditions that cause pain become more common. But pain is not normal. Good pain relief is possible for all types of pain.
"The nurses and nurse assistants are so busy — I don't want to bother them by asking for pain medication."	The nurses and nurse assistants want to know about your pain. The staff want to provide the best treatment possible.

Misconceptions About Pain	Facts About Pain
"If my pain medicine doesn't work as well as it used to, it means I am getting immune or addicted to it."	Sometimes people get used to a medicine. This is called tolerance — not addiction. If tolerance happens, staff can increase the dose or change to a different pain medicine.
"It is better to save pain medicine for when the pain gets really bad."	If a resident waits too long to take pain medicine, they may actually need a stronger medicine or higher dose. Taking pain medicine on a regular schedule may help prevent pain.
"It's easier to cope with the pain than with the side effects of pain medication, especially constipation."	Pain medicine, particularly narcotics, can cause constipation. But constipation can be prevented and treated with stool softeners and laxatives. Worries about side effects should not stop the resident from taking pain medicine for their pain.

Used with permission, University of Colorado Health Sciences Center, Denver, Colorado. Development of pamphlet was supported by AHRQ grant U18-HS11093-3.

Pain Treatment

The most common treatment for pain is medication. Many drugs are available to treat various types of pain. Typically, a combination of drugs is used to manage pain caused by cancer or chronic illness. The physician and other members of the team select which drugs to use.

Your input about the resident's experience is a key part of this decision. The team must clearly understand what type of pain the resident is experiencing and other information about the resident's pain.

You also are responsible for reporting any side effects (undesired effects) of the pain medication. Possible side effects are shown in Box 13-1.

In addition to pain medication, other therapies are used to help manage pain, keep the resident more comfortable, and improve their sleep. Complementary or alternative therapies often help the resident feel more in control. The choice of treatments or therapies depends in part on the resident's preferences, beliefs, flexibility, and mobility. For example, techniques such as progressive

muscle relaxation and meditation can help release tension and reduce pain (Figure 13-2). Box 13-2 describes some nondrug therapies commonly used to help relieve residents' pain.

BOX 13-1

POSSIBLE SIDE EFFECTS OF PAIN MEDICATION

- Constipation
- Diarrhea
- Nausea and vomiting
- Sleeping too much
- Complaints of stomach pains
- Rash
- Slowed respiratory rate
- Dizziness when standing or changing position

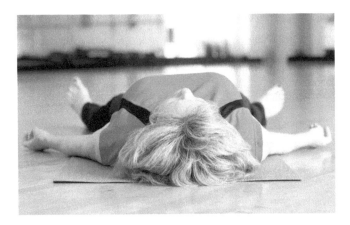

Figure 13-2 Various types of complementary and alternative therapies may be used to help relieve residents' pain.

Your role assisting with nondrug therapies depends on your experience. The charge nurse or physical therapist will train you in techniques used in your facility. The charge nurse and other team members decide which alternative or complementary therapies to use for each resident. You will likely be asked to report how effective the treatment is in comforting the resident and/or relieving pain.

BOX 13-2

NONDRUG THERAPIES FOR PAIN

- **Heat/cold application** involves using dry or moist heat or cold on a specific area to relieve pain or increase the resident's comfort.

- **Vibration** can be used to promote comfort or help relieve pain. This form of electrical massage is applied lightly or with pressure on various body areas. Different types of vibrating devices are available for different parts of the body.

- **Massage** is a method of relaxation that can be used to help residents relax both physically and mentally. A three-minute backrub using slow, rhythmic strokes is a safe and effective way to decrease pain and promote relaxation.

- **Acupuncture** is an ancient Chinese healing method. The acupuncturist inserts very thin needles in specific body sites. Acupuncture is said to allow energy to flow to or from areas that do not have enough energy or have too much energy. Acupuncture is believed to help restore and regulate the body's energy balance.

- **Distraction** is a technique used to direct a resident's attention away from pain. With distraction, the resident deliberately focuses on something other than the pain and thus responds less to it. Talking, books, movies, and social activities are all distractions.

- **Humor** is an enjoyable and often effective form of distraction that can be used to get the resident's mind off their pain.

- **Relaxation** techniques are methods that help reduce anxiety, muscle tension, and pain. Such techniques include meditation, music, massage, and deep breathing.

- **Guided imagery** is a healing technique that uses words and sometimes music to bring the body and mind to a relaxed and focused state.

- **Animals** provide relaxation and companionship and help distract a resident's attention from pain.

Promoting Comfort and Sleep

Research has shown that frequent sleep disturbances, such as getting up to go to the bathroom, may affect the body's natural pain inhibitors and cause more pain.

This is especially so with women. Getting enough sleep is important to our overall health and well-being.

According to the CDC, not getting enough sleep is linked with many chronic diseases and conditions, such as, type 2 diabetes, heart disease, obesity, depression, and an increased risk of falls.

You may care for residents with sleep disorders, which can put them for an increased risk for health problems. Some common sleep disorders are:

- Insomnia is where a resident may have difficulty falling and or staying asleep.

- Restless Legs Syndrome (RLS) is a condition that causes an uncontrollable urge to move the legs. This typically occurs in the evening and at night causing difficulty with falling and staying asleep.

- Sleep apnea occurs when a resident's breathing repeatedly starts and stops during sleep. Some symptoms include, loud snoring, gasping for air during sleep, being tired during waking hours, and difficulty staying asleep.

You are responsible for helping all residents feel as comfortable as possible and get enough sleep. The techniques listed in Box 13-2 can be used to help promote comfort and sleep in addition to relieving pain.

It is helpful to encourage residents to use the bathroom before going to bed at night.

You may also want to encourage them to rest during the day. This can mean quiet time reading or listening to music. Understanding how each resident likes to relax and prepare for sleep will help you know what to do to assist them.

You can also help control the resident's environment to keep them comfortable and promote sleep:

- Make sure that the room it is not too hot or too cold. Ask the resident how the room temperature feels to them. Remember that what you consider a comfortable temperature may be different from what the resident finds comfortable.

- Be sure there are extra blankets nearby in case they get cold during the night. If residents cannot pull up additional covers on their own, be sure to check on them throughout the night.

- Limit noise at night. Do not talk to others in the resident's room or outside their door.

- Lower the lights in the hallways. Close the resident's door, if appropriate.

- Be sure to pull window shades and close curtains at night so outside lights do not shine in the resident's window.
- Pay attention to any odors. Empty bedpans, change soiled linens, and manage incontinence in a timely manner.

End of Life

Facing the end of life is a very difficult time for the resident and their loved ones. Your role as a nurse assistant is to support them through this phase with as little pain and discomfort as possible. People nearing the end of life generally have comfort needs in these areas:

- Physical comfort
- Mental and emotional needs
- Spiritual issues
- Practical tasks

Physical Comfort

There are things that can be done to help a dying person be more comfortable. Some residents may be uncomfortable due to pain, breathing problems, skin irritation or breakdown, digestive issues, temperature sensitivity, or fatigue. Always reinforce the importance of the resident reporting the first sign of increased pain so measures can be taken to help control it. Some breathing problems can be relieved with positioning, fans, and oxygen therapy. Dryness in the eyes and mouth are a source of discomfort and can easily be relieved with lip balms, damp cloths, moistened cotton swabs, or ice chips (as tolerated).

Skin irritation and breakdown occur when the ability to move is limited. Constant pressure can result in pressure sores (see Chapter 9). Changing position and providing proper skin care help to relieve the pressure. Additional pads, mattresses, and protectors can be used to help relieve the pressure and prevent skin damage.

Common digestive problems are constipation, nausea, vomiting, and loss of appetite. The cause and treatments for these symptoms are individualized and may be a combination of interventions. Adjustments may be made in diet and medications to try to alleviate the problem. Loss of appetite is a normal part of the dying process. Forcing food when the resident does not want it may cause the resident more discomfort than not eating.

People who are dying may not be able to communicate their needs. It is important to observe the resident for clues. Repeated attempts to push back the blanket

may indicate that they are too hot. Shivering, hunching shoulders, and pulling up covers may indicate that they are cold. Your role is to recognize the clues and intervene.

Fatigue is common in people nearing the end of life. Keep activities simple and provide convenient alternatives such as a bedside commode and shower chairs.

Mental and Emotional Needs

Death is a natural stage in life, but most people do not like to talk about it. When we face the death of another person, we are reminded that we, too, will die someday. Many people fear death because they are afraid of the unknown. The dying person realizes that they will have no more chances to do things they wanted to do. At this time, people ask themselves many questions, such as "What is the meaning of life?" or "What have I done that has made a difference or that will be remembered after I'm gone?" You as a nurse assistant can help residents face their fears and deal with negative emotions such as regret or sadness.

Spiritual Issues

People at the end of life may have spiritual needs that are as important as their physical needs. Finding meaning and peace in the process are very important. You will need to inform the charge nurse if arrangements need to be made for a social worker, spiritual counselor, or clergy member to visit the resident. Many people find solace in their faith or spiritual beliefs at the end of life. It is important to honor their wishes and beliefs.

Practical Tasks

Residents at the end of life may worry about practical tasks. They may be concerned about what will happen to loved ones left behind and who will take over the daily chores and tasks that they have been responsible for. Final wishes and details of responsibilities should be discussed to provide reassurance and comfort to the dying person.

Advance Directives

An **advance directive** is a legal document communicating a person's wishes in regard to health care decisions in the event he or she becomes unable to make those decisions. There are two general types of advance directives: the living will and the durable power of attorney for health care. The federal Patient Self-Determination Act requires all health care facilities to inform residents with information on advanced directives. This usually take place at the time of admission. Residents have a right to accept or reject treatment. Different states use different forms, but all have the same purpose.

A living will states the resident's wishes about withdrawing or withholding life-sustaining procedures if the person becomes terminally ill. The document also specifies which medical treatments the person accepts or rejects. A living will must be written while the individual is mentally competent. The resident can revoke it at any time by notifying the physician or other health care provider or by destroying the original document.

A durable power of attorney for health care is a legal document that designates someone, usually a family member, close friend, or an attorney, to make health care decisions if the person becomes incapacitated and unable to make decisions for themselves.

Other forms can be used for a resident to express their wishes, such as a Physicians Orders for Life-Sustaining Treatment (POLST), also known as Portable Medical Orders or a Do Not Resuscitate (DNR). Either of these forms can be revoked or changed by the resident at any time. The POLST Physicians Orders for Life-Sustaining Treatment (POLST) is a medical order that is typically initiated for those who are seriously ill. The POLST provides specific wishes regarding health care decisions that carries over to all health care providers. A POLST may include information such as the resident's wishes regarding cardiopulmonary resuscitation (CPR), use of antibiotics or IV fluids or if they want to be transferred to a hospital. A DNR form acknowledges the resident's wishes regarding CPR. If a resident has a DNR, CPR will not be initiated if they stop breathing or their heart stops.

You do not need to understand all the legal issues related to these documents, but you should know your facility's general policy about advance directives. You should also know which residents in your care have them.

Feelings About Dying

Elderly residents have experienced the death of loved ones and friends. Because of this, they may think more about life and death. Their spiritual needs often become more important as they review their lives. How people feel about their approaching death varies greatly. These feelings are usually based on their life experiences and spiritual beliefs. Cultural background also plays a role in what a person believes and how they respond to dying.

Some welcome death as a release from pain and suffering. Many have positive expectations based on their religious beliefs. Following are some common beliefs:

- There is a life after death that is free of pain and hardship.
- One will be reunited with loved ones who have already died.
- One will be reincarnated into another body or form.

To support a resident throughout the dying process, you need to understand their beliefs about death. For example, some dying residents fear dying alone, even though they may accept death as positive or freeing. If a resident seems fearful of being alone, develop a plan to be with them as needed. Be sure to respond when they ask for you. Many people fear a painful death. Ask the charge nurse to discuss pain management with the resident.

Residents may also have concerns related to how they lived their lives. For example, they may:

- Feel that they have unfinished business, such as resolving a dispute with a family member.
- Feel unhappy about how they lived their lives. They may feel they failed to achieve all they wanted.
- Feel guilty about something they did or did not do. For example, they may feel that they were not supportive enough of a family member or friend.

The process of life review is very important. Be supportive, open, and nonjudgmental. Always listen to the resident. Think about basic human needs as you care for a dying resident and try to meet as many of their needs as possible. Be sure to report to the charge nurse any information the resident communicates to you so that other members of the team can also provide support.

Stages of Grief

Regardless of individual differences in attitudes and spiritual beliefs, most dying people go through similar feelings about the process. Dr. Elisabeth Kübler-Ross, a psychiatrist who worked with many dying patients, described five stages of grief or loss. These stages apply to the dying person and to those experiencing loss, such as the loss of a loved one. The five stages are denial, anger, bargaining, depression, and acceptance. While called "stages," these emotional states do not necessarily occur in a linear order. They may overlap, and people may move back and forth between several stages for a period of time.

- **Denial** — When people first learn that they are dying, most experience a "not me" reaction. They may refuse to talk about death or to acknowledge physical evidence that they are dying.

- **Anger** — The person asks, "Why me?" They may lash out at family members, caregivers, or even at God. Often they are looking for someone to blame.
- **Bargaining** — The person may try to bargain with physicians or a higher power to gain time to complete unfinished business.
- **Depression** — This occurs when the individual acknowledges that death is coming. They experience sadness and are beginning to mourn their loss of self.
- **Acceptance** — The dying person has worked through most of their earlier feelings and reached a state of calm or peacefulness. Typically, a person who has reached the acceptance stage focuses on living each day to its fullest. A dying resident may work to help friends and family work through their feelings of grief and loss over their approaching death.

Residents may ask you to help their loved ones accept that they are dying. They may evaluate their lives and come to accept both the good and bad aspects. Letting a dying resident talk and being an active listener are key to caregiving at this time. Make sure the resident knows it is all right to talk to you about their feelings.

Almost everyone who is terminally ill knows that their death is inevitable. You may hear family members or staff say that a resident hasn't been told about their approaching death. This does not mean that they do not know.

Often it means only that the person is not yet ready to talk with loved ones about their feelings. You may need to tell family members and other staff about clues you notice about the resident's attitude. Encourage them to listen carefully to what the resident says.

End-of-Life Care

End-of-life care involves a team effort. This includes support for the resident in their decision making, symptom management, and bereavement support. The goal is to meet the resident's individual needs. The resident and family make choices about how the resident wants to be cared for as they approach death.

A critical part of end-of-life care is maintaining the resident's dignity at all times. Their choices are to be honored and their symptoms relieved. If the resident does not want medical care in an effort to prolong life, it will not be given. End-of-life care that focuses on providing comfort and emotional and spiritual support is known as palliative care.

End-of-life care is typically discussed with residents and family members as part of the admission process.

Decisions do not have to be made immediately but thinking about these decisions is encouraged. The residents need time to make choices, discuss their fears, and address any issues. It is better to introduce residents to this subject as a necessary planning stage. This planning ensures that each resident's wishes will be honored when the time comes. Think about media coverage you've seen of legal battles and families torn apart because of disagreements about what the person's wishes were. Planning and documenting the resident's wishes at an early stage will prevent these problems.

Your role in this process is to get to know residents. Know their likes and dislikes. Listen to what they say about their fears. Then tell other members on the team about issues they need to address. Always report any changes you observe. Your observations and reports will ensure early intervention for residents' symptoms. Giving comfort and emotional support can make a huge difference in how they experience the end of their lives. Creating a positive relationship with terminally ill residents is important.

Spend time with them. Do not rush your care. If you feel you need more time with a resident than your other duties allow, discuss this with the charge nurse.

Hospice

Many people think of hospice care simply as end-of-life care, but hospice is a specific program that involves a specially trained health care team. Hospice services focus on palliative care.

Medicare includes a benefit that covers hospice services for eligible people in hospitals, home, and long term care settings. The Medicare benefit applies only when life expectancy is six months or less. This is often a problem in LTC facilities for residents who want and need palliative care but who have a longer life expectancy. For example, residents with end-stage Alzheimer's disease may live much longer than six months but would benefit greatly from hospice services.

Some facilities have special units for residents receiving hospice care. Many people are admitted specifically for this service. You will be asked to work with the hospice team as you follow the resident's care plan.

Helping Dying Residents Cope with Their Feelings

The dying process can be brief or may last a long time. When death is approaching soon, the resident may need more help coping with their feelings. Often the resident becomes restless because of their fear. Report this to the nurse so that anti-anxiety medication may be given, if appropriate. Stay calm to avoid adding to the resident's fear.

For most people, listening is the best thing you can do. If you stay calm and listen carefully, you will know what they need. Your physical presence helps reassure them that they are not dying alone.

Use the communication technique of reflection to encourage residents to talk about their fears and feelings. Ask open-ended questions such as "What are you most worried about?" If a resident is worried about their care, ask what they would like to have done. Assure them they will be made as comfortable as possible. Tell them they will not be left alone. Take time to sit with a dying resident and hold their hand (Figure 13-3). Sometimes a simple touch can comfort the resident. Often you do not have to say anything.

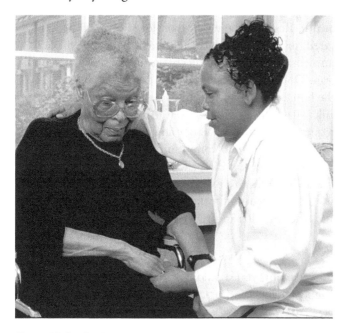

Figure 13-3 Residents must feel able to talk about their fears of dying.

If a resident seems to be denying their impending death, do not try to force them to "face reality." The person is not ready to deal with that realization. You can do more harm than good by forcing the issue. Let the resident adjust at their own pace.

Residents may blame caregivers for not providing enough treatment or not keeping them comfortable. They may be short-tempered with everyone, including other residents and even devoted family members. Do not take personally any anger directed your way. Do not try to talk a resident out of being angry; acknowledge

the person's feelings. You might say "What you're going through is really hard, isn't it?"

A resident experiencing the bargaining stage may say things such as "I just want to be able to hold my grandson one more time." Relay their wishes to the family. Help in any way you can to meet their request for "one more." The resident may be concerned about "unfinished business." If the person can complete whatever that is, they may be able to more easily accept their situation.

You may see signs of depression such as withdrawal from others, crying, or a lack of interest in anything but themselves. Your role is, as always, to be supportive. Be there and accept the resident's need to work through these feelings. You might acknowledge their feelings by saying "You seem very sad" or "I can see that you're having a hard time today." Even if they do not answer, you have communicated your concern and your willingness to listen.

When a resident reaches the stage of acceptance, they usually become calmer. They can more easily talk about dying. They often want to talk about what they want done with their belongings, how they want to be cared for at death, and even their funeral arrangements. In our culture, people are often uncomfortable talking about these things with a dying person. Family members may refuse to talk about death directly with the resident. You and other staff members may be the only people residents can talk to openly if they want to avoid upsetting family members. Keep listening.

Comfort Measures

Earlier in this chapter you learned how to promote sleep and comfort and your role in pain management. Apply this knowledge when caring for a dying resident. Do everything you can to ensure that the resident is comfortable and to provide for their privacy. Follow these guidelines:

- Keep the room well lighted and well ventilated. To offset noises, play soothing music or their favorite music. Offer the resident and family privacy as needed. Keep distracting conversations away from the resident's area.

- Identify yourself frequently. Explain everything you are doing, even if the person is not responsive.

- Offer food and fluids if the resident can tolerate them.

- Change the resident's position frequently. Use pillows for supportive positioning unless ordered not to. Sometimes repositioning is painful, such as, residents with bone cancer. Sometimes a catheter is used to reduce the need for frequent repositioning.

- Change the resident's clothing and bedding when it is soiled by perspiration, urine, or feces.
- Keep the resident well groomed. Help the resident live as well as possible while dying. (Figure 13-4) Keeping them well-groomed can lift their spirits.

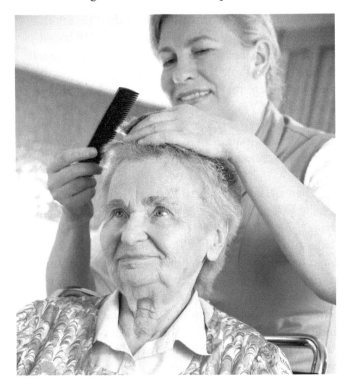

Figure 13-4 Help the residents to look and feel their best.

- Give skin care to prevent or reduce skin breakdown.
- Because dying people often breathe through their mouth, give mouth and lip care frequently.
- Take the resident's vital signs as directed and notify the nurse of any changes. Also immediately report to the nurse any changes in the resident's pain or other changes such as increased restlessness.
- Spend time talking with and listening to the resident. Let the resident know how special you feel to be with them. Share memories and stories from the resident's family and loved ones. Remember that because hearing is the last sense to fade, the resident may be listening even when they do not seem to be fully conscious.

Helping the Family

Family members go through the same stages of grief as the dying person but may not move through the stages at the same time. You may have to assist the communication between family members and the resident.

Some family members are not able to move beyond the denial stage while their loved one is still alive. They may refuse to talk with the person about their wishes for care or funeral arrangements. If you see this behavior, tell the charge nurse. The charge nurse may need to schedule a meeting with the family to address their fears and the resident's wishes.

Some family members express their anger and guilt by insisting on giving all the care to their loved one. Or they may be very critical of the care you provide. Other family members may withdraw and not visit the person because they are unable to express their feelings directly.

While it's appropriate to encourage family members to participate as much as they can in the resident's care, you may have to remind them to take some time for themselves. They need to rest and take care of their own health. Reassure them that their loved one will be well cared for in their absence. Tell them the nurse will call immediately if there is any change in the resident's condition. Do not take personally any criticism or complaints the family makes during this time. Give them time to talk — and listen, listen, listen. If a family member requests to be notified about any change in the resident's condition, be sure to communicate that to other staff.

When a resident dies, allow the family time alone with the body. Offer to sit with them. Pray with them if they ask and you feel comfortable doing so. Give them privacy and offer to call a spiritual counselor.

Religious and Cultural Practices

At this point, you should be familiar with the resident's religious beliefs and practices and those of family members. You will know their wishes for any rituals at the time of death. Many residents want to have religious symbols, medals, statues, or pictures with them. You may be asked to read from the Bible or another religious text or to pray with them. Do this if you are comfortable doing so. If not, make an attempt to find another staff member who can assist.

A rabbi, priest, minister, or other spiritual counselor may visit the resident and family regularly. Their presence is often requested at the time of death. The resident may want to talk with their spiritual counselor when they know death is near. Be sure to provide privacy for these visits.

Take care to understand the concerns of family members at the time of death. A family member may insist on staying with the body. Sometimes this is due to their difficulty accepting the death, but often it involves traditional religious or cultural practices of caring for the body after death.

Family members want to know that their loved one's body will be treated with respect. Reassure them. Explain what will happen with the body. If the family wants to bathe the body or perform another ritual, let them do so if their request is appropriate and allowed by facility policy. This participation is often important for their emotional healing.

Helping Other Residents Cope with Their Loss

A resident's death affects all residents. For some, it is a reminder that their own death is not far away. For others, the death means the loss of a good friend. Residents should always be informed of another resident's death.

Encourage them to talk about their feelings, and reminisce with them about the resident who died. A memorial service held in the facility provides a way for residents and staff to talk about their loss and to remember the good things about the person who died (Figure 13-5).

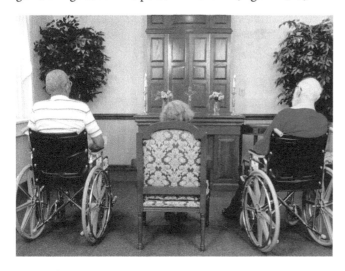

Figure 13-5 Attending a memorial service gives residents an opportunity to talk about their feelings and to honor and remember the friend they have lost.

Often, other residents want to know how the person died. Were they in pain? Was someone there when they died? These questions may arise from their concern for how they will be treated when their time comes. Answer their questions as completely as you can without violating confidentiality rules.

Managing Your Own Feelings

You will often develop close relationships with residents. Before or after they die, you may experience the same feelings as the family and other residents. You are trying to help the resident, family, and other residents deal with their feelings, but who will help you deal with yours?

If you are really listening to the dying resident, you can learn much from them. They may be offering support in various ways to everyone involved. If you have helped the person to have a peaceful death, take comfort in that knowledge.

Identifying your own feelings is the first step in resolving them. Knowing that others also feel the loss helps. Talking with other staff members is a good step. You will probably find that they have similar feelings. Also realize that it is okay to cry sometimes.

Signs of Approaching Death

There are usually physical signs that death is approaching. You may see the following signs hours or minutes before a person dies:

- Decreased blood circulation causes the hands and feet to feel cold to the touch. The face becomes pale or gray. The skin looks spotted.
- The resident's eyes may stare blankly into space, with no eye movement, even when you pass your hand in front of their face.
- Breathing becomes irregular, sometimes rapid and shallow, at other times slow and heavy.
- Heavy perspiration is common.
- Loss of muscle tone causes the body to seem limp. The jaw may drop and the mouth may stay partly open.
- You will hear what is sometimes called the "death rattle," a gurgling sound when the resident breathes.
- The pulse becomes rapid, weak, and irregular.
- Just before death, respiration and pulse stop.

When you recognize the signs of impending death, notify the nurse immediately. The family should be contacted if they are not already present. If you had advance knowledge of the resident's approaching death, you should have already spoken with the resident or the family about their final wishes. Make every effort to meet the resident's and family's requests concerning the last hours of life. Family members will remember their last interaction with their loved one for a long time. That experience will have a lasting effect on their emotional health.

Physical Care of the Body

Every facility has specific procedures for caring for the body after death. Postmortem means after death, and these procedures are usually outlined in a policy called Postmortem Care. Box 13-3 lists common practices. Your facility may include other procedures in postmortem care. Be sure to read and follow your facility's policy.

BOX 13-3

CARING FOR THE RESIDENT'S BODY AFTER DEATH

1. Treat the body gently and with respect.
2. If the resident has a roommate who is aware of their surroundings, arrange for the roommate to go somewhere else until the body is removed.
3. Close the door or pull the curtain for privacy.
4. Ask the nurse to remove tubes and dressings as necessary.
5. Put the resident's body in a flat position with the limbs straight. Place one pillow under the head to prevent their face and neck from becoming discolored.
6. Put their hands on their chest.
7. Put their dentures in their mouth.
8. Wash the body as you would when giving a bed bath. Place a fresh dressing over any open or draining wounds.
9. Comb their hair.
10. Cover their perineal area with a pad to absorb any drainage.
11. Put a clean gown on their body.

- The nurse assistant must accept what residents say about the pain they feel and report their pain as they describe it.
- A person's level of pain can be measured using a numerical or visual pain scale to express how they feel.
- Signs that a resident is experiencing pain include tense or negative facial expressions, abnormal movements or lack of movement, and sounds such as crying or moaning.
- Possible side effects of pain medications include constipation, diarrhea, nausea, vomiting, stomach pain, rash, confusion, slowed respiratory rate, dizziness when standing or changing position, and excessive sleeping.
- Complementary and alternative therapies commonly used to manage pain include massage, acupuncture, guided imagery, meditation, and other relaxation techniques.

- You can help promote comfort and sleep for residents by making sure that the environment is comfortable and quiet, bathroom needs have been met, and the resident feels safe and is not in pain.
- An advance directive communicates wishes in regard to health care decisions in the event a person becomes unable to make those decisions.
- The Kübler-Ross five stages of grief (or loss) are denial, anger, bargaining, depression, and acceptance.
- End-of-life care involves a team that works to support the resident in regard to decision making, symptom management, and facing eventual death. End-of-life care that focuses on providing comfort and emotional and spiritual support is known as palliative care.

> ## Key Terms

advance directive — legal document that specifies a person's wishes in regard to health care decisions if he or she becomes incapacitated and unable to make those decisions

bereavement — period of mourning after the death of a loved one

endorphins — natural morphine-like substances produced in the nervous system that reduce the sensation of pain

hospice — program that provides palliative care for the terminally ill and support services for the patient and the family

insomnia — is where a resident may have difficulty falling and/or staying asleep

living will — legal document that specifies a person's wishes in regard to withdrawing or withholding life-sustaining procedures and which medical treatments the person accepts or rejects

pain — unpleasant sensation caused by stimulation of specialized nerve endings

palliative care — care that focuses on providing comfort and improving quality of life by relieving pain and other symptoms

Physicians Orders for Life-Sustaining Treatment (POLST) – is a document that provides specific wishes regarding health care decisions that carries over to all health care providers.

restless legs syndrome (RLS) — is a condition that causes an uncontrollable urge to move the legs.

sleep apnea — occurs when breathing repeatedly starts and stops during sleep

1. **What can a nurse assistant do to promote comfort and sleep for residents?**

   a. Make sure the radio and television are playing at a loud volume to drown out the background noise

   b. Make sure that the room temperature is cold, this will encourage the resident to stay in bed

   c. Ask the nurse to put in a urinary catheter, this will prevent them from needing to get up to go to the bathroom once they are in bed

   d. Make sure that the environment is comfortable and quiet, that their bathroom needs are met, and that the resident feels as comfortable as possible

2. **Possible side effects of pain medication include:**

   a. Constipation

   b. Diarrhea

   c. Vomiting

   d. All of these

3. **Natural morphine-like substances released by the brain during exercise that can alter one's feeling of pain are called:**

   a. Norepinephrine

   b. Epinephrine

   c. Insulin

   d. Endorphins

4. **What is considered the fifth vital sign?**

   a. Pain

   b. Sleep

   c. Hearing

   d. Unconsciousness

5. **A legal document used by a resident to communicate their wishes about the care they want if they become incapacitated and cannot make decisions is called:**

   a. Death Certificate

   b. Living will/advance directive

   c. Residents Rights

   d. Palliative Agreement

6. **Bereavement is:**

   a. An abnormal response to anything one cannot control

   b. The final stage of the grieving process

   c. A process nurse assistants use to comfort a dying resident

   d. A period of grief after a loved one dies

7. **The five stages of grief in order are:**

   a. Denial, anger, bargaining, depression, acceptance

   b. Anger, denial, depression, bargaining, acceptance

   c. Depression, anger, denial, bargaining, acceptance

   d. Bargaining, anger, denial, acceptance, depression

8. **What Medicare benefit may cover residents in a long term care setting with a life expectancy of six months or less?**

   a. Hospice

   b. Medicare Part D benefits

   c. Medicaid

   d. Ancillary benefits

9. **What is the role of a nurse assistant in pain management?**

   a. To only report the resident's pain during report at the end of the shift

   b. To report information about the resident accurately and in a timely manner as well as perform other strategies such as assisting the resident with repositioning

   c. To limit direct resident care, since this can increase pain

   d. To let families know what medications the resident is on for pain

10. **Comfort measures for a dying resident may include:**

    a. Keeping their room well lit and well ventilated

    b. Telling everyone including family members to stay away

    c. Keeping the resident in the same position in bed

    d. Keeping the television on for company

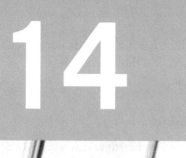

14

Ethics, Law, and Regulatory Guidelines

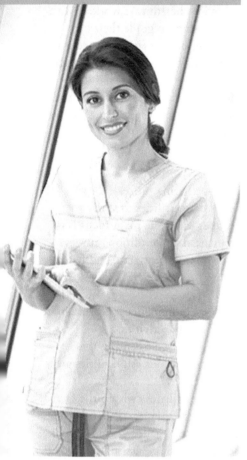

Excellence in care starts with caring about the individuals who have been entrusted to your care. Think of how you would want your loved one to be cared for as you carry out your daily tasks. In this chapter, we discuss ethical decision making in health care settings. We also outline the regulatory process associated with long term care facilities.

Ethics and the Law in Long Term Care

It is important to understand the difference between ethics and laws. **Ethics** are moral principles that govern a person's behavior or the activities of an organization. **Laws** are the rules and regulations that govern the affairs of a community, state, or nation. When laws are violated, there are specific penalties and consequences. Ethical principles and laws set standards for how a particular society defines acceptable and legal behavior by its citizens.

Ethics in the Workplace

Ethical decision making involves doing the right thing and making appropriate choices in the work environment. Workplace ethics involve your actions, judgment, and behavior, including aspects such as how you dress, how you present yourself, how you speak, what you say, and how you treat others. Nurse assistants are expected to maintain a professional appearance, practice good hygiene, and be honest, kind, and considerate when interacting with others. It is important to complete tasks in a timely manner, do your best to fulfill your duties, and treat others with respect at all times. In health care facilities and within health care professions, expectations for ethical behavior are often incorporated into a formal document known as a Code of Ethics or Code of Conduct.

Code of Conduct

The health care setting requires ethical decision making every day. Most facilities incorporate **Code of Ethics** or **Code of Conduct** training during orientation to all new employees. This code covers the basic standards and expectations for how employees are to act with integrity in the workplace. The code defines how staff members are to treat residents, families, other employees, organizational stakeholders, vendors, contractors, and members of the community. All employees are expected to follow the standards set forth in the Code of Conduct.

Health care organizations are required to comply with all laws and regulations pertaining to the provision of services. They must make every effort to identify any risks for noncompliance and to take action to correct any deficiencies. The code supports these efforts by promoting ethical and legal behavior and transparency across all parts of the organization. The code addresses general areas related to compliance concerns and in most facilities, detailed policies and procedures provide specific guidance on how to handle various situations that may occur. In situations in which neither the code nor policies provide adequate guidance, you should consult your supervisor for clarification.

The Regulatory Process

The Code of Conduct provides health care workers with a framework of professional ethics to guide their caregiving, and the laws governing patient rights protect the patients who are receiving care. The provision of services by facilities who receive Medicare and Medicaid funding is regulated by the federal Centers for Medicare and Medicaid Services. State-level personnel conduct surveys of long term care providers.

What Is a Survey?

A survey is an information-gathering process. Surveys are conducted in long term care facilities to verify that residents are receiving proper care. The main focus is to observe residents and evaluate their condition. Surveys help ensure that the facility is following state and federal guidelines for operation. As you know, all skilled nursing facilities that receive payments from Medicare and Medicaid must meet certain requirements. These requirements serve as the basis for survey activities.

Written survey guidelines are used to ensure that surveys are conducted in a fair manner. All facilities are evaluated based on the same criteria.

The survey process evaluates all areas within the facility. Every department must meet a set of standards when inspected. All staff must work together as a team to make the survey process a success. As a nurse assistant, you will have an active role in some parts of the process. During a survey, the physical environment is observed and information is gathered from many sources, including residents, families, staff members, and medical records.

Remember the minimum data set (MDS) and quality indicators discussed in an earlier chapter. They are used as indicators of potential problems or concerns that need further investigation during the survey process. Quality indicators measure information about the residents' health and well-being. Your facility's results are compared to other facilities in your state, and then nationally, to determine if there is a potential problem.

Many areas are assessed in a survey, and they are all important. The survey examines staffing on each shift, how staff members carry out tasks (such as giving medications at the right time), and the cleanliness and condition of residents' equipment and environment. Surveyors observe how laundry is done and how soiled items are handled. The surveyors want to see that staff members understand infection control and carry out the proper procedures, such as handwashing, to prevent the spread of infection.

Surveyors look at the physical structures to see that they meet standards listed in the *Life Safety Code* published by the National Fire Protection Association. The Code is a set of standards for building safety widely used in the United States to specify construction, protection, and occupancy features necessary to minimize danger to life in the event of a fire. Inspections include fire drills and safety checks and focus on the physical plant, maintenance, and the operation of systems within the facility (Figure 14-1).

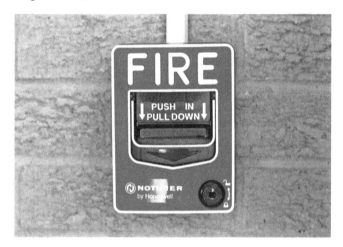

Figure 14-1 As part of a survey, safety inspections are performed to ensure that all systems, such as fire alarms, are in working order.

Surveyors observe residents, review charts, and ask staff questions about the care being provided. The facility is toured to observe safety and cleanliness. Surveyors review employee records to ensure that staff have the proper credentials. Surveyors check that staff members have received the in-service education and health screenings required by each state. They watch staff at work to verify that care is being given in compliance with all regulations. They interview residents and families to find out how they perceive the care they are receiving.

Long Term Care Survey

The Long Term Care Survey is required for every facility that accepts Medicaid or Medicare payments for resident care. This type of survey is conducted every nine to 15 months.

A survey visit can occur at any time of the day or night, including the weekend. Surveyors come to the facility unannounced and spend several days or up to a week. The length of the survey depends upon the size of the facility and any areas of concern found in their first few days. If surveyors find severe care issues, they may stay even longer. An extended survey can potentially be very serious for the facility, and the surveyors will explore their focus areas in more depth to ensure resident safety.

Optional surveys are conducted by accrediting organizations. Facilities choose to be reviewed by other organizations to receive an additional "stamp of approval." Accredited facilities are viewed as providing higher-quality care. Accrediting organization surveys are usually scheduled in advance, but there still may be an unannounced visit. In addition, some surveys are required if a facility has a contract with an agency such as the U.S Department of Veterans Affairs.

Reasons for Surveys

A facility can receive a survey for three main reasons:

- An annual survey is required in every state for all facilities that provide long term care services. These surveys are conducted by the state's Department of Health and Human Services.

- A survey may be conducted based on a complaint about the facility. If a family member, staff, or visitor files a complaint, the state agency will assign surveyors to investigate. This type of survey is unannounced and is usually a day visit at the facility.

- A survey may be done as a follow-up to the annual survey, usually conducted 30 to 45 days after the annual survey. Follow-up visits are made to ensure that any deficiencies found in the annual survey have been corrected and that compliance is being maintained.

Steps in the Survey Process

Several steps are involved in the survey process. Some happen before the survey team arrives, and others are conducted on site. The following sections describe these steps and how you may be involved.

Survey Preparation

Surveyors want to see what care is like on a normal day. Staff should behave as if every day is a survey day. The facility must remain clean, the residents must have their needs met, and the documentation must be up-to-date and accurate. If these processes are consistently maintained, the results will be positive.

Before visiting a facility, the surveyors review the facility's history and quality indicator documents. These reports include information about the type of residents in the facility, any complaints that have been made, and any past problems. Surveyors look for issues that may show a pattern of concern, such as weight loss, falls, or pressure ulcer development.

Initial Interview

Once in the facility, the surveyors first see the administrator. They introduce the members of their team and explain their roles and the reason for the survey. You may be asked to show the surveyors to the administrator's office or to gather additional staff together. Remember to greet everyone with a smile, and offer to show them where the restrooms are located or other areas of the facility. Offer to bring a drink of water or anything else they may need as they settle into the location where they will be working. Your customer service skills are very important during this time.

During the initial interview, the surveyors explain the reason for their visit and any complaints that they will be reviewing. One surveyor may conduct this interview while other team members begin rounds to inspect the nursing units.

It is important that you keep providing care to residents as you normally do. Keep doing frequent rounds and answering call lights and requests promptly. Make sure that your residents are clean, happy, and content.

Surveyors typically post a sign in the facility to let everyone know they are available. They will make time to speak with anyone who wants to meet with them to discuss care in the facility.

Facility Tour

Surveyors usually begin their facility tour shortly after their arrival. In their initial tour, they observe residents and the environment. It is common for survey team members to split up and tour various areas and units. This prevents staff from trying to correct any problems before the survey begins.

The surveyors take notes and later compile them to look for areas of concern. Their first impressions are very important! What they see, hear, smell, and experience on that first round will set the tone for the rest of their visit. The initial tour is designed to:

- Make an initial review of the facility, residents, and staff

- Make an initial evaluation of the environment, the residents' equipment, and the facility's kitchen

- Confirm or resolve any concerns based on earlier reports and any new concerns that arise once in the facility

During their tour, the survey team will focus on the following quality-of-life issues:

- Residents' grooming and dress, including cleanliness and appropriate shoes and slippers

- Staff members' interaction with residents in regard to residents' dignity, privacy, and care needs, including the availability and responsiveness of staff to residents' requests for assistance

- How staff members talk to residents, the nature and the manner of their interactions, and whether they speak with residents when giving care

- Scheduled activities and how appropriate they are for residents

- Equipment in proper working order and in good repair

- Alarms used for residents' safety in proper position and functioning

Another focus is the residents' emotional state and behaviors and the interventions of staff:

- Resident behaviors such as crying out, disrobing, acting agitated, rocking, or pacing

- How staff address these behaviors, including response time, availability, and methods of dealing with residents who are experiencing behavioral issues

Surveyors also focus on care issues such as:

- Breaks in infection control procedures
- Skin conditions, such as being too dry or wet
- Mouth care, including clean teeth and moist lips
- Skin tears, bruising, or evidence of fractures that need investigation
- Dehydration risk factors, including the availability of water for most residents, and other factors such as the amount and color of the urine in tubing and collection bags, how much residents depend on staff, strong urine odors, and residents' complaints of dry mouth and lips
- Clinical signs such as edema, emaciation, and contractures

- Functional risk factors such as poor positioning and use of physical restraints
- Side effects of any antipsychotic drugs
- The presence of any infections, including antibiotic-resistant strains of bacteria, urinary tract infections, skin rashes (especially if they are spreading, undiagnosed, or not responding to treatment), respiratory infections, and gastroenteritis (including diarrhea)
- Medications given correctly as ordered by the doctor
- Perineal and catheter care performed correctly
- Pressure sores, old scars from pressure sores, or evidence of surgical repair of pressure sores
- Amputations
- Significant weight loss
- Use of feeding tubes or improper positioning for feeding
- Use of ventilators, oxygen, and intravenous therapies

Surveyors evaluate facility environment and safety issues:

- Infection control practices, such as handwashing, glove use, and isolation procedures
- Functioning, clean equipment, including kitchen equipment
- Maintenance of a clean and homelike environment
- Availability, use, and maintenance of assistive devices
- Staff knowledge of disaster and emergency preparedness plans

It is important that you know the facility's policies and procedures related to all these focus areas. How you handle your care and interactions with residents will play a major role in the survey outcome. If the initial tour reveals problems, the surveyors may immediately begin an extended survey. As a nursing assistant, your actions will be examined throughout the survey process, so it is important that you are prepared.

After the tour, the surveyors will interview residents and more closely examine the resident records. They want to ensure that documentation is consistent and accurate.

Resident Interviews

Surveyors observe and interview residents individually and in groups. The group interview usually happens during a meeting with the resident council. This is another reason why it is important to always pay attention to concerns raised in the resident meetings. If the facility has been responsive and has taken care of issues reported by residents, that positive service will be seen in this interview.

Surveyors measure the facility's care standards in part through resident observations and interviews. They want to know how residents feel about the care that they are being given. You can never be sure how residents will answer the surveyors' questions, so it can be helpful to know what questions may be asked. Common questions include:

- Can you choose what you wear?
- What choices do you have about when you get up and go to bed?
- Have you ever been treated roughly by staff?
- Have you ever felt afraid here?
- Do you participate in activities when you wish to?
- Do you have any problem getting to activities?
- Can you choose your food preferences?
- Is the food served the way you like it?
- Do you get things to drink between meals?
- How do staff members act toward you when they take care of you?
- Do you have choices about when and how your care is provided?
- Do you feel that staff members treat you with respect and dignity?
- Have you lost any personal items? Did you tell a staff member? What did he or she do?
- How promptly do staff members respond to your call signal?
- During evenings and at night, are sounds too loud and distracting? If yes, have you told a staff member about this? How did he or she respond?
- How do staff members react to residents who repeatedly ask for help?
- Is your mail sealed when you get it?
- Do you have privacy when you want to use the telephone?
- Can you meet with your visitors in private?
- Do you have enough light in your room to read?
- Is your room cool enough in the summer and warm enough in the winter?
- Have you seen any bugs or rodents in the facility or in your room?

These are just a small sample of the questions that residents may be asked during a survey. You can have a positive impact on the survey by helping make sure that residents can answer all of the above questions positively. That is done by assuring that residents are respected and well cared for every day (Figure 14-2).

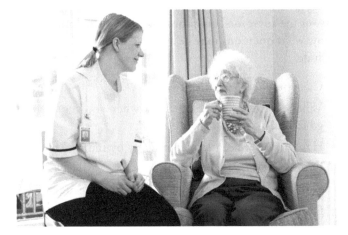

Figure 14-2 You play a role in creating a comfortable, homelike environment for residents, and this can be observed by surveyors.

Family Interviews

Family interviews are an important part of the survey process. Surveyors will ask family members many of the same questions they ask residents. They want to ensure that families have a choice in the care that their loved one is getting. It is important that family members have had positive interactions with staff that they can talk about with the surveyors. If you and other staff are responsive to the needs and concerns of the family, then those actions will become known to the surveyors. You should always pay attention to the family's concerns and solve problems as they arise.

Staff Interviews

When it is your turn to be interviewed, be proud of what you do and answer questions with confidence. If you are asked a question that you cannot answer, don't guess. It is okay for you to say that you are not sure about something. If you do not understand the question, then say so. Making up an answer will only cause a bigger problem. Be sure to tell the surveyor that you will be glad to find the answer for them. Report these questions to your charge nurse, who can help find the answers.

Surveyors may ask you questions such as:

- What would you do in case of a fire?

- What would you do if you thought a resident was being abused?

- How do you know what your facility's policies are?

- What can you tell me about your facility's quality improvement program?

- How are changes in residents' care communicated to you? How do you communicate changes in residents?

- How do you know what equipment is needed to care for your residents?

- How do you know if a resident is on special isolation precautions?

Here are some tips for a successful interview:

- Make sure that you know your facility's policies and procedures for abuse, fire safety, disaster plans, and reporting issues.

- When responding to a surveyor's questions, avoid over-sharing. Answer questions simply and stick to the facts.

- Don't try to impress the surveyor. Be professional and polite and use appropriate language. Do not try to impress them with all that you know.

- Don't blame others or bring up problems that you may have had with other staff members or other departments.

- Don't complain. If you have a legitimate problem, you should discuss it with your supervisor, not the surveyor.

- Smile. Surveyors like to see nurse assistants who are smiling and interacting pleasantly and respectfully with residents and families.

- Be polite in your interactions with residents, families, staff, and visitors. This is always part of good customer service.

- Don't let stress get the best of you. Take a minute to refocus. Take your scheduled breaks to give yourself time to relax and decompress.

- Keep a positive attitude, and the surveyors will have a good understanding of how valuable you really are.

Resident Monitoring and Reviews

Surveyors will carefully review residents' medical records and plans of care. They may also ask specific questions about a resident you are caring for. You should know what is documented in your resident's record and care plans. Surveyors will watch staff to ensure that activities in the care plan are actually being done.

Surveyors also review incident reports, fall records, and injury reports. From this they will determine whether staff are doing all they can to prevent injuries and maintain safety for residents.

Surveyors want to make sure that staff protect residents' rights during caregiving. They will observe care activities such as range of motion exercises, splinting, and special feeding techniques. They will take note of how staff members communicate with residents while giving this care. Surveyors are always looking for the outcome of all care activities. They want to make sure the facility is offering services that will maintain residents' current level of functioning and improve their condition. Any decline in function needs to be prevented, if possible.

Meal service is another focus of this monitoring. Surveyors inspect the cleanliness of the kitchen and review documentation about meals. They examine menus, temperature logs for refrigerators, dietary assessments, and weight records. They watch staff serve the food to ensure that the correct portion size and consistency of food is provided as ordered for specific residents. If a resident does not eat the provided food, the staff should request alternatives for the resident. Surveyors will taste food items and monitor food temperatures and preparation techniques. They will look for positive staff interactions with residents during meals.

Surveyors will observe for any breaks in infection control techniques. They will watch to make sure that residents' hands are cleaned before and after meals, that any spilled foods are removed, and that clothing is changed after meals, if needed. They will watch meals being served at different times and in different areas of the facility. They want to ensure that meal service is consistent throughout the facility.

Surveyors also observe specialty items and procedures, such as use of catheters, oxygen, restraints, or special dressings. They will pay special attention to pressure ulcers, tube-fed residents, IV solutions, and tracheotomy care. They will want to see how these specialty care procedures are performed and will review techniques used, the safety of procedures, and infection control practices. Surveyors will watch to ensure that the resident's dignity and privacy is maintained throughout all of these procedures.

Throughout the survey process, surveyors will investigate any concerns identified during the tours, observations, interviews or found while reviewing the medical records or facility documents.

Exit Conference

At the end of the survey, the surveyors hold an **exit conference** with the administrator and leadership team. The ombudsman and officer of the resident council are invited to attend the exit conference. This conference serves as a preliminary verbal report of the survey results. In this meeting, surveyors describe any items of concern that they found (Figure 14-3). The final written report will describe in more detail any areas that do not meet the minimum standards for long term care facilities.

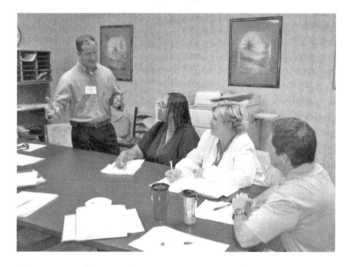

Figure 14-3   The on-site survey concludes with an exit conference.

Final Report and Follow-Up

After leaving the facility, the surveyors produce a report of their findings. They use standard measures for the level of deficiencies that they will cite. A **deficiency** is cited when the facility did not meet the minimum standard for a specific area. Deficiencies in the areas of resident rights, quality of care, and quality of life are the most serious.

The results of the survey are calculated using a rating system. Long term care facilities are rated from one to five stars. The stars are determined by the survey results, staffing patterns, and quality indicators. Every facility has the goal of having a five-star rating.

The final official report is sent to the facility. If the survey found a number of serious problems, the facility may not be allowed to hold nurse assistant training programs, admit new residents or may be fined or even closed — depending on the seriousness of problems found. The facility's interdisciplinary team develops a plan to correct any problems and notifies the surveying agency of this plan. The agency may accept the facility's plan, ask for revisions, or reject it outright. If this happens, the facility has to start over and make an alternate plan for correction.

When the facility's plan is accepted, a time frame is set for the correction of problems. At the end of that time, a follow-up visit is conducted to ensure that the facility has corrected the problems.

All long term care survey results are a matter of public record and are published on the Medicare.gov Nursing Home Compare website. The facility must also post a copy of the most recent survey results in an area where the public and residents can view it.

Your Role in the Survey Process

You may be asked questions by the surveyors or asked to gather information to help with the survey process. Your exact role depends on the surveyors' requests. Follow these general guidelines:

- Do not call in sick (unless you really are sick)
- Look professional at all times
- Smile and say hello
- Carry out your assignments as usual
- Be confident in yourself when you are asked questions
- Do not try to tell the surveyors what you think they want to hear
- Help housekeeping by notifying them of any spills
- Keep work areas neat and clean, even if they are not your areas
- Make sure that the break room is not dirty or cluttered
- Be observant of everything going on around you
- Make sure you know your facility's policies

If you have any questions before, during, or after the survey, be sure to talk to the charge nurse. If you are not certain about a policy or process, it is very important to let your supervisor know before the survey. He or she will be glad to explain it to you to prevent any confusion during the survey.

If you wish, you can request a copy of your facility's survey results. Remember, you are a vital part of the health care team. Your role is very important and can make a huge difference in the survey results.

Nurse Aide Training Regulations and Competency Testing

The Omnibus Budget Reconciliation Act of 1987

The Omnibus Budget Reconciliation Act of 1987 (OBRA 87), also known as the Nursing Home Reform Act, contains provisions designed to assure delivery of quality care to long-term care facility residents. This act established minimum standards for nursing facilities. The act included the requirement that each state must establish nurse aide training programs with minimum requirements for competency. These laws and regulations apply to all nursing facilities that are funded by Medicare and Medicaid. In most states, you must complete a nurse aide training program that has been approved by the state in order to take the state test nurse aide competency exam.

Nurse Aide Registries

Federal regulations require each state to establish and maintain a registry of individuals who have completed training and who the state finds to be competent to function as nurse aides. Nurse aide registries must include information on any substantiated finding of abuse, neglect, or misappropriation of property made by the State survey agency related to an individual. The purpose of the registries is to prevent unemployable individuals from being employed in long-term care facilities. Federal regulations require states to update the nurse aide registry records within 10 working days of substantiating findings against an individual. States also must remove from the registry the records of nurse aides who have not performed nursing or nursing-related services for a period of 24 consecutive months, unless the records include substantiated findings. Those records must remain on the registry indefinitely, except under specific circumstances, such as notification of the death of the individual.

State Nurse Aide Regulations

Each state has specific regulations related to nurse aide training, some of states exceed the minimum Federal requirements. Each nursing facility and nurse aide training program must operate within both Federal and State regulations. Most states require all nurse assistants to complete a state-approved nurse aide training program. Some states allow candidates to challenge the competency evaluation without taking a state-approved class if specific requirements are met.

What is Required to Get a Job as a Nurse Assistant

In order to work in a nursing facility as a nurse assistant you must have taken and successfully passed the state nurse aide competency evaluation, frequently referred to as the "state test". You are eligible to take the state test after you successfully complete your nurse assistant training or have met the state specific requirements for challenging the test. Check with your state office that oversees nurse assistant testing or certification to learn more about eligibility and documentation requirements for challenging the test. All candidates must pass the state specific background check and screening requirements.

How to Apply to Take the State Competency Evaluation

Once you are ready to take the state test you must register with the testing entity in your state. You can ask your instructor about the process for applying to take your state test. If you have taken a course though a nursing facility, they can give you guidance on how to apply to take the test. Some facilities will assist you with the registration process.

Online registration is a common process. Once your test is scheduled, they will provide you the specific directions including the location of the test site, the date of the test, what time you should arrive, what documents you should bring with you, and what you should wear. Most testing entities prohibit candidates from having electronic devices, including smart watches turned on during the test.

Some testing entities will provide directions for scheduling a test, provide sample test questions, step by step skill procedures, and information on what is expected of you, including dress code and documentation that you will be required to bring the day of testing.

Make sure that you read and understand the information provided by the testing entity. If you do not follow their policies or fail to bring the required documentation to the testing site, you may not be able to test.

Preparing for the Competency Evaluation

Most testing entities provide candidates with a handbook that provides information on registering for and taking the test. If a handbook is provided, make sure that you read the material so you will know what to expect. Some handbooks can be found online on the testing entity's website. Some testing entities provide testing for multiple states; make sure that you are viewing information for your state.

The state test consists of two parts: knowledge and skills. For the knowledge portion you will take a written test; it is typically multiple choice and can be computer-based or paper-and-pencil. For the skills portion of the test, you will demonstrate your ability to perform the personal care skills that you learned during your class.

The best way to prepare for the written part of the test is to do well in your nurse assistant training. The information needed to succeed is in your training materials. Study all training materials as you are waiting to take the state test. To study for the skills portion of the test, make sure that you are familiar with the skills that you will be tested on. If the testing entity has provided a handbook that lists the skills, practice these skills, and know them well.

Some states provide sample tests that you can take to help you practice for the test. There are also tests available online, keep in mind that these tests may not be specific to your state and may contain information that does not meet your state requirements.

Depending on your state, you may not be able to test immediately after completing your nurse assistant training course. If this is the case, it is important that you continue to study until you take the state test.

Here are some tips for taking the written portion of the test:

- Review what you have learned in your nurse assistant training program.
- Ask your instructor for a sample test and become familiar with the types of questions that may be on the test.
- Answer the questions to the best of your ability.

Tips for taking the skills part of the test:

- Review all the skills you learned in your nurse assistant training program. If you have a handbook for the testing entity practice all of the skills listed. If you do not have a handbook, ask your instructor if they can provide you with skills to study.
- Practice each skill with other students or family members. Ask your instructor, charge nurse, or staff development coordinator at your facility to help you with anything that you are having difficulty with or do not understand.
- Always remember to include all preparation and completion steps.

General tips for taking the state test:

- Get a good night's sleep before the test.

- Eat a well-balanced meal before the test.

- Make sure you know the correct address and directions to the test site. Drive there ahead of time if you have doubts or are anxious about finding the location.

- Be on time; if you are late, they may not allow you to test.

- Make sure that you have read and understand the rules of the testing site.

- Show up prepared with all of the necessary documents and tools needed to take the test.

- Before starting, take a few deep breaths to help release stress and tension.

How do I get the results of my test?

The testing center will notify you on how and when you will receive your test results. In some states you will know within a day and other states may take up to several weeks.

Requirements for In-service Education

In-service education is an important part of quality care. It keeps staff updated as residents' needs change, technology improves, and with current nursing care practices. In-service education involves a learning process that may be either formal or informal. Long term care facilities are required to offer nurse assistants a minimum of 12 hours a year of in-service education. The staff educator will typically post upcoming classes.

In-service education gives you an opportunity to grow, change, and improve. It is a good way to stay challenged and motivated. It is one of your most valuable employee benefits. Attending in-service education classes in your facility is the most efficient way to gain new hands-on information. Taking additional classes, subscribing to professional magazines, and joining professional organizations are other ways to continue your education and improve the quality of your care.

Each state has specific requirements related to in-service education, including how many hours are required to renew your nurse assistant certification or license in order to continue working and remain on the registry. It is your responsibility to make sure you meet your minimum state requirements.

How to Remain on the Nurse Aide Registry

Each state has different requirements for maintaining on the nurse aide registry, in addition to the required in-service education hours. Each state has a renewal period, this is typically every two years. Make sure that you are familiar with your states renewal process. If you do not renew timely, you will not be able to work in a nursing facility.

Points to Remember

- Ethics are moral principles that govern a person's behavior. Laws are the rules and regulations that govern the affairs of a community, state, or nation.

- Ethical decision making involves doing the right thing and making appropriate choices every day as you carry out your duties and care for residents.

- The Code of Ethics or Code of Conduct is introduced during orientation, and all employees are expected to follow the standards for quality care and proper behavior outlined in this document.

- Surveys are conducted to ensure that facilities meet established standards of care. The process includes survey preparation, initial interview with the administrator, a facility tour, and interviews with residents, families, and staff members. Residents and caregiving routines are observed, and residents' records are examined.

- Survey results reveal any deficiencies (problems) that have been discovered, and the facility must develop a plan to correct all deficiencies.

- Getting ready for a survey is what you do every day. If you give the highest possible level of care, are attentive in your work, and know your residents, then you should feel proud. Those are exactly the qualities and behaviors that surveyors want to see during their visit.

- As you are preparing to take your state test, make sure you review your specific state requirements for testing and maintaining an active status on the state registry.

Key Terms

Code of Ethics or Code of Conduct — covers the basic standards and expectations for how employees are to act with integrity in the workplace

deficiency — weakness, problem, or noncompliance issue identified during the survey process

ethics — moral principles that govern a person's behavior or the activities of an organization

exit conference — a preliminary verbal report of the survey results

laws — rules and regulations that govern the affairs of a community, state, or nation

long term care survey — periodic survey required of all facilities that receive payment from Medicare or Medicaid

1. **What is the best way to prepare to take the state nurse assistant exam?**
   a. Study your How to be a Nurse Assistant textbook and review skills you have learned
   b. Read three or four other nursing textbooks
   c. Ask an experienced nurse assistant if they remember what was on the test
   d. Spend a day volunteering and helping nurses in a hospital

2. **Surveys are conducted to ensure:**
   a. That family members visit frequently
   b. All staff members are receiving insurance benefits
   c. That facilities meet established standards of care
   d. That staff are adhering to the facility dress code

3. **Which of the following is an environmental issue included in a survey?**
   a. Weight loss
   b. Positioning
   c. Dehydration
   d. Cleanliness of rooms

4. **Which of the following may be a reason for a survey?**
   a. Family complaint
   b. Reported abuse of resident
   c. Complaint about an unexplained injury
   d. All of these

5. **The state certification test for nurse assistants has two (2) parts:**
   a. Knowledge and Skills
   b. Mental and Practical Applications
   c. Statistics and Outcomes
   d. Quality and Utilization

6. **What is the purpose of the nurse aide registry?**
   a. To make sure staff works a set number of hours every week
   b. To prevent unemployable individuals from being employed in long-term care facilities
   c. To prevent overstaffing in the facility
   d. To ensure that facilities follow the required federal regulations

7. **What act included the requirement that each state must establish nurse aide training programs with minimum requirements for nurse aide competency?**
   a. State regulations
   b. The Unemployment Act
   c. OBRA 87
   d. HIPAA

8. **What decision making process involves doing the right thing and making appropriate choices in the work environment?**
   a. Code of Conduct
   b. The Quality Assurance process
   c. Ethical decision making
   d. Directive decision making

9. **Laws are:**
   a. Rules and regulations that govern the affairs of a community, state, or nation
   b. A decision based on a selected group
   c. Guidelines for only a collective group to follow
   d. Are not necessary at the facility level

10. **The code that covers the basic standards and expectations for how employees are to act with integrity in the workplace is:**
    a. The code of ethics
    b. The code of integrity
    c. The code of conduct
    d. The code of confidentiality

Appendix A: Glossary

A

abuse — cruel or inhumane treatment that causes physical and/or psychological harm; threats made to a person

accommodation — resolving conflict by giving in to the wishes of another person

accreditation — process of certifying that a facility meets certain quality and performance standards

acquired immunodeficiency syndrome (AIDS) — severe disorder of the immune system caused by the human immunodeficiency virus (HIV)

activities director/coordinator — staff member who plans and directs activities for residents

activities of daily living (ADL) — tasks that are required for daily living, such as bathing, dressing, personal hygiene, and eating

acute — problem that begins rapidly and lasts for a limited period of time

administrator — general manager of a facility

admissions director/coordinator — staff member who coordinates the process of admitting new residents

advance directive — legal document that specifies a person's wishes in regard to health care decisions if he or she becomes incapacitated and unable to make those decisions

advocate — someone who takes the side of another person and speaks for them

agenda behavior — actions that follow a certain agenda, often a past routine

aggression — hostile, threatening, or violent behavior toward others

airborne precautions — measures taken to prevent the airborne transmission of pathogens

airborne transmission — infection spread by microorganisms contained in particles or droplets suspended in air

allegation — a person's statement that someone has done something wrong or illegal

alveoli — air sacs in the lungs

Alzheimer's disease — progressive brain disease that causes memory loss, other cognitive impairments, and behavioral changes

Alzheimer's unit — unit that provides care for residents with Alzheimer's disease and other types of dementia

antibiotic — drug that inhibits the growth of or kills certain microorganisms

antibody — protein produced by the body to fight infection or illness

anxiety — a feeling of uneasiness, worry, fear or dread

apnea — temporary cessation of breathing, especially during sleep

aphasia — communication disorder that results from damage to parts of the brain responsible for language; affects ability to speak and understand speech and ability to read and/or write

arteries — blood vessels that carry oxygenated blood to all parts of the body

arthritis — joint inflammation that causes pain and limits movement

artificial airway — tubular device placed into the respiratory tract to facilitate breathing or the removal of secretions

asepsis — the absence of bacteria

aspiration — when fluid or foreign material is inhaled into the lungs

assessment — evaluation of a patient or condition

assignment — a specific set of tasks that an employee is expected to perform

assistant director of nursing — senior nursing professional who reports to the director of nursing

assisted living facilities (ALF) — residential facilities that provide a limited amount of assistance with daily activities

attending physician — directs and provides the primary care of individual residents

aura — a sensation that often precedes a seizure

auscultation — using a stethoscope to hear sounds produced by internal organs (such as heart, lungs, or bowels)

Autism Spectrum Disorder (ASP) — a disorder that affects a person's ability to communicate and interact with others

autonomy — ability to act independently and make decisions for oneself

avoidance — staying away from a person or issue instead of dealing with a conflict

awareness — consciousness of one's environment

B

bacteria — single-celled microorganisms; some are beneficial and others may cause infection (singular = bacterium)

baseline — initial measurement or observation used for later comparison

behavioral symptoms — actions caused by a disease or condition

benign prostatic hyperplasia (BPH) — enlargement of the prostate gland

bereavement — period of mourning after the death of a loved one

biohazardous waste — waste containing blood or other potentially infectious substances; includes needles, blades, and other sharps

biologicals — medical products made from living organisms, such as vaccines or blood components

Bipolar disorder — a condition that causes severe fluctuations in mood, energy levels, concentration and affects their ability to carry out function of daily living

blood pressure (BP) — measurement of the pressure of blood in the arteries

bloodborne pathogens — pathogen present in blood that can be transmitted via blood or body fluids

body language — nonverbal communication that includes posture, gestures, and facial expressions

body mass index (BMI) — measurement that estimates the percentage of fat tissue in the body

body mechanics — principles of proper body movement for efficiency and injury prevention

body system — group of organs and structures that work together to perform vital functions

bowel or fecal incontinence — the inability to control bowel movement, causing leakage from the rectum

brace — device that supports and strengthens a body part

bradycardia — slower than normal pulse rate

bradypnea — slower than normal respiratory

bronchi — two main air passageways (right and left) into the lungs; singular form is bronchus

bronchioles — branches of each bronchus

C

call system — system that enables residents to signal that they need assistance from staff

cancer — group of diseases characterized by the uncontrolled growth of abnormal cells

capillaries — tiny blood vessels that connect the smallest arteries and veins; the site of gas exchange

cardiac arrest — complete cessation of heart activity (no heartbeat)

cardiopulmonary resuscitation (CPR) — emergency procedure to restore cardiopulmonary function

care plan — written document created after the resident assessment is completed that outlines the goals of care, nursing interventions (actions and approacheswhat care is to be provided), and the time frame for accomplishment and evaluation

cataract — clouding of the lens of the eye that reduces vision

Centers for Medicare and Medicaid Services (CMS) — the agency responsible for surveying and certifying long term care facilities as approved to receive federal funding

Cerebral palsy (CP) — a disorder that affects movement and posture

cerebral vascular accident (CVA) — condition that occurs when blood flow to the brain is interrupted; also called a stroke

chain of infection — process by which infection is spread

charge nurse — nursing professional with day-to-day responsibility for supervising resident care

chemical restraints — medications used to sedate a resident, slow their muscle activity, or change their behavior

chemotherapy — type of drug therapy used as a treatment for disease, especially cancer

cholesterol — fatty substance produced by the body and ingested in food

chronic — problem that usually begins gradually and lasts for an extended period of time

chronic obstructive pulmonary disease (COPD) — chronic inflammatory disease of bronchial passages and lungs; three most common types are bronchitis, emphysema, and asthma

circulatory system — body system that includes the heart, blood vessels, and lymphatic tissues and vessels

clarity — clearness of communication

cleaning — removing soil from a surface or object

Code of Ethics or Code of Conduct — covers the basic standards and expectations for how employees are to act with integrity in the workplace

Code of Federal Regulations (CFR) — set of rules published in the Federal Register by the departments and agencies of the U.S. government

cognitive impairment — measurable decline in memory and thinking skills

collaboration — working together to accomplish a task or resolve a conflict

comatose — describes a person who is a coma (unconscious)

communication — sending and receiving messages verbally, nonverbally, in writing, or through symbols

compassion — sympathetic understanding of another person's suffering or situation coupled with a sincere desire to help

communication board — a device used for those who have difficulty communicating verbally, it is customized with signs, symbols or pictures that help the resident communicate their needs.

competition — challenge or contest in which there is a winner and a loser

compromise — resolving conflict by both parties agreeing to something less or different than they originally wanted to achieve a peaceful resolution

conflict resolution — process for settling a dispute or disagreement

congestive heart failure (CHF) — condition that occurs when the heart muscle weakens and becomes ineffective in moving blood throughout the body

constipation — - difficulty in emptying the bowelsdifficulty in moving bowels

contact precautions — measures taken to prevent the spread of infection caused by microorganisms transmitted by direct or indirect contact

context — the entire situation, background, or environment that provides meaning to a person's words

continuing care retirement community — facility that provides several tiers of care: independent living, assisted living, and skilled nursing care

contracture — abnormal shortening of muscle tissue due to lack of movement or improper positioning

contraindicated — when a condition is present that provides a reason for not recommending a medical treatment

coronary artery disease (CAD) — condition in which the major blood vessels that supply the heart become damaged or diseased, often due to plaque build-up and/or inflammation

corporal punishment — physical punishment, such as spanking or slapping

cuing — prompting a resident to begin a task or activity by telling or showing

culture — the collective customs, attitudes, and beliefs of a particular group of people; may relate to ethnic or religious background and/or social groups

customer service — the actions involved in serving a customer's needs

customs — traditional practices of a particular group of people

D

defensiveness — being overly sensitive to perceived criticism from others

deficiency — weakness, problem, or noncompliance issue identified during the survey process

dehydration — serious condition that results from excessive loss of water from the body; can occur due to inadequate fluid intake

delegate — to give or entrust someone with a task or job

delusion — false thought that a person believes to be real

dementia — mental disorder characterized by memory loss, impaired reasoning, and personality changes

denial — ignoring or blocking true feelings or the truth about a situationavoiding an issue or problem instead of dealing with it directly

depression — a common mood disorder that causes a persistent feeling of sadness and loss of interest

dermatitis — inflammation of the skin

dermis — inner layer of the skin beneath the epidermis

developmental disability — chronic condition caused by physical and/or mental impairment that affects language, learning, mobility, and the activities of daily living; may prevent a person from living independently

diabetes — disease in which the body either doesn't produce enough insulin or doesn't use insulin properly, resulting in high blood glucose

dialysis — process of filtering and removing waste products from the blood used when the kidneys are not functioning properly

diarrhea — feces passed frequently and in liquid form; loose stool

diastolic pressure — number that reflects the pressure when the heart is at rest between beats

digestive system — body system involved in processing food, providing nutrients to the body, and expelling waste

dignity — a sense of pride and self-respect; being worthy of honor and respect

direct transmission — spread of infection from one person to another or when infected blood or body fluids come in direct contact with broken skin or mucous membranes

director of nursing — senior nursing professional who directs the approach for care and determines staffing requirements

director of staff development — staff member who develops and oversees nursing education programs

discrimination — an unfair or unjust treatment of people or groups of people

disinfection — process that kills or inhibits the growth of virtually all microorganisms on objects and surfaces

documentation — written and/or digital reports maintained by the facility relating to a resident's care and condition

Down syndrome — also known as trisomy 21, is a genetic disorder caused by the presence of all or part of a third copy of chromosome 21

droplet precautions — measures taken to prevent the spread of infection caused by microorganisms transmitted by droplets produced by coughing, sneezing, talking, or performing procedures

droplet spread — infected oral or nasal secretions transmitted via the eyes, nose, or mouth of another person, most commonly passed through coughing, sneezing, or talking

dysphagia — difficulty swallowing food, liquid, or medication

dyspnea — difficult or labored breathing

E

edema — swelling of the legs and ankles due to excess fluid in body tissues

electronic medical record (EMR) — digital version of the patient chart and medical record

elimination — process of ridding the body of waste products via urine and stool

emesis — the action of vomiting

empathy — ability to understand and share the feelings or perspective of another person

endocrine system — body system made up of glands that secrete hormones

endorphins — natural morphine-like substances produced in the nervous system that reduce the sensation of pain

enteral nutrition — providing liquid nourishment using a nasogastric tube or a tube surgically inserted through the abdominal wall into the stomach

epidermis — surface (outer) layer of the skin

epilepsy — sometimes called a seizure disorder, a disorder in which the seizures are not caused by a temporary medical condition

ergonomics — study of the interaction of workers and their environment; its principles drive the design of equipment and work environments

ethics — moral principles that govern a person's behavior or the activities of an organization

exit conference — a preliminary verbal report of the survey results

exposure — being in the vicinity of or in contact with an infectious microorganism

expressive aphasia — communication disorder that involves difficulty communicating but the person can usually comprehend what is being said to them

external customer — residents, families, and customers who are outside of the long term care facility

external evacuation — moving residents out of the facility to another site for safety

F

face sheet — one-page summary of important information about a patient/resident

fainting — a temporary loss of consciousness caused by decreased blood flow to the brain

fall — unintentionally coming to rest on the ground, floor, or other. lower level, but not as a result of an overwhelming external force

fever — elevated body temperature

flow sheet — document used to record health and activity information about a resident over a period of time

Fowler's position — lying on the back with the head of the bed raised 45 to 60 degrees

fracture — break in a bone or other hard tissue

functional incontinence — occurs when the bladder doesn't fully empty causing constant or frequent dribbling

fungus — type of microorganism that can cause infection; examples are yeast and mold (plural = fungi)

G

gait belt — also known as a transfer belt, used to help steady a resident during transfers or walking

gastroesophageal reflux disease (GERD) — a digestive disorder that occurs when stomach contents leak back into the esophagus

gerontology — scientific field focused on the study of aging

goal — a desired result or outcome

grievance — formal complaint of a wrong, injury, or injustice

H

hallucination — false sensory experiences (visual images, sounds, smells, etc.) that appear to be real

healthcare-associated infection (HAI) — infection contracted while in an inpatient, outpatient, or residential health care facility

Heimlich maneuver — emergency procedure to dislodge food or an object obstructing the airway

hemodialysis — type of dialysis in which blood is removed from the body and filtered through a machine that removes waste products and excess fluid and returns the blood to the body

hemorrhage — excessive or uncontrolled bleeding

hepatitis — viral infection of the liver

history — information about a resident's previous health status, lifestyle, and medical treatment

history and physical (H&P) — patient/resident history combined with a physical exam

hospice — program that provides palliative care for the terminally ill and support services for the patient and the family

hospice care — care for terminally ill patients that aims to provide comfort and alleviate pain

human immunodeficiency virus (HIV) — virus that attacks the body's immune system

hydration — supplying water to the body to maintain fluid balance

hyperglycemia — abnormally high blood sugar

hypertension — high blood pressure

hypodermis — layer of fatty tissue beneath the epidermis

hypoglycemia — abnormally low blood sugar

hypotension — low blood pressure

hypoxia — state in which not enough oxygen is reaching body tissues

I

immunization — administration of a vaccine to prevent a specific infectious disease

incontinence — inability to voluntarily control urination or defecation

Incontinence Associated Dermatitis (IAD) — is a form of dermatitis caused by frequent exposure from urine and/or stool

indirect transmission — infection spread when a microorganism is transferred from one person to another via a vehicle (inanimate object) or a vector (living host such as a tick or mosquito)

infection — invasion and multiplication of microorganisms such as bacteria and viruses that are not normally present in the body; may or may not produce symptoms

inflammation — cellular and tissue response to injury and infection

influenza — viral respiratory infection; also called the flu

in-service education — educational programs provided for employees while on the job

insomnia — is where a resident may have difficulty falling and/or staying asleep

inspection — careful observation of the resident's body to determine health status

integumentary system — body system made up of the skin, nails, and hair

interdisciplinary team — staff members from various departments who work together to plan and implement care

intermediate care facility — facility that provides care for people with intellectual disabilities and works to promote their functional status and independence provides nursing and supportive care to residents who have a variety of mental or physical disabilities

internal customer — customers who are part of the same organization; supervisors and coworkers

internal evacuation — moving residents to another location within the facility for safety

involuntary seclusion — the isolation of a resident against their will, such as locking them alone in a room

isolation precautions — measures taken to prevent the spread of infection from an infected resident to other people

J

Joint Commission — nonprofit organization that accredits and certifies U.S. health-care facilities and programs; full name is The Joint Commission

K

ketones — substances made when the body breaks down fat for energy

kiosk — centrally located electronic device used to input patient/resident data

L

latent — in a resting or dormant state

laws — rules and regulations that govern the affairs of a community, state, or nation

level of care — classification based on the intensity of medical and nursing services provided in a health-care setting

licensed practical nurse (LPN) — health professional who provides basic nursing care under the supervision of a registered nurse or physician

licensed social worker (LSW) — licensed professional who usually has a master's degree in social work and who counsels residents and families

licensed vocational nurse (LVN) — health professional who provides basic nursing care under the supervision of a registered nurse or physician

living will — legal document that specifies a person's wishes in regard to withdrawing or withholding life-sustaining procedures and which medical treatments the person accepts or rejects

long term care — a range of medical and nonmedical services provided for people who have a chronic illness, disability, or cognitive impairment that affects their ability to perform everyday tasks

long term care survey — periodic survey required of all facilities that receive payment from Medicare or Medicaid

M

malignant — cancerous tumor or cells that grow uncontrollably and spread to other parts of the body

managed care — type of health insurance coverage that monitors quality of care and is designed to contain costs

MDS coordinator — staff member who assesses residents' functional capabilities and determines the appropriate level of care; also called a nurse assessment coordinator

Medicaid — joint federal-state health insurance program for low-income individuals and families

medical asepsis — reduces the number of microorganisms, also known as clean technique

medical director — senior staff physician who directs medical care in a facility

Medicare — federal health insurance program for individuals age 65 and older and certain people with disabilities

mental abuse — any action that makes a resident fearful, such as threatening them with harm or threatening to tell others something they do not want them to know

mentally competent — capable of rational decision making and being responsible for one's actions

microorganisms — organisms that cannot be seen with the naked eye; some are capable of causing infection

misappropriation of resident property — includes deliberately misplacing a resident's belongings or money, or using a resident's belongings without his or her permission or theft

mixed incontinence — is a combination of stress and urge incontinence

mobility — ability to move freely

mode of transmission — the means by which a microorganism is transferred from one carrier to another

multidrug-resistant organism (MDRO) — describes microorganisms that have evolved in a way that makes them resistant to the action of antibiotic

multiple sclerosis — progressive disease that affects nerve fibers

musculoskeletal system — body system made up of bones, muscles, tendons, ligaments, and joints

myocardial infarction — damage to an area of the heart due to lack of blood supply and oxygen; commonly called a heart attack

N

natural flora — microorganisms that are always present, that usually do not cause disease

nausea — an uneasy or sick feeling in the stomach

neglect — failure to provide proper care

negligence — failure to act in the same way that a reasonable person with the same training would act in the same situation

nervous system — body system made up of the brain, spinal cord, and nerves

nonpathogenic — describes microorganisms that do not cause infection

nonverbal communication — sending and receiving messages without using words

NPO — abbreviation for nil per os, Latin for "nothing by mouth." Used to designate a period of time during which a person cannot eat or drink before surgery or some other type of medical procedure.

nurse practitioner (NP) — works with the interdisciplinary team to direct and provide primary care for residents

nursing staff — trained members of the nursing team; includes LPNs/LVNs, registered nurses, and nurse assistants

nutrition — nourishment obtained from food

O

objective information — factual information gathered through observation

obsessive-compulsive disorder (OCD) — a condition that is characterized by unwanted, repetitive thoughts (obsessions) or behaviors (compulsions) that they feel needs to be repeated over and over

occult — hidden; not able to be seen

Occupational Safety and Health Administration (OSHA) — federal agency responsible for protecting worker health and safety

occupational therapist (OT) — licensed health professional who works with residents to improve their ability to perform everyday tasks

ombudsman — official or designated person who investigates and resolves complaints; advocate for resident rights

open-ended question — question that requires a more complex answer than a simple "yes" or "no."

orthosis — equipment or device, such as a brace or splint, used to provide support to a weak or injured part of the body

osteoarthritis — degenerative joint disease caused by wear and tear of the joint

osteoporosis — bone disease that involves loss of tissue; bones become weak and brittle and prone to fractures

ostomy — surgical procedure that creates an opening from the intestine to outside the body for the discharge of wastes

outbreak — sudden increase in cases of a disease within a certain geographic area

ovaries — female reproductive glands that secrete sex hormones and produce eggs

overflow incontinence — occurs when the bladder doesn't fully empty causing constant or frequent dribbling

P

pain — unpleasant sensation caused by stimulation of specialized nerve endings

palliative care — care that focuses on providing comfort and improving quality of life by relieving pain and other symptoms

palpation — physical examination conducted by touching the resident's body with the fingers and/or hands

parasite — organism that lives in or on another organism

Parkinson's disease — neurological disease that affects motor skills

pathogen — microorganism or substance that can produce disease

percussion — tapping on a body area (chest, back, abdomen) to hear the sound produced; used to determine the status of internal tissues and organs

perineal care — cleaning and care of the area between the anus and external genitals

peripheral vascular disease (PVD) — condition that causes diminished blood flow to the extremities

peritoneal dialysis — type of dialysis in which waste and fluid are removed from the blood using a surgically placed catheter in the abdominal (peritoneal) cavity

personal care — care provided for residents that includes bathing, mouth care, hair care, grooming, and dressing

personal health record (PHR) — an individual health history kept by the patient, usually in electronic form

personal protective equipment (PPE) — is equipment worn to minimize exposure to hazards that cause serious workplace injuries and illnesses

pharynx — tube extending from the back of the nasal passages and mouth to the esophagus

physical abuse — any action that causes physical harm

physical examination — an organized examination of the body to determine health status; includes visual inspection, auscultation, palpation, percussion, and smell

physical restraints — any devices that limit a resident's movement or access to their body.

physical therapist (PT) — licensed health professional who uses methods that include exercise, heat, massage, mobilization, and manipulation to reduce pain and improve mobility

Physicians Orders for Life-Sustaining Treatment (POLST) — is a document that provides specific wishes regarding health care decisions that carries over to all health care providers.

plaque — fatty deposit on blood vessel walls

pneumonia — serious bacterial or viral lung infection

podiatrist — physician specializing in the care and treatment of the feet

policies and procedures (P&Ps) — guidelines and procedures established by a facility for daily operations and emergency/disaster situations

portal of entry — the opening by which a microorganism enters the host

portal of exit — the place where a microorganism leaves the reservoir

positioning — assisting a resident in changing position

post-acute care unit — unit that provides a high level of care for residents; may include rehabilitative services

postoperative — period of time after surgery

preoperative — period of time before surgery

preoperative orders — physician orders prior to surgery

prone position — lying in a face down position on the abdomen

prostate cancer — cancer of the prostate gland in males

prosthesis — an artificial body part

protocol — an official or standard way of doing something, usually put in writing

psychosocial — relating to the psychological and social aspects of mental health

pulse — measure of heart rate taken by feeling the expansion of an artery as blood is pushed through when the heart contracts

pus — thick yellowish-white fluid formed in infected tissue

R

radial pulse — pulse measurement taken by feeling the radial artery at the wrist

radiation therapy — treatment for cancer or other disease using x-rays or other forms of radiation

reflection — restating in your own words what another person has said to be sure that you understand the speaker's meaning and feelings

registered dietician (RD) — staff member who develops food plans and special diets for residents

registered dietician nutritionist (RDN) — staff member who develops food plans and special diets for residents

registered nurse (RN) — health professional who provides an advanced level of nursing care and may supervise other nursing staff

regulated waste — contaminated waste that must be disposed of according to facility policies and government regulations

rehabilitation — process of regaining a former state of health or function

rehabilitation unit — unit that provides specialized care designed to help residents return to a previous level of physical functioning after an illness or injury

relocation stress syndrome — stress and anxiety experienced by a person relocating to a new environment, such as a resident entering a long term care facility

reproductive system — body system made up of reproductive organs and glands

reservoir — person, animal, or environment in which an infectious agent lives

resident — person admitted to a long term care facility

Resident Assessment Instrument (RAI) — assessment tool used in long term care facilities to document key information about residents, including care plans and outcomes

resident-centered care — focuses on the resident's individual preferences and needs with the resident being an active participant in their care.

respiration — exchange of oxygen and carbon dioxide between the atmosphere and body cells; breathing

respiratory rate — measurement of the number of breaths per minute

respiratory system — body system that allows for the exchange of oxygen and carbon dioxide in the body

respite care — care provided for residents who enter a facility for a temporary stay until their regular caregivers become available

Restless Legs Syndrome (RLS) — is a condition that causes an uncontrollable urge to move the legs.

restorative — activities designed to help a person be as independent and functional as possible

restorative nursing — nursing care designed to promote a resident's ability to achieve the highest level of function and to live as independently as possible

retaliation — the act of getting revenge or punishing a person for doing something

rheumatoid arthritis — autoimmune disease that causes inflammation of the joints

routine care — daily care activities

S

safety data sheet (SDS) — sheet containing information about products and chemicals; includes guidelines for safe handling and emergency response

sanitation — promotion of hygiene and prevention of disease by maintaining clean conditions

schizophrenia — a severe mental disorder that affects how a person acts, thinks and behaves

sebaceous glands — microscopic glands in the skin that secrete an oily substance called sebum

secretions — substances such a saliva, mucus, perspiration, tears, etc. that come out of the body

seizure — abnormal electrical activity in the brain that causes sudden, involuntary muscle movements

self-determination — freedom to make your own choices and choose your own activities

service mentality — dedication to making sure that customers' needs are satisfied

sexual abuse — any sexual act where the resident does not or cannot give consent

sexually transmitted disease (STD) — infectious disease transmitted through sexual contact

shift — scheduled period of work for a group of employees (as in day, evening, and night shifts)

shock — medical emergency in which body tissues and organs are not receiving adequate blood and oxygen

side-lying position — (lateral) positioned on either side with knees slightly bent

sims position — the resident is positioned on their left side with the hip and lower leg slightly bent and the right hip and knee bent

sitz bath — bath in a tub or special basin in which only the perineum and buttocks are immersed

skilled nursing care — care for residents needing post-acute care from both nursing and rehabilitation services; care performed by or under the supervision of a licensed nurse

sleep apnea — occurs when breathing repeatedly starts and stops during sleep

special senses — vision, hearing, equilibrium (balance), smell, taste, and touch

specimen — sample of fluid or tissue taken for examination and/or testing

speech-language pathologist (SLP) — highly trained professional who works with residents who have swallowing, speech, language, or other communication problems

spiritual counselor — staff member who coordinates religious services and provides counseling for residents and families

splint — device to use to support or immobilize a body part

sputum — material coughed up from the lungs and expelled through the mouth; contains mucus, cellular debris, microorganisms, and may also contain blood or pus

standard precautions — evidence-based practices designed to prevent transmission of infectious disease

sterilization — process that completely eliminates all microorganisms from a surface or object

stoma — surgically created opening that is kept open for drainage or the removal of waste

stool — feces; solid waste from the bowel

stress incontinence — occurs when pressure is put on the bladder like coughing, sneezing, laughing, lifting or exercising

stroke — condition that occurs when blood flow to the brain is interrupted; also called a cerebral vascular accident (CVA)

subcutaneous — under the skin

subjective information — information based on an assumption, opinion, or on what the resident says about how they feel

substance use disorder — occurs when the recurrent use of alcohol and/or drugs causes clinically significant impairment, including health problems, disability, and failure to meet major responsibilities at work, school, or home

suicide — when death is caused by self-harm with the intent to die

sundowning — worsening of symptoms of Alzheimer's disease and other types of dementia that occurs in the late afternoon or evening; also known as sundown syndrome

supine — lying on the back

surgical asepsis — known as sterile technique, eliminates all microorganisms

susceptible host — a person who at risk of developing an infection from a microorganism

systolic pressure — number that reflects the pressure in the artery when the heart is pumping

T

tachycardia — faster than normal pulse rate

tachypnea — faster than normal respiratory rate

temperature — measurement of the degree of heat in the body

terminal conditions — illnesses from which a patient is not expected to recover; death will likely occur within a short period of time

testes — two oval glands that produce sperm cells and secrete male sex hormones; also called testicles

The Joint Commission — nonprofit organization that accredits and certifies U.S. health-care facilities and programs

themes of care — core principles that form the basis for all care provided to residents

therapeutic — referring to a treatment

therapeutic diet — special diet used as a treatment for a disease or condition

time management — the ability to plan and prioritize tasks and perform activities efficiently to make the best use of available time

total parenteral nutrition (TPN) — nutrition administered intravenously

tracheostomy — creation of an opening into the trachea to facilitate breathing; also known as a tracheotomy

trapeze — suspended horizontal bar used to help position a person in bed

traumatic brain injury unit — unit that specializes in rehabilitative care for residents with traumatic head injuries

U

urge incontinence — is a sudden strong urge to urinate, followed by urinary leakage

urinalysis — physical, chemical, and microscopic examination of a urine sample

urinary incontinence — condition in which a person cannot voluntarily control urination

urinary system — body system that helps maintain fluid balance and eliminates liquid waste

urine — liquid waste produced by the kidneys and stored in the bladder

V

validation therapy — approach that validates and supports a person's perception of the world; used in treatment of Alzheimer's disease and related conditions

vector — living agent that transmits infection

vehicle — some type of inanimate object that acts as a carrier for microorganism

veins — blood vessels that carry deoxygenated blood from the body back to the heart and lungs

verbal abuse — using profanity or other words that attack, insult, threaten, bully, or humiliate another person

verbal communication — sending and receiving messages using spoken or written words

virus — a type of microorganism that survives only in living things

visual communication — using symbols, such as traffic lights, road signs, memes, and emojis

vital signs — measurements of temperature, pulse, respiration, and blood pressure

void — to empty the bladder; urinate

vomiting — also known as emesis, is when stomach contents exit through the mouth

vulnerable resident — someone in need of special care, support, or protection because of age, disability, or risk of abuse or neglect

Appendix B: Common Medical Abbreviations

ā — before
abd — abdomen
a.c. or āc — before meals
ADL — activity of daily living
ad lib — as desired
Adm — administrator
AM — morning
amb — ambulate
amt — amount
AP — apical
ASAP — as soon as possible
bid 2 — two times a day
BM — bowel movement
B/P or BP — blood pressure
BR — bedrest
BRP — bathroom privileges
BSC — bedside commode
C — Celcius
c̄ — with
cath — catheter
cc — cubic centimeter
CHF — congestive heart failure
c/o — complains of
CPR — cardiopulmonary resuscitation
CVA — cerebrovascular accident; stroke
DC or D/C — discontinue, stop
DNR — Do not resusitate
DNS — Director of Nursing Service

DON — Director of Nursing
drsg or dsg — dressing
dx — diagnosis
F — Fahrenheit
FBS — fasting blood sugar
FF — force fluids
ft. — foot, feet
FWB — full weight bearing
h or hr — hour
H20 — water
HA or H/A — headache
HOH — hard of hearing
hs — hour of sleep; bedtime
ht — height
I&O — intake and output
ICP — interdisciplinary care plan
IV — intravenous
kg — kilogram (2.2 kg = 1 lb)
L or lt — left
lb — pound
MD — medical doctor
midnoc — midnight
ml — milliliter (1 ml = 1 cc)
NA — sodium (salt)
NAS — no added salt
neg. — negative
NKDA — no know drug allergies
noc — night

NPO — nothing by mouth
NWB — non weight bearing
02 — oxygen
OD — right eye
OOB — out of bed
OS — left eye
OT — occupational therapy
p̄ — after
p.c. or p̄c — after meals
PM — afternoon or evening
PO — by mouth
PR — per (or by) rectum
PRN — as needed
PT — physical therapy
PWB — partial weight bearing
q — every
qd — every day
qhs — every hour of sleep
qid — four times a day
qod — every other day
q2h, q3h, etc. — every 2 hours, 3 hours, etc.
R or rt — right (R can also mean rectal)
RCP — resident care plan
res — resident
ROM — range of motion
s̄ — without
SOB — shortness of breath
spec — specimen
Stat — immediately
tid — three times a day
TPR — temperature, pulse, respiration
u/a or U/A — urinalysis
VS — vital signs
W/C — wheelchair
wt — weight
x — times

Appendix C: Common Medical Prefixes and Suffixes

Prefix/suffix	Translation	Example
a-, an-	without, lack of	anemia (lack of blood)
ab-	away from	abduct (move extremity away from body)
ad-	toward, near	adduct (move extremity toward the body)
-al	pertaining to	dermal (pertaining to the skin)
-algia, -algesia	pertaining to pain	myalgia (muscle pain)
ante-	before, forward	antecubital (before or in front of the elbow)
anti-	against	antidepressant (drug to counter depression)
arter-	artery	arteriosclerosis (hardening of arteries)
auto-	self	autoinfection (infection by organism already in the body)
bi-	twice, double	bifocal (two points of focus)
bio-	life	biology (study of living things)
brady-	slow	bradycardia (slow heart rate)
-cele	herniation, pouching	mucocele (cavity containing mucus)
cent-	hundred	centimeter (hundredth of a meter)
-centesis	puncture and aspiration	thoracentesis (puncture through thoracic cavity to remove fluid)
-cid(e)	cut, kill	germicide (kills germs)
-cise	cut	incise (cut into)
circum-	around	circumcision (incision removing foreskin around penis)
con-	with	concurrence (agree with)
contra-	against, opposite	contraception (against conception)
-cyte	cell	erythrocyte (red blood cell)
de-	down, away from	dehydrate (remove water)
dia-	across, through	diameter (distance across a circle)
dis-	apart from, separate	disinfection (apart from infection)
dys-	difficult, abnormal	dysfunctional (not functioning normally)
ecto-	outer, outside	ectoderm (outer layer of tissue)
-ectasis	dilation	telangiectasis (dilation of capillaries)
-ectomy	removal of	tonsillectomy (removal of tonsils)
-emia	blood condition	anemia (lacking iron in blood)
en-	in, into, within	enclave (tissue enclosed inside other tissue)
endo-	inside	endoscope (instrument for looking inside the body)
epi-	over, on	epidermis (outer layer of skin)
eryth-	red	erythrocyte (red blood cell)
-esthesia	sensation	paresthesia (abnormal sensation)
ex-	out, out from	extract (to remove)
extra-	outside of	extracellular (outside the cell)

Prefix/suffix	Translation	Example
-genesis	development	pathogenesis (development of disease)
-genic	producing	pathogenic (disease-causing)
-gram	printed recording	arteriogram (diagnostic picture of an artery for visualization)
-graph	instrument for recording	audiogram (device to evaluate hearing)
hemi-	half	hemiplegia (half of body paralyzed)
hyper-	over, excessive	hypertension (high blood pressure)
hypo-	below, deficient	hypoglycemic (low blood sugar)
-iasis	condition of	nephrolithiasis (condition of having kidney stone)
il-	not	illegible (not readable)
in-	into, within or not	injection (forcing liquid into)
inter-	between	intercostal (between the ribs)
intra-, intro-	within	intravenous (within the veins)
-ism	a condition	rheumatism (condition of having rheumatoid arthritis)
-itis	inflammation	appendicitis (inflamed appendix)
-logy	the study of	psychology (study of the mind)
-lysis	destruction of	hemolysis (destruction of blood cells)
leuk-	white	leukocyte (white blood cell)
macro-	large	macromastia (abnormally large breasts)
mal-	illness, disease	malabsorption (inadequate absorption of nutrients)
-megaly	enlargement	acromegaly (enlargement of head, hands, and feet)
-meter	measuring instrument	spirometer (instrument that measures breathing)
-metry	measurement	telemetry (measurement using remote transmitter)
micro-	very small	microorganisms (very small organisms)
mono-	one, single	monoplegia (paralysis of one extremity)
neo-	new	neoplasm (tumor growing new cells)
non-	not	noninflammatory (not causing inflammation)
olig-	small, scanty	oliguria (low excretion of urine)
-oma	tumor	granuloma (tumor consisting of granulation tissue)
-oscopy	look into	gastroscopy (look into the stomach)
-osis	condition	fibrosis (condition of fibrous tissue formation)
-ostomy	opening into	colostomy (opening into the colon)
para-	abnormal	paralgesia (abnormal painful sensation)
-pathy	disease	myopathy (disease of muscle)
-penia	lack	leukopenia (lack of enough white blood cells)
per-	by, through	perfusion (passage of fluid through an organ)
peri-	around, covering	pericardium (the sac around the heart)
-phasia	speaking	aphasia (speaking or language disorder)
-phobia	exaggerated fear	hydrophobia (fear of water)
-plasty	surgical repair	myoplasty (repair of a muscle)
-plegia	paralysis	quadriplegia (paralysis of arms and legs)
poly-	much, many	polyuria (much urine)
post-	after, behind	postoperative (after surgery)
pre-, pro-	before, in front of	preoperative (before surgery)
-ptosis	falling, sagging	ptosis (drooping eyelid)

Prefix/suffix	Translation	Example
re-	again, back	reinjure (injure again)
retro-	backward	retrograde (moving backward)
-rrhage	excessive flow	hemorrhage (heavy bleeding)
-rrhaphy	suturing	colporrhaphy (surgical suturing of vagina)
-rrhea	profuse discharge	diarrhea (heavy discharge of watery stool)
-scope	examination instrument	microscope
-scopy	examination using a scope	endoscopy (looking inside body with endoscope)
semi-	half, part	semi-reclined (partly lying down)
-stasis	control, stop	hemostasis (stopping bleeding)
-stomy	creation of opening	colostomy (opening of bowel to abdomen)
sub-	under	subcutaneous (under the skin)
super-	above, excessive	superinfection (excessive infection occurring during the treatment of another infection)
tachy-	fast, rapid	tachycardia (fast heartbeat)
-tomy	incision	sinusotomy (incision of a sinus)
trans-	across	transdermal (across the skin)
uni-	one	unilateral (one side)
-uria	condition of the urine	polyuria (passing abnormally large amount of urine)

Appendix D: English-Spanish/Spanish-English Glossary of Basic Long Term Care Terms

ENGLISH-SPANISH GLOSSARY

abdomen — abdomen
ache — dolor
afternoon — tarde
angry — enojado
ankle — tobillo
arm — brazo
back — espalda
bandage — venda
bathroom — cuarto de baño
bathtub — bañera
bed — cama, lecho
bedpan — chata
black — negro
blanket — manta
blood — sangre
blouse — blusa
blue — azul
bottom — fondo
bread — pan
breakfast — desayuno
brother — hermano
brown — castaño
butter — mantequilla
cane — bastoón
chair — silla
chest — pecho
chew — masticar
child — niño
chin — barbilla
clean (adjective) — limpio
clear — transparente
clothes — ropa; men's suit: traje,
  woman's dress: vestido
coffee — café
cold (adjective) — frío
comfort — consuelo
constipation — estreñimiento
cough (noun) — tos
cream — crema
cup — taza or vasa
dark — oscuro
daughter — hija
day — día
depressed — depresivo
dinner — cena
dirty — enlodado

disease — enfermedad
doctor — doctor
door — puerta
dress (clothing) — vestido
drink (verb) — beber
drink (noun) — bebida
dry — seco
ear — oreja
eat — comer
eggs — huevos
elbow — codo
emergency — emergencia
exercise — ejercicio
eye — ojo
eyeglasses — lentes
face — cara
family — familia
fever — fiebre
finger — dedo
fire — fuego
floor — suelo
flu — influenza
foot — pie
forehead — frente
fork — tenedor
friend — amigo
fruit — fruta
green — verde
hair — pelo
hairbrush — cepillo (para el pelo/
  cabello)
hallway — pasillo
hand — mano
hat — sombrero
head — cabeza
hearing aid — audífono
help! — ¡socorro!
here — aquí
hot — caliente
hungry — hambriento
husband — marido
ice — hielo
infection — infecccíon
juice — jugo
knee — rodilla
knife — cuchillo

left — izquierdo
leg — pierna
light — luz
lonely — solitario or solo
lunch — almuerzo
man — hombre
meat — carne
medicine — medicina
milk — leche
morning — mañana
mouth — boca
move — mover
music — música
neck — cuello
need (noun) — necisidad
night — noche
nightgown — camisón
no — no
noon — mediodía
nose — nariz
nothing — nada
nurse — enfermera
oxygen — oxígeno
pain — dolor
painkiller — analgésico
pajamas — piyamas
pants — pantalones
pantyhose — media
pardon me — perdóneme
pepper — pimienta
pillow — almohada
plate — plato
please — por favor
potatoes — papas
preference — preferencia
priest — sacerdote
red — rojo
right (opposite of left) — derecho
roommate — compañero de cuarto
sad — triste
salt — sal
sheet — sábana
shirt — camisa
shoes — zapatos
shoulder — hombro
shower — ducha

sister — hermana
sit — sentarse
skin — piel
skirt — falda
sleep (noun) — sueño
sleep (verb) — dormir
snack — bocado
sneeze (noun) — estornudo
socks — calcetínes
son — hijo
sorry — lo siento
spoon — cuchara
spouse — cónyuge
stand — estar de pie
stomach — estómago
stool (feces) — excremento
sugar — azúcar
sunlight — luz del sol
swallow — tragar
table — mesa

talk — hablar
teeth — dientes
telephone — teléfono
television — televisión
thanks — gracias
thermometer — termómetro
thirsty — sediento
toast — tostada
today — hoy
toes — dedos del pie
toilet — taza
toilet paper — papel higiénico
tomorrow — mañana
toothbrush — cepillo de dientes
toothpaste — pasta dentífrica
underclothes — ropa interior
urinal — orinal
urinate — orinar
urine — orina
vegetable — verdura(s), vegetal(es)

vomit (noun) — vómito
wake (verb) — despertar
walk (verb) — andar, caminar
walker — andador
want (verb) — desear
wash (verb) — lavar
water — agua
weigh — pesar
wet — mojado
wheelchair — silla de ruedas
when? — ¿cuando?
where — ¿donde?
white — blanco
wife — esposa
window — ventana
woman — mujer
wound — herida
wrist — muñeca
yellow — amarillo
yes — sí

SPANISH-ENGLISH GLOSSARY

abdomen — abdomen
agua — water
almohada — pillow
almuerzo — lunch
amarillo — yellow
amigo — friend
analgésico — painkiller
andador — walker
andar — walk (verb)
aquí — here
audífono — hearing aid
azúcar — sugar
azul — blue
bañera — bathtub
barbilla — chin
bastoón — cane
beber — drink (verb)
bebida — drink (noun)
blanco — white
blusa — blouse
boca — mouth
bocado — snack
brazo — arm
cabeza — head
café — coffee
calcetínes — socks
caliente — hot
cama — bed
caminar — walk (verb)
camisa — shirt
camisón — nightgown
cara — face
carne — meat
castaño — brown

cena — dinner
cepillo (para el pelo/cabello)
    — hairbrush
cepillo de dientes — toothbrush
chata — bedpan
codo — elbow
comer — eat
compañero de cuarto — roommate
consuelo — comfort
cónyuge — spouse
crema — cream
¿cuando? — when?
cuarto de baño — bathroom
cuchara — spoon
cuchillo — knife
cuello — neck
dedo — finger
dedos del pie — toes
depresivo — depressed
derecho — right (opposite of left)
desayuno — breakfast
desear — want (verb)
despertar — wake (verb)
día — day
dientes — teeth
doctor — doctor
dolor — ache
dolor — pain
¿donde? — where
dormir — sleep (verb)
ducha — shower
ejercicio — exercise
emergencia — emergency
enfermedad — disease

enfermera — nurse
enlodado — dirty
enojado — angry
espalda — back
esposa — wife
estar de pie — stand
estómago — stomach
estornudo — sneeze (noun)
estreñimiento — constipation
excremento — stool (feces)
falda — skirt
familia — family
fiebre — fever
fondo — bottom
frente — forehead
frío — cold (adjective)
fruta — fruit
fuego — fire
gracias — thanks
hablar — talk
hambriento — hungry
herida — wound
hermana — sister
hermano — brother
hielo — ice
hija — daughter
hijo — son
hombre — man
hombro — shoulder
hoy — today
huevos — eggs
infeccíon — infection
influenza — flu
izquierdo — left

jugo — juice
lavar — wash (verb)
leche — milk
lecho — bed
lentes — eyeglasses
limpio — clean (adjective)
lo siento — sorry
luz del sol — sunlight
luz — light
mañana — morning, tomorrow
mano — hand
manta — blanket
mantequilla — butter
marido — husband
masticar — chew
media — pantyhose
medicina — medicine
mediodía — noon
mesa — table
mojado — wet
mover — move
mujer — woman
muñeca — wrist
música — music
nada — nothing
nariz — nose
necisidad — need (noun)
negro — black
niño — child
no — no
noche — night
ojo — eye
oreja — ear
orina — urine

orinal — urinal
orinar — urinate
oscuro — dark
oxígeno — oxygen
pan — bread
pantalones — pants
papas — potatoes
papel higiénico — toilet paper
pasillo — hallway
pasta dentífrica — toothpaste
pecho — chest
pelo — hair
perdóneme — pardon me
pesar — weigh
pie — foot
piel — skin
pierna — leg
pimienta — pepper
piyamas — pajamas
plato — plate
por favor — please
preferencia — preference
puerta — door
rodilla — knee
rojo — red
ropa — clothes
ropa interior — underclothes
sábana — sheet
sacerdote — priest
sal — salt
sangre — blood
seco — dry
sediento — thirsty
sentarse — sit

sí — yes
silla — chair
silla de ruedas — wheelchair
¡socorro! — help!
solitario — lonely
solo — lonely
sombrero — hat
suelo — floor
sueño — sleep (noun)
tarde — afternoon
taza or vasa — cup
taza — toilet
teléfono — telephone
televisión — television
tenedor — fork
termómetro — thermometer
tobillo — ankle
tos — cough (noun)
tostada — toast
tragar — swallow
traje — men's suit
transparente — clear
triste — sad
vegetal(es) — vegetable
venda — bandage
ventana — window
verde — green
verdura(s) — vegetable
vestido — woman's dress
vómito — vomit (noun)
zapatos — shoes

Appendix E: Weights and Measures

Weights and Measures

There are two commonly used measurement systems, the house hold or US Customary System and the metric system. Each unit of weight and measures can be converted between the two systems.

Measurement — Length

1 foot (ft.) = 12 inches

1 yard (yd.) = 3 feet

1 foot (ft.) = 0.30 meters (m)

1 inch (in.) = 2.54 centimeters (cm)

1 centimeter (cm) = 10 millimeters (mm)

1 meter (m) = 100 centimeters (cm)

Weight and Volume

1 gram (g) = 1,000 milligrams

1 kilogram (kg) = 1,000 grams

1 liter (L) = 1,000 milliliters (ml)

1 milliliter = 1 cubic centimeter (cc)

1 ounce (oz.) = 29.574 milliliters/cubic centimeters

1 gallon (gal) = 3.78541 liters (L)

1 quart (qt) = 32 fluid ounces (fl oz)

1 pint (pt) = 473.176 milliliters (ml)

1 cup = 8 fluid ounces (fl oz)

1 tablespoon (tbsp) = 14.7868 milliliters (ml)

1 teaspoon (tsp) = 4.92892 milliliters (ml)

To convert milliliters or cubic centimeters to ounces, multiply by 0.0338

To convert ounces to milliliters or cubic centimeters, multiply by 29.57

1 kilogram (kg) = 2.2046 pounds (lbs.)

To convert kilograms to pounds, multiply by 2.2046

To convert pounds to kilograms, divide by 2.2046

Weight conversion examples:

A resident weighs 150 lbs but you have to record the weight in kilograms. How many kilograms does this resident weigh? To determine the weight you will divide the weight in pounds by 2.2046.

1150 ÷ 2.2046 = 68.039. The resident's weight would be 68.039 kg (this can be rounded to 68.04 kg).

If you needed to convert kilograms to pounds you would use the following formula: kg = lbs × 2.2046.

Your resident weighs 75 kilograms, how many pounds does your resident weigh?

75 × 2.2046 = 165.345. The resident's weight would be 165.345 lbs.

To accurately measure the volume of a substance:

1. Pour the substance into the graduate container
2. Place the container on a flat surface
3. Looking at eye level, use the measurement at the lowest point of liquid surface (the center of the meniscus)
4. Record the measurement using the appropriate abbreviations

Measuring example:

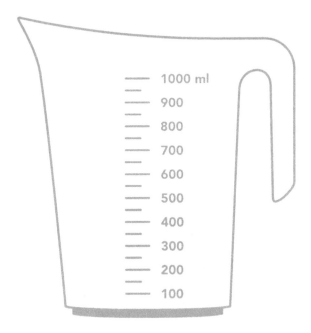

How many milliliters or cubic centimeters are in this graduated cylinder?

Use the conversion factor: 1 ml = 1 cc

There are 500 cc or 500 ml in this graduated cylinder.

Temperature

To convert Celsius to Fahrenheit, divide by 5, then multiply by 9, then add 32

Example: 36°C ÷ 5 = 7.2

7.2 × 9 = 64.8

64.8 + 32 = 96.8° F

To convert Fahrenheit to Celsius, subtract 32, then multiply by 5, then divide by 9

Example: 80°F − 32 = 48

48 × 5 = 240

240 ÷ 9 = 26.6667°C

Telling Time- Standard & Military

There are two systems used for telling time:

1. Standard time (also called civilian time) splits the 24-hour day into 12-hour increments, also known as am and pm

   A.M. = midnight until noon

   P.M. = noon until midnight

2. Military time is a 24-hour clock with four digits and no colon

   The clock starts at one minute after midnight (0001) and ends at midnight (2400) which shows the 24-hour circulation of a day

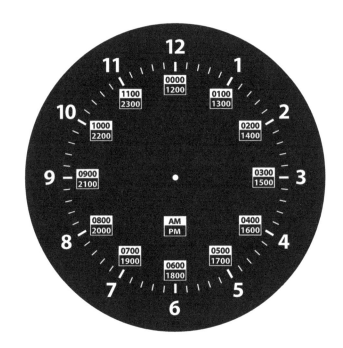

Time Conversion Table

Standard Time	Military Time
12:00 am (midnight)	0000
1:00 am	0100
2:00 am	0200
3:00 am	0300
4:00 am	0400
5:00 am	0500
6:00 am	0600
7:00 am	0700
8:00 am	0800
9:00 am	0900
10:00 am	1000

Standard Time	Military Time
11:00 am	1100
12:00 pm (noon)	1200
1:00 pm	1300
2:00 pm	1400
3:00 pm	1500
4:00 pm	1600
5:00 pm	1700
6:00 pm	1800
7:00 pm	1900
8:00 pm	2000
9:00 pm	2100
10:00 pm	2200
11:00 pm	2300
12:00 midnight	2400

Examples of time conversions:

7:59 am in standard time would be 0759 in military time

7:59 pm in standard time would be 1959 in military time

3:30 pm in standard time would be 1530 in military time

Index

Page numbers in **boldface** refer to key text references. Numbers followed by *b, f,* and *t* indicate boxes, figures, and tables.

A

Abbreviations, 138, 140, 355
Abuse, **58**
definition of, 62, 347
 mental, **58,** 62, 351
 physical, **27,** 37, **58,** 62, 352
 preventing, 60–61
 right to be free from, 58
 sexual, **58,** 62, 353
 signs of, 60
 types of, 58–60
 verbal, **27,** 37, **58,** 62, 354
Abuse-prevention programs, 58, 59*t*
Academy of Sleep Medicine, 15
Acceptance, 328
"Access to Employee Exposure and Medical Records Standard" (OSHA), 117
Accommodation, **28,** 36, 347
Accreditation, **7,** 16, 347
Acquired immunodeficiency syndrome (AIDS), **108, 288**
 breaking the chain of infection, 77
 definition of, 130, 290, 347
Active assistive ROM (AAROM) exercise, 199
Active listening, 22
Active ROM (AROM) exercise, 198–199
Activities
 and quality of life, 35, 35*f,* 47–48, 47*f*
 restorative, **194**–197, 207, 353
Activities director/coordinator, **5,** 16, 347
Activities of daily living (ADLs), **2**
 aids for, 197
 definition of, 16, 347
 equipment to help with, 111*t*
 techniques for, 313–316
Acupuncture, 325*b*

Acute problems, **248**
Adaptability, 30*t*
Administrator, **5,** 16, 347
Admission, transfer, and discharge rights, 57–58
Admission of residents, 152–155, 152*f,* 154*f*
Admission papers, 134
Admissions director or coordinator, **5,** 154, 347
Adolescents, 40, 41*t*
Adrenal glands, 282, 282*f*
Advance directives, **326**–327, 333, 347
Advocacy groups, 61
Advocates, **57,** 57*f,* 62, 347
AEDs (automated external defibrillators), 122
Agenda behavior, **310,** 318, 347
Age-related macular degeneration (AMD), 279
Aggression, **27**
 definition of, 36, 347
 guidelines to help you remain calm and protect yourself and your residents, 27, 27*f*
Aging, 248
 changes in circulatory system with, 263*t*–264*t*
 changes in digestive system with, 269*t*
 changes in ear with, 280*t*
 changes in endocrine system with, 283*t*
 changes in eye due to, 277*t*
 changes in female reproductive system with, 287*t*
 changes in integumentary system with, 250*t*–251*t*
 changes in male reproductive system with, 286*t*
 changes in musculoskeletal system with, 256*t*
 changes in nervous system with, 275*t*
 changes in other senses with, 281*t*
 changes in respiratory system with, 260*t*

 changes in urinary system with, 273*t*
Agitation, 312*t*
AIDS (acquired immunodeficiency syndrome), **108, 288**
 breaking the chain of infection, 77
 definition of, 130, 290, 347
Airborne precautions, **80,** 104, 347
Airborne transmission, **67**
 breaking the chain of infection, 77
 definition of, 104, 347
Alcohol-based hand rub, 68, 70
Allegation, 62, 347
Alternative ways to provide care, 49–50, 50*f*
Alveoli, **259,** 259*f,* 290
Alzheimer's disease, **306**–307, 307*f,* 311
 behavioral symptoms exhibited by residents with, 312, 312*t*–313*t*
 definition of, 318, 347
 guidelines for dressing residents with, 315
 guidelines to help residents remain continent, 313–314
 guidelines to help residents with bathing, 315–316
 guidelines to help residents with eating, 314
 guidelines to help residents with hydration, 314
 guidelines to make grooming easier and more pleasant, 316
 nurse assistant's role in providing care, 308–309
 stages of, 308, 309*b*
 strategies to assist with behavioral symptoms, 312*t*–313*t*
 techniques for activities of daily living, 313–316
Alzheimer's unit, 16, 347
American Heart Association, 147*t*
Anger and resentment, 44
 signs and symptoms to look out for, 280*t*
 stage of grief, 328
Animals, 325*b*
Ankle
 movements of, 198*b*

Information gathering, 134–135, 139
Information sharing
    with family members, 44, 44*f*
    guidelines for, 56
    OSHA requirements, 109
    reporting information, 136
    right to information, 55–56
    right to notification of change, 57
    types of reporting, 136
Injury prevention, 110–112
    for equipment-related injuries, 197
    for pressure injuries, 253
    for residents, 27
Inner ear, 279, 280*f*
In-service education, **10**
    definition of, 16, 350
    requirements for, 344
Insomnia, **325**
    definition of, 333, 350
    strategies to assist residents with, 312*t*
Inspection, **140**, 166, 350
Insurance, **6**
Intake and output (I&O), 218
Integumentary system, **250–255**
    age-related changes, 250*t*–251*t*
    definition of, 290, 350
    preventing skin problems, 251, 251*t*–252*t*
    signs and symptoms to look out for, 251*t*
    structures of, 250, 250*f*
Intellectual disability, 305–306, 305*b*
Interdisciplinary approach
    to resident admission, 154
    to resident discharge, 164
    to resident transfer, 163
Interdisciplinary team, 4, 4*f*
    definition of, 16, 350
    guidelines for working with, 11, 11*f*
    team members and responsibilities, 4–6
Intermediate care facility (ICF), **3**, 16, 350
Intermittent peritoneal dialysis (IPD), 298
Internal customers, **30**, 37, 350
Internal evacuation, **118**, 130, 350
Interviews
    family, 340
    Long Term Care Survey, 338–340
    resident, 339–340
    tips for success, 340
Inventory forms, 155, 156*f*
Involuntary seclusion, **59,** 62, 350
Iris, 277, 277*f*
Islets of Langerhans, 282

Isolation precautions, **79**–80, 79*f*, 105, 350
"I" statements, 28

J

J canes, 195*t*
Job description, 7, 8*f*
Job requirements, 343–344
The Joint Commission, **7**, 17, 350, 354
Joints, 197–198, 256, 256*f*
    movements of, 197, 198*b*
    signs and symptoms to look out for, 257*t*
    types of, 197–198, 198*f*

K

Ketones, **239**
    definition of, 245, 351
    testing urine for, 243
Kidney disease, 274
Kidneys, 272, 273*f*
Kiosk, **135**, 166, 351
Knee
    movements of, 198*b*
    range-of-motion exercises for, 204, 204*f*
Knee-ankle-foot orthosis (KAFO), 196
Knee braces, 196
Kneel drop procedure, 119
Kübler-Ross, Elisabeth, 327–328

L

Labeling residents' belongings, 157
Labeling residents' clothes, 156, 156*f*
Labeling specimens, 139, 140*f*
Lacerations, 255
Language
    body language, **21,** 21*f,* 36, 348
    important points to remember, 20–21
Large intestine, 268, 268*f*
Latent infection, **249**–250
Lateral (side-lying) position, **172**
    positioning residents, 182–183, 182*f*–183*f*
    turning residents from supine to, 178, 178*f*
Laughter, 311, 311*f*
Laundry, 5, 156–157
Law(s), 335, **336,** 345, 351
    Elder Justice Act of 2010, 58

Health Insurance Portability and Accountability Act (HIPAA), 55, 135
    Nursing Home Reform Act, 342
    Older Americans Act, 61
    Omnibus Budget Reconciliation Act of 1987 (OBRA '87), 54, 342
Legal rights, 54–61
Leg exercises, 204, 204*f*
Lens, 277, 277*f*
Lesion, 255
Level of care, 17, 351
Licensed practical nurse (LPN), **10,** 17, 351
Licensed social worker (LSW), **5,** 17, 351
Licensed vocational nurse (LVN), **10,** 17, 351
Life Safety Code (NFPA), 337
Lifestyle, healthy, 13
Lifestyle preferences, 42, 42*f*
Lift scales, 151, 151*f*
Ligaments, 256
Linens, 73, 73*f*
Liquid diets, 212
Listening, 311
    active, 22
    for conflict resolution, 29
    in difficult situations, 33
    with empathy, **22**
Liver, 268, 268*f*
Living will, **327,** 333, 351
Long term care (LTC), 2–3
    alternative ways to provide care, 49–50
    basic terms, 361–363
    definition of, 17, 351
    ethics and law in, 335–336
    insurance plans for, **6**
    nurse assistant roles in, 7–11, 7*f*
    oversight, 6–7
    payment for, 6
    resident-centered care, **48**–49, 48*f*
Long term care facilities, 2–3, 2*f*
    abuse-prevention programs, 58, 59*t*
    accreditation, 7
    activities director or coordinator, **5,** 16
    administration, 7
    administrator, **5,** 16
    admission of residents to, 3–4, 152–155, 152*f*, 154*f*
    admissions director or coordinator, **5,** 154
    assistant director of nursing, **10,** 16

R

RACE directions for fire response, 121
Radial pulse, **144**
    definition of, 166, 352
    procedure for taking, 147, 147*f*
Radiation therapy, **249,** 291, 352
RAI (Resident Assessment Instrument), **135**–136, 136*f,* 166, 353
RAI utilization guidelines, 136
Range-of-motion (ROM) exercises, 198–199
    active (AROM), 198–199
    active assistive (AAROM), 199
    guidelines for, 199–200, 199*f*
    passive (PROM), 199, 199*f*
    to prevent skin problems, 252, 252*t*
    procedure, 201–205, 201*f*–205*f*
Range-of-motion (ROM) machines, 111*t*
Reading glasses, 24, 24*f*
Reagent sticks/test strips, 239
Reassurance, 308
Recreational therapy, 7
Rectal glass thermometers, 141*t*
Rectal temperature, 141, 141*t,* 143
Reflection, **23,** 37, 352
Reflux, gastroesophageal, **270**–272, 290, 350
Registered dietitian (RD), **5,** 17, 352
Registered dietitian nutritionist (RDN), 17, 352
Registered nurse (RN), **10,** 17, 352
Registries, 342, 344
Regulated waste, **110,** 130, 352
Regulations
    for LTC facilities, 336–337
    for nurse aide training, 342
    state nurse aide, 342–343
Rehabilitation, **3, 194,** 207, 352
Rehabilitation units, **3,** 17, 353
Rehabilitative care, 2*t,* 6
Relaxation techniques, 325*b*
Relief, 44
Religious practices, 41–42, 330–331
Relocation stress syndrome, **152,** 166, 353
Renal diets, 211–212
Reporting information, 136
    "by a certain time" reporting, 136
    immediate reporting, 136, 137*f*
    to prevent skin problems, 252*t*
Reproductive system, **284, 286**
    definition of, 291, 353
    female, 286–288
    male, 284–286
Resentment, 44

Reservoir, **66**
    breaking the chain of infection at, 77
    definition of, 105, 353
Resident Assessment Instrument (RAI), **135**–136, 136*f*
    definition of, 166, 353
    RAI utilization guidelines, 136
Resident care conferences, 45, 45*f*
Resident care plan, **136**
Resident-centered care, **48**–49, 48*f*
    alternate ways to provide care, 49–50
    definition of, 51, 353
Resident rights, 53–63
Residents, 4, 4*f,* 40–42
    admission of, 43–44, 152–155, 152*f,* 154*f*
    aggressive, 27, 27*f*
    assessing, 135–136
    assistance needs, 81
    assisting, 13*b*
    autonomy, **9**
    with behavioral problems, 26–27
    care services provided in long term care facilities, 2*t*
    cognitively impaired, 25
    communicating with, 24–26, 25*f,* 26–27
    cultural differences, 9, 9*f*
    definition of, 17, 353
    depressed, anxious, or discouraged, 25–26
    discharging, 164–165
    dying, 328–329, 329*f*
    expectations of nurse assistants, 31
    factors that influence care, 11
    family members and significant others, 4, 4*f*
    food preferences, 211
    guidelines for effective communication with, 23
    hearing-impaired, 24
    history, 40–42
    honoring, 47, 47*f*
    as individuals, 9, 9*f*
    infections in, 78, 78*t*–79*t*
    Long Term Care Survey interviews, 339–340
    misappropriation of resident property, **59**–60, 62, 351
    monitoring of, 340–341
    new, 154
    perceptions of care, 32–33, 33*f*
    personal funds and belongings, 57, 155–156, 156*f*
    personal preferences, 81
    personal products, 83

    personal resources, 6
    positioning and moving, 169–208
    preferences and routines, 13
    preparation for, 154
    protection from injury, 27
    psychosocial needs in isolation, 80
    relationships with, 45–46, 46*f*
    safety rules, 111–112
    as sources of information, 134
    speech-impaired, 24–25
    transferring, 111–112, 163, 163*f*
    treatment-resistant microorganism threats to, 79
    visually impaired, 24
    vulnerable, **60,** 62, 354
Residents' Bill of Rights, 54, 54*f,* 56
Resiliency, 30*t*
Resources to help you provide care, 310
Respect
    for peers and supervisors, 34
    for residents, 48
    for residents' privacy, 157
Respiration, **146, 259**
    abnormal patterns, 146
    definition of, 166, 291, 353
Respirators, 72–73
Respiratory distress, 294
Respiratory rate, **146**
    definition of, 166, 353
    procedure for taking, 148
Respiratory system, **259**–262
    age-related changes, 260*t*
    definition of, 353
    positioning for easier breathing, 296, 296*f*
    signs and symptoms to look out for, 260*t*
    structures of, 259, 259*f*
Respite care, **3,** 17, 353
Responsibility, 30*t*
Restless legs syndrome (RLS), **325,** 333, 353
Restorative activities, **194**–197, 207, 353
Restorative nursing, **3,** 17, 353
Restraints, 60, 115
    chemical, **59,** 62
    physical, **59,** 62, 352
    right to be free from, 58
Retaliation, **57,** 62, 353
Retina, 277, 277*f*
Rheumatoid arthritis, **257,** 291, 353
Rights
    admission, transfer, and discharge, 57–58
    to be free from restraint and abuse, 58
    to choose, 56